The Clinical Practice of
# Complementary, Alternative, and Western Medicine

# The Clinical Practice of
# Complementary, Alternative, and Western Medicine

# W. John Diamond, M.D.

**CRC Press**
Boca Raton   London   New York   Washington, D.C.

## Library of Congress Cataloging-in-Publication Data

Diamond, W. John, 1948-.
  The clinical practice of complementary, alternative, and Western medicine / W. John Diamond
        .    p.   cm.
     Includes bibliographical references and index.
     ISBN 0-8493-1399-6 (alk. paper)
     1. Alternative medicine. 2. Internal medicine. I. Title.
  R733 .D47 2000
  615.5—dc21                                                                                          00-010343
                                                                                                              CIP

© 2001 by CRC Press LLC

No claim to original U.S. Government works
International Standard Book Number 0-8493-1399-6
Library of Congress Card Number 00-010343
Printed in the United States of America  1  2  3  4  5  6  7  8  9  0
Printed on acid-free paper

# Dedication

To South Africa, the country that nurtured and educated me, and to the United States of America, the country that gave me the opportunity to do this work. To my loyal patients who held the keys to the knowledge and allowed me to open the door.

# Author

**William John Diamond** was born in Johannesburg, Republic of South Africa on March 28, 1948. He was educated at Parktown Boys' High School where he injured his back in a diving accident, an event that changed his future plans to be a mining engineer. He served his military training at the Army Gymnasium in Pretoria, was a member of the State President's Guard, and received a B.Sc. (anatomy and embryology) in 1970, B.Sc. (Hons) (physiological chemistry) and M.B., B.Ch. in 1973 from the University of the Witwatersrand Medical School, in Johannesburg, Republic of South Africa. His internship was served in medicine, and obstetrics and gynecology at the Edendale Hospital, Pietermaritzburg, Republic of South Africa, and his residency in clinical pathology (clinical hematology and clinical chemistry) was at the Groote Schuur Hospital of the University of Cape Town Medical School in 1975 and 1976.

In July 1976, he emigrated with his family to the United States and became a resident in anatomical pathology in the Department of Pathology and Cytopathology at the Montefiore Hospital and Medical Center of the Albert Einstein College of Medicine in the Bronx, New York. He was a clinical fellow at the Clinical Center of the National Institutes of Health in Bethesda, Maryland in 1978–1979 and later became Scientific Director of the American Red Cross Blood Services, Syracuse, New York, and was an associate professor of clinical pathology at the State of New York Health Sciences Center, Upstate Medical Center, Syracuse, New York.

In 1980 he moved to Reno, Nevada and became an attending pathologist with Laboratory Medicine Consultants, a large pathology group serving Northern Nevada and Western California. In 1988 he left pathology and opened the Triad Medical Center to offer "Alternative Medicine" to the citizens of Northern Nevada having received his training in acupuncture at the UCLA Medical Acupuncture for Physicians course. In 1990–92 he received his homeopathic training at the Pacific Academy of Homeopathy in Berkeley, California. Master Chinese herbalist Anastacia White was his teacher in Traditional Chinese Medicine and herbology from 1992 to 1998. Dr. Diamond was medical editor of *Biological Therapy*, and Medical Director of BHI and Heel, USA in Albuquerque, New Mexico and of the Botanical Laboratories in Ferndale, Washington during the years 1992–1996. He was the lead author of *Alternative Medicine, a Definitive Guide to Cancer*, published in 1997.

At the moment he conducts a busy Integrated Medicine practice and is medical director of Integrated Medicines, LLC, a company dedicated to research and development of innovative medications based on natural and energetic principles.

# Acknowledgments

There are many people to thank for their interest, help, and encouragement. I wish to thank the following people who did more than they had to, and were key to formulating my thinking and outlook on life and medicine: Elliot Wolfe, my English and Latin teacher, for standing by me when things looked grim; Professor Phillip Tobias, for teaching me the scientific method; Dr. John Cosnett for teaching me clinical medicine and to appreciate the human body; Professor Leopold Koss for teaching me pathology and being my first mentor; Dr. Bob Milne and Dr. Yiwen Y. Tang for teaching me energetic medicine; Dr. David Tansley for opening my mind to the possibilities of esoteric medicine; and Professor William A. Tiller for showing me that it was real; Dr. Joseph Helms, for teaching me acupuncture; and Joe Daley and Lynn Amara, for teaching me homeopathy.

I am deeply indebted to Anastacia White, Master Herbalist, for her years of insightful tuition and guidance, without whom the reflections of TCM and herbal prescribing found in Chapter 6 would not have been possible. The bulk of the herbal patterns discussed there are taken from her detailed lectures, which I encourage all serious students to attend.

I need to offer great thanks and kudos to Dr. Gary Holt, my very supportive partner, who was the first doctor to experience if the system could be taught. He must be a good learner, because he is great at it! Thanks also to his assistants Joanne and Darlena.

I could not have written this book without the help and encouragement of two wonderful friends: Ron Kendall, who rescued my crashed computer disk multiple times and supplied me with jokes on e-mail to keep me going, and my dear late friend Stephen Poe, who dared and challenged me to write this book and egged me on even when he was not feeling well.

I want to thank my clinic staff, receptionists Judy and Cathy and my extremely efficient, loyal, and long-suffering medical assistant Patty, who have come along for the whole journey. Without them it would not have been possible, and the patient healing would not have been as complete. To Vauna, thanks for teaching me about allergy.

Mothers hold the world together, and I wish to thank mine for always seeing the best in me and allowing me to be an inquisitive child.

Children are the future of the world, and I wish to thank David, Jane, and Rory, my wonderful children, for teaching me what it was all about. I apologize for always having a book in my hand and a faraway look in my eye. To my beloved wife, Barbara, who never faltered one step of the way, but has been heard to say, "There must be a special place in heaven for wives of homeopaths."

To Barbara Norwitz, Publisher, and CRC Press for having the courage, patience, and foresight to publish this book.

Last, but not least, to the State of Nevada, Board of Medical Examiners, thank you for being open-minded and nonjudgmental.

# The Modalities and Assessment of the Patient

*"There are two types of physicians — those that are free men and those that are slaves. The slaves, to speak generally, are treated by slaves, who pay them a hurried visit, or receive them in dispensaries. A physician of this kind never gives a servant any account of his complaint, nor asks him for any; he gives him some imperial injunction with an air of finished knowledge, in the brusque fashion of a dictator, and then is off in haste to the next ailing servant .... The free practitioner attends free men, treats their diseases by going into things thoroughly in a scientific way; and takes the patient and his family into his confidence. Thus he learns something from the sufferers, and at the same time instructs the invalid to the best of his powers. He does not give his prescriptions until he has won the patient's support .... Now which of the two methods is that of the better physician or director of the bodily regimen?"*

Plato, 2500 years ago.

# Contents

## *Section I: Integrated Medicine — Background*

## *Section II: Traditional Chinese Medicine (TCM)*

**Chapter 6**

## Chapter 7

# Section III: Other Forms of Alternative Medical Treatment

**Chapter 8**

## Section IV: The Practice of Integrated Medicine

# Section I

Integrated Medicine — Background

# 1 Introduction

## A NEW PARADIGM

In defining a new paradigm it is difficult to know where to begin. How do you take fifteen years of medical practice in pathology and ten years of clinical observation utilizing the theories of traditional Chinese medicine, acupuncture, homeopathy, and therapeutic nutrition and meld them into a model of biological understanding and medical practice? The answer is actually quite simple — start from the beginning and build a convincing model based upon sound physics, physiology, pathology, and clinical medicine and see if the model fits the expected outcome. If it does, you have proven your point and advanced the medical understanding of biology; if it does not, it opens the way to suggestions of a better model and a new direction of inquiry.

Most of what will follow was derived from a combination of fundamental training in the "alternative" modalities and pure clinical observation of 10,000 patients in a general family practice over a period of ten years. As my experience grew, further training was incorporated into the model and the process refined to present you with this still evolving account. Although I am a trained laboratorian and feel that I have an objective and logical mind, I make no excuses for occasional scientific lapses and for some of the personal bias that is interjected into some topics, such as the emotional component of disease and the concept of goal-oriented biology. In many of the sections, especially those regarding the concepts of disease and the energetics of disease, I will be nauseatingly repetitive, looking at the same facts from several different contexts. The reason for this redundancy is that I am giving you thoughts that have had ten years to ferment into a fine wine. These thoughts, to the uninitiated, will have the quality of Kool-Aid, at best, refreshing but without much substance. To take the quantum leap from the comfort of the known deterministic and linear concepts of Western medical concepts and disease, to the swirling chaos of energetic ambiguity and the nonlinear dynamics of functional biology, requires much thought, reflection, faith, and perseverance.

I hope that this book will take you on a journey to a new insight and understanding of human biology at all its levels of complexity and integration, and in the end leave you with more questions than it can possibly answer.

## PERSONAL HISTORY

In order to follow my logic over the years and the historic background that brought me to this quantum change in my medical practice, I think I had better start from the beginning.

I feel that I was short-changed during my medical education. I was adequately taught the prevailing concepts of Western medical thought, which, although marvelous in focused acute and traumatic situations, left me puzzled and inept when these principles were applied to complex chronic and multiorgan disease. Inadequate answers to my probing questions of the biological anomalies that were so blatant to me led me to leave my medical training after my third year of medical school and pursue the more pristine sciences of physiological chemistry, gross anatomy, and embryology. I was very fortunate to have had as my mentor Professor Philip Tobias, the great anatomist and anthropologist, who saw to it, that I was trained in critical and independent thinking first and second, that I completed my medical training second. It was hard to go back to the soft sciences of medicine and I probably openly expressed as much. However, I did complete my medical training, and although I graduated in the top ten percent of my class of 220, I was banished to another province to complete my obligatory internship, a happening that was to change my understanding of disease and medicine forever. I will recount these happenings and their outcomes in the section under energetic medicine.

Many years later, after a frightening personal medical experience, which led me to reexamine my medical beliefs about the origins and interrelatedness of disease, I decided at last to seek out the truth and go back to the only enduring source of all medical knowledge — the clinical patient. To accomplish this task I left the intellectual, financial, and emotional safety of pathology and opened up a general medical practice — my very own laboratory. The medical modalities of treatment I learned and practiced were chosen based solely on the modality's representing a complete system of healing within itself, and having a complete philosophical and spiritual aspect to its nature. The medical modalities fulfilling these criteria were homeopathy; traditional Chinese medicine, including acupuncture and herbology; and hypnosis, psychotherapy, and Ayurvedic medicine. The initial documentation of the patient response in the early years was, to say the least, obsessive–compulsive. I would call patients three to four times a day, every day, until I saw them again two weeks later. As confidence and an understanding of the modalities and the individual patient responses began to crystallize and fall into predictable patterns, the frequency of inquiry abated. There were many trials and tribulations, some involving my peers, most of whom thought I was going through a midlife crisis and looked upon me with absolute disdain, and some involving my family and friends who were the unwitting and involuntary victims and guinea pigs of many of my outlandish ideas and newly acquired skills. There were times when I doubted my own sanity, but always my patients brought me back to the observed reality of their biological progress and the positive changes occurring as together we peeled back the layers of disease. Without their support and participation I would still be a doctor with a theory and an idea, instead of a physician with some concrete ideas of what the new biology really represents. The therapeutic concepts to be presented are the result of meticulous clinical observations of approximately 10,000 patients followed longitudinally over ten years and treated individually with an integrated medical approach.

# 2  Principles of Integrated Medicine

## DEFINITION OF INTEGRATED MEDICINE

Integrated medicine is the holistic practice of medicine in which the patient, not the disease, is placed at the center of the healing process; the disease is defined by both the patient and the doctor; the patient is assessed as a spiritual, emotional–mental, and physical being; and all modalities of healing are appropriately integrated to produce, not just a medical cure, but a deeper healing of the patient on his or her own terms.

As a result of this information coming from real patients with common diseases, you will recognize your patients and your therapeutic dilemmas among the information presented. Integrated medicine is based on the clinical and scientific observation and rational application of human biology, working with the physiology of the body and not against it. To make this quantum leap we have to take our knowledge of the laws of physics, physiology, pathology, and pharmacology and apply it solely to the individualized biology of the patient in front of us, with only a passing acknowledgment of double-blind studies. The patient you see in front of you and how you treat him or her *is* the clinical trial. Arthur M. Young, the inventor of the Bell Helicopter, in his book "The Reflexive Universe — Evolution of Consciousness," made the point rather well. I will paraphrase his words: One has to master the science of one's profession. But, having done that, follow not the constraints of that science blindly, but strike out to new territories and make your mark.[1]

Take the plunge! Integrate and individualize your approach to treatment. You and your patients will be pleasantly surprised. This integrated approach will afford you a feeling of scientific accomplishment and emotional satisfaction that will enhance your medical experience and lead to new avenues of learning and personal discovery. Please join me so that we can all benefit from a broader integrated biomedical approach.

## BACKGROUND CONCEPTS

We are all products of our social and family backgrounds and environments. The way we see ourselves and others, including our patients, is governed largely by these early learned perceptions of reality. We are not drawn to an examination of our relationship to the cosmos or anything larger than our immediate surroundings until we are faced with a traumatic life event, such as a personal illness or the death of a friend or loved one. It is during these times of induced introspection, usually on the meaning of life in general or even our own lives, that we first face the dilemma of the meaning of our existence and our place in the universe.

During one such traumatic circumstance in my own life, I first looked to external events as the cause of my physical dis-ease, but was eventually forced to look within for the primary cause. Although I was certainly a willing victim of the stressful macrocosm of my surroundings — family, occupation, community, and country — the cause of my disease was eventually found to be in the microcosm of my internal illusion of "fear of failure." "As above, so below" is the saying: One could also add, "as without, so within." We can define holistic biological medicine in terms of the relationships between the outer, revealed symptoms and the inner, internalized causes of disease. David Bohm, Professor of Theoretical Physics at Birkbeck College in London, has, through the medium of theoretical physics, defined his concept of wholeness as an unfolding flow of our manifested and hidden realities. He introduced the notion in which any element (the explicate order or symptomatic manifestation) contains within itself the totality of the universe, which includes both matter and consciousness (the implicate order or causes of disease).[2] This is also true of the human condition. The macrocosm and microcosm of man are but reflections of each other. Both the external and internal milieus need to be assessed as the cause of dis-ease and in the search for wellness. Until now, doctors have been preoccupied with the external milieu and its manifestations — the explicate order or symptoms. It is time to integrate both the explicate and implicate orders, the outside and the inside, the effects and the causes. It is not enough to document and adjust the manifest symptoms of the disease, we have to understand the origins of the symptoms and why the body is using them for its own ends. We need this holistic medical attitude to really assess and treat the root cause of disease.

## HOLISM

The term *holism* was coined by a fellow countryman, Field Marshal General Jan Christian Smuts (1870–1950). He was a South African soldier, statesman, and philosopher and the first person credited with conceptualizing the modern concept of *holism*. He came to this philosophical construct based on his need to accommodate both British and Boer political interests after the South African Boer War and more on the idea that South Africa, as a socioeconomic unit, was more than its parts. This idea of looking at the good of the whole rather than its components culminated in the formation of the Union of South Africa in 1910. This concept was developed in his writings and activities and extended to the relationships between countries and peoples. Assistance in the formation of the United Nations was one of his major accomplishments. It is somewhat ironic that his political party's defeat in 1948 by the Nationalist Party lead to the establishment of apartheid and the social reverse in South Africa of the very "holism" to which he ascribed.

In the context of disease and healing, this definition of *holism* can be taken to encompass all levels: the person as an integrated biological whole, not just a collection of organ systems encased in skin and connected by nerves and vessels; the person as body–mind–soul, an extended, more mystical, and metaphysical concept of the whole; the person as a integral part of his or her environment and surroundings including the universe. However, the meaning of holism in medicine relates to the interrelatedness, dependence, and connectedness between all parts of the human being: separate cells, organ systems, mind and body, and body and soul. The human whole is more than the sum of his or her parts and cannot be meaningfully dissected to understand the whole. One is reminded of the story of the blind men who came upon an elephant in the jungle. They could not see what this creature was, so they attempted to reconstruct its image by each examining a portion of the animal. One had the trunk, one the tail, one the tusk, one a leg, etc. Each blind man came to a different conclusion as to the nature of the beast.

This circumstance is not unlike medical specialists looking at the same patient as an isolated organ system reflecting their specialist training. I recently had a very frustrating interaction with a cardiologist. The patient in question had experienced rather severe palpitations with a history of irregular menses, insomnia, and hyperthyroid disease. My question to the cardiologist was: does this patient have organic cardiac disease, or did he think that the irregular menses, insomnia, and palpitations were all part of her thyroid presentation? The answer was that she did not have any organic cardiac disease. When I questioned him about the thyroid component of her disease I was told to send her to a gynecologist, order a sleep study, and have her see an endocrinologist. This incident probably represents an extreme case, but you can see my point.

Regular medicine is based on reductionistic thought and a physicochemical paradigm of linear cause and effect. While there is nothing inherently wrong with taking this approach to understand the pathophysiology of the body, biology does not operate under these stylized steady-state, linear (cause-and-effect) objective conditions. So, although medicine as we know it is able to explain in minute detail, chromosomal deletions or inborn errors of metabolism, it has not been able to adequately define *life*, *health*, or *healing*, when looking at the total biology of the patient. These concepts belong to the paradigms of thermodynamically open, nonlinear, and chaotic systems that respond to energy, consciousness, and emotions. What is even more surprising is that recent advances that have started to explain the interrelationship between body and mind, such as psychoneuroimmunology, even if proven and published in acceptable journals, are rarely accepted and integrated into the philosophy and practice of medicine. Breakthrough advances in conceptually different scientific disciplines, such as physics, psychology, and general biology, are rarely part of medical education, which seems to have a life and direction of its own. My greatest insight into the causes of manifest disease was stimulated while reading Ernest Rossi's book on Jungian therapeutic hypnosis, *The Psychobiology of Mind-Body Healing*.[3] It is this kind of cross-pollination of the open mind that leads to new paradigms of understanding. However, very little scientific cross-fertilization takes place between disciplines. Scientific inquiry has also been reduced to its parts. The mind-set of reductionism is convenient, comfortable, and intellectually satisfying, and so, the status quo is maintained. It seems that any change in an established system can only be made from a structure of thoughts emanating from outside the confines of the system. Thomas S. Kuhn in his landmark 1962 treatise *The Structure of Scientific Revolutions*[4] comments on this fact: "Unanticipated novelty, the new discovery, can emerge only to the extent that his anticipation [the scientist's] about nature and his instruments prove wrong." If the scientist believes he is always right, then no progress or discovery can be made. It is for this reason that the resurgence of nontraditional medicine is being spearheaded by the lay public and nontraditional thinkers in medicine. It is also improbable that integrated medicine will evolve or be championed in any revolutionary sense, within established academic medical institutions. Medical schools as a whole have only offered lip service to alternative medicine, with most courses being elective courses and consisting of the soft, noncontroversial subjects of guided imagery, simple herbalism, or therapeutic touch.

The most damaging medical concept propagated by reductionistic thinking is the separation of the mind from the body. In one fell swoop the body–mind was removed from contention and the dismembered and decorticate human could now conveniently be dealt with piecemeal. The body was further dissected into organ systems and the mind was only of therapeutic importance in mental illness. This very dilemma of what constitutes psychiatry and mental disease was eloquently argued by Dr. George Engel of the University of Rochester School of Medicine in his landmark paper in April 1977, "The Need for a New Medical Model: A Challenge for Biomedicine."[5] In this wonderful and insightful discussion he contrasts two schools of thought as to what represents psychiatry: the "Medical Model" limits psychiatry's field to behavioral disorders consequent to brain dysfunction, and the "Behavioral Model" of psychiatry is concerned with behavioral disorders consequent on psychosocial issues and the problems of living, social adjustment reactions, character disorders, dependency syndromes, existential depressions, and various social deviancy syndromes. He goes on to say:

> To provide a basis for understanding the determinants of disease and arriving at rational treatments and patterns of healthcare, a medical model must also take into account the patient, the social context in which he lives, and the complementary system devised by society to deal with the disruptive effects of illness, that is, the physician role and the health care system. This requires a *biopsychosocial model*. Its scope is determined by the historic function of the physician to establish whether the person soliciting help is "sick" or "well"; and if sick, why sick and in which ways sick; and then to develop a rational program to treat the illness and to restore and maintain health.
>
> The boundaries between health and disease, between well and sick, are far from clear and never will be clear, for they are diffused by cultural, social, and psychological considerations. The traditional biomedical view, that biological indices are the ultimate criteria defining disease, leads to the present

paradox where some people with positive laboratory findings are told that they are in need of treatment when in fact they are feeling quite well, while others feeling sick are assured that they are well, that is, they have no "disease." A biopsychosocial model that includes the patient as well as the illness would encompass both circumstances. The doctor's task is to account for the dysphoria and the dysfunction that lead individuals to seek medical help, adopt the sick role, and accept the status of patienthood."

Engel ends with a very thought-provoking discussion concerning grief as a disease. "Are the fatigue and weakness of the woman who recently lost her husband conversion symptoms, psychophysiological reactions, manifestations of a somatic disorder, or a combination of these?" (pp. 129–130). It turns out, on pure clinical observation, that the mind is the cause and biological projection of the majority of bodily ills. We will deal further with these issues when we combine the observable biological truths from medicine, psychology, psychoneuropharmacology, and bioenergetics into an integrated whole.

## THE ENERGETIC COMPONENT OF MEDICINE

My first introduction to the energetic component of medicine was during my early experiences with the Zulu nation as a medical intern in the South African province of Natal. I had been banished there because I was thought not worthy of being educated any further in the academic hospital centers in Johannesburg. I was, as one famous professor (an expert in iron metabolism) put it, "a lost cause." However, in Pietermaritzburg in a 2000 bed hospital I was able to think in an unfettered manner and carefully examine my new charges — the men, women, and children of the Zulu nation. The Zulu, a fierce, proud warrior tribe, had a strong belief in spirits and the afterlife. At times, during internecine feuds, spells would be cast on opposing parties by the sangoma or witch doctor. These spells would result in my seeing patients with no adverse clinical or laboratory findings, who literally wasted away and died in front of me in spite of all the modern medical marvels I had at my disposal. Many of the victims were unaware that a spell had been cast and this fact was only discovered by members of his immediate family after the demise of the unfortunate individual. One of the inexplicable findings with respect to these spells was that all the malicious activity was done at a distance remote from the victim, but still seemed to have an effect. Much the same sort of energy transfer is seen in the voodoo cult of Haiti and in the laying on of hands and the effect of prayer, albeit negative energy in the first instance and positive in the second two instances.

In integrated medicine, both acupuncture and homeopathy exhibit elements of supersensible energetic transformation of the body–mind. Professor William Tiller, Professor Emeritus of the Department of Material Sciences and Engineering at Stanford University alluded to this area of unseen and unmeasurable energy in his recent book, *Science and Human Transformation*:[6] "It has often been stated that physics has always concerned itself with the nature of things, that is, real objects. By real objects is meant those objects perceived by the physical sensory system since this is the only sensory system that is fully operational in the general mass of present-day humanity. However, those objects perceived by other sensory systems in a much smaller segment of present-day humanity, are no less real. Rather, they are objects for which statistical consensus does not presently exist. Almost a century ago Steiner wrote about these supersensible domains of nature and how one might proceed to develop self towards cognition of the vast information territories of these supersensible domains" (p. 179). These phenomena will be explained in more detail under the section dealing with the alternative modalities.

If there are energetic as well as physical components to illness, then these clinical observations should be supported by the more fundamental constructs of our existence on this planet, namely, physics. The theoretical evidence for our existence as both physical and energetic beings comes from the discipline of quantum mechanics and the relationship between matter, energy, and consciousness (information). It is clear from these models that we are dealing with a body–mind immersed in a matter–energy–time–informational model. These concepts are superbly outlined in the Big Sur Dialogues that are chronicled in Fritjof Capra's books, *The Web of Life* and his earlier work *The Tao of Physics*.[7,8]

The jump from regular medicine to the concepts of integrated medicine, although seemingly strange and unsubstantiated at first, becomes so much more logical and fulfilling for patient and physician as one sees the wisdom of biology, its underpinnings in physics, and its natural movement toward healing. What was strange and seemingly out of place becomes familiar and part of a solid, clinically based approach as the bigger, holistic picture of biology becomes apparent.

It is not the drugs or modalities used that labels the practice of medicine as holistic or reductionistic, but rather the attitudes of the patient and the doctor to the disease and its biological purpose.

## HISTORICAL AND BIOLOGICAL CONCEPTS OF INTEGRATED MEDICINE

In order to explain the sudden renewal of interest in, and rediscovery of, complementary and alternative medicine, we first have to retrace some medical history. As I mentioned earlier, I was privy to the activities of the witch doctors of the Zulu nation. These shrewd and intuitive shamans were able to use native herbs as well as psychology and superstition to treat illness and influence tribal politics. Both physical and psychic approaches are characteristic of most "primitive" societies. In the early ages of our civilization these two aspects of healing separated into the herbalists who cared for the physical body (mechanists) and the priests who cared for the psyche (vitalists). The mind–body split had already begun.

In modern times, physical disease has been more or less conquered (so we have been led to believe), and there is a renewed interest in the psychic or spiritual side of our being. In a search for the vitalistic roots of our medical heritage, healers and patients have gone back to the modalities that have retained their dual mechanistic and vitalistic character. The modalities that fit this definition are homeopathy, traditional Chinese medicine, Ayurveda, Native American tradition, and other societal, religious, and aboriginal traditions.

The common ties that hold these healing traditions together are founded in the appreciation of the human as being an integrated mind, body, and soul. For most holistic modalities, health represents an internal and external self-regulating dynamic balance of the whole body whereas disease represents a departure from this balance. Healing is the return to balance aided by the body's natural self-regulating healing ability and the partnership of the directed patient-centered activities of the healer and the patient.

All these concepts can be realized in a more Western scientific approach by the principles of *biological and functional medicine*. In this broad conceptual framework, human physiology and pathophysiology are looked upon as an integrated whole over time, where a change in one system is characterized by compensatory changes in all systems and the individuality of a person's physiology is of paramount importance. Roger Williams first drew attention to patient biochemical individuality and diversity in his landmark 1956 publication *Biochemical Individuality*.[9] The principle underlying these concepts relates to a patient-centered, not disease-centered, homeodynamic balance. These principles have been fostered and carried on by Geoffrey Bland, Ph.D. in his many books and lectures.[10] Herein lies the beginning of an integrated concept of health and disease.

In Western medicine (allopathic medicine) disease is characterized by the patient's symptoms and elicited signs that together make up a diagnosis. A treatment is chosen based on the diagnosis and, if appropriate, the symptoms and signs disappear, the patient is cured, and all is well. Integrated medicine is very interested in the allopathic diagnosis because of its prognostic and pathophysiological information. The diagnosis provides a framework within which other modalities may be used therapeutically in an integrated manner. However, symptoms are not looked upon by most patient-centered modalities as being the ultimate problem, but rather the body's response to the problem — a balancing act to achieve thermodynamic homeostasis, where the symptom represents a small bodily sacrifice to balance the whole. Apart from the schism of the body–mind, this is the most important distinction separating allopathic and holistic medical philosophy.

Many different terms have been bantered about relating to holistic medical thought and practice. *Alternative medicine*, *complementary medicine*, *holistic medicine*, and *natural medicine* have all been used to indicate either a philosophy, metaphor, or positioning in regards to Western medicine. There is, however, only one medicine — that which heals and puts the whole patient in the center of care. A very pertinent question to ask is: Is all complementary medicine holistic? I have certainly seen allopathic clinicians who were holistic in everything they did for a patient, without knowing any acupuncture, homeopathy, or the like. I have also seen classical homeopaths who embodied the very worst of narrow and rigid idealized medical thought who had absolutely no place in the healing of any patient. From this question it follows that a holistic approach derives more from the attitude of the practitioner than the modality of medicine. An appreciation of the differences between orthodox and integrated medicine can be seen in Table 2.1. *Integrated medicine* is defined as a philosophical biomedical approach, based on scientific laws and clinical observation, that uses all appropriate modes of healing for the benefit of the patient at all levels of his or her being. The key to integrated medicine is to use the least intrusive and suppressive input, encouraging the body's natural self-regulating healing process, and to heal the root cause of disease, not only its manifestation.

## WHO PRACTICES OR USES INTEGRATED MEDICINE?

If asked about their interest in complementary or alternative medicine (CAM), physicians will fall into three basic categories: (1) not interested, (2) intellectually interested in what they are, or (3) interested in learning and using some CAM techniques. These three categories give some insight into the actual physician issues regarding CAM at this time.

**TABLE 2.1**
**Comparison of Orthodox and Integrated Medicine.**

| Category | Orthodox Medicine | Integrated Medicine |
|---|---|---|
| Philosophy | Reductionistic; linear cause and effect; specialization; cure as end | Holistic; multicausal and dimensional; interrelational |
| Disease | Organ and pathology specific; external causation | Patient-centered; functional; pattern of dysfunction |
| Diagnosis | Based on clinicopathological parameters; often lab dependent | Based on patient pattern of imbalance; multidimensional |
| Treatment | Based on diagnosis; little individualization; drug based; material; either suppressive or ablative; treats symptom not cause | Based on patient picture, no diagnosis necessary; individualized; works with biology; treats cause; all modalities |
| Patient | Passive and dependent; a victim of circumstance; compliant | Active participant; responsible for outcomes; informed |
| Doctor | Authoritarian and detached; responsible only for the elements of the disease presented | Nonjudgmental; connected yet not enabling; responsible for the entire patient presented |
| Lifestyle | Of secondary importance to primary treatment | Of primary importance to disease modification |
| Emotional–Mental Issues | Of secondary importance, especially if not drug amenable | The primary event in disease causation |

The uninterested physicians are either totally ignorant of these issues or have already taken a position regarding CAM without actually having investigated it to any extent. There is really nothing more to say about this group other than if they are in control of an institution or decision making, CAM has no chance at all. Presentation of scientific data or patient results will have no effect on them, as the decision they have made is emotional and not based on logic or scientific data.

The intellectually curious are physicians who keep up to date with medical trends and knowledge and do so both for their own and their patient's benefit. They are interested in order to be knowledgeable about what herbs and medications their patients are taking and to whom they may refer patients if deemed appropriate. They can be coaxed to move into the next group as trends and times change.

The last group of doctors has had enough experience to realize that much of the chronic disease seen does not respond to traditional therapy. They feel that they are at a therapeutic impasse. It is unsettling for them to exhaust therapeutic possibilities, and so they search for more satisfying ways of addressing these problems. CAM appears to them to be a reasonable therapeutic alternative. CAM also allows for some creativity and self-reliance when dealing with the pharmaceutical companies. The most difficult issues for these doctors are how to explain this approach to their peers and administrators and how to get adequately trained in CAM modalities. Explaining therapeutic alternatives to their patients is usually not a problem. Other issues relate to clinical practice guidelines, competency, and credentialing. These issues have hardly been addressed at this time, although Woolf et al.[11] have proposed guidelines for evidence-based trials of CAM therapies.

Patients access CAM for many different reasons. However, the movement towards CAM has been motivated primarily by the ensconced attitude of the medical system, which is too rigid and technical and has reduced the patient's autonomy to a therapeutic choice of drugs or surgery. Modern medicine is also too physician-centered, in that the doctor, not the patient, defines the nature and boundary of the patient's problems. The doctor values his diagnostic skills above his patient interactive skills. Most patients are not upset with their regular doctors, but are just seeking more options and a wider interpretation of their problems. Some patients are pragmatically just trying to address unsolved medical issues by whatever means necessary, while others have a serious intellectual and sometimes emotional commitment to CAM for a variety of personal reasons. For some patients sensitivity to many medications is an issue; for others the drastic nature of some orthodox treatment is unacceptable. Many patients are now computer literate and will do extensive online searches on the Internet or through the National Library of Medicine's database and choose a CAM therapy after assessing orthodox therapy. Many times the patient is more knowledgeable than the doctor on a particular topic. In almost all cases, however, the complementary practitioner is chosen by word of mouth. There are extensive networks of patients in every community who act as medical resources and referral centers.

Patients receiving CAM are quite happy to pay out of pocket as evidenced by two studies by Eisenberg.[12,13] The 1993 original paper surveyed 1539 adults about their use of "alternative medicine" in the past year. Fully one third (34%) had used one form of alternative therapy, and one third of those had seen an alternative medicine provider. Extrapolation to the entire U.S. population showed that there were an estimated 425 million visits to alternate providers with expenses totaling $13.7 billion, of which $10.3 billion was paid for out of pocket. The second paper in 1998 looked at trends in alternative medicine from 1990–1997 and showed a marked increase in alternative therapy use by the general population as compared with the original study. The rate had increased from 33.8% to 42.1% and the likelihood of a patient's seeing an alternate provider had increased from 36.3% to 46.3%. Some patients with chronic diseases, for example HIV, tend to use alternative therapies at a very high rate (73%). The extrapolated estimates of visits to alternative care providers had gone up from 427 million visits in 1990 to 629 million visits in 1997, thereby exceeding total visits to all U.S. primary care physicians. Estimated yearly expenses had also increased to $21.1 billion, of which $12.2 billion was out of pocket. The actual out-of-pocket expenditure figure for 1997 was $27 billion, which exceeded the 1997 out-of-pocket expenditures for all U.S. physician services. This out-of-pocket payment is quite substantial and cannot be ignored by anyone practicing medicine in the HMO and managed-care environment. At a time when remuneration is being squeezed and payments are dwindling, CAM offers the physician a financial shot in the arm with a cash practice — a fair payment for a fair service.

At this time more and more insurers and HMOs are embracing CAM as part of their offered services. This is not because of any altruistic bent on the part of these third party payers, but because their customers are demanding it, or changing to suppliers who offer it, and because it seems, at least on preliminary data, to save money and decrease hospitalizations. In fact, I spent an entire year, at the request of a childhood friend, treating the chronic patients of a large Medicare HMO. All patients had failed or were refractory to conventional therapy. The patients were treated with acupuncture, homeopathy, and Chinese herbs, and the root causes and pathophysiology of their diseases were explained to them. Each patient was individually instructed on the specific emotional, day-to-day life processes and drug contributions to their disease status and manifestation. They were taught to take responsibility for their disease and its daily status and learned to match their behavior patterns with the exacerbations or improvements in their diseases. Patients were monitored both energetically by Meridian Stress Assessment (see The Energetic Exam) and by a daily diary with gross physiological measurements, such as daily weighing for patients with congestive heart failure (CHF) and daily peak flow volumes for patients with asthma or chronic obstructive pulmonary disease (COPD). Cutoff numerical criteria for coming into the clinic for assessment were established, and each patient had command and control of his or her clinical condition based on the above parameters. I eventually had to stop traveling to the center because of an overwhelming patient load that left my own patients complaining and shortchanged.

Hospitals are getting into CAM to differentiate themselves from their competition and to try to offer a full service to the community, which can include health spas, gyms, health information, preventative medicine, and lifestyle classes. The market for CAM and CAM-associated products has boomed in the past two years. The herbal market in the United States is experiencing unprecedented growth. Herbal sales increased 59% in 1997 to $3.24 billion with almost 60 million Americans taking some herbal medication that year. Health food stores, drug stores, supermarkets, pharmacies, and professionals have become purveyors of these products. Now, even pharmaceutical firms have entered the market.

The market for CAM has changed significantly in the last 3 to 5 years. From a "Mom and Pop" cottage industry, it has suddenly blossomed into a mature market with leading players, evolving consumers, and intense competition. The market has been almost exclusively patient driven. This change has been mediated by patient empowerment and equal access to medical information on the Internet. The main therapeutic modalities have been acupuncture and chiropractic, probably because of the number of practitioners involved. Herbology and homeopathy come in way behind, and all other modalities follow them. Some historical issues have skewed the market in an interesting way. Because of the popularity of single Western herbs, e.g., St. John's Wort and Echinacea, the real strength and sophistication of Chinese herbology has been overlooked. In addition, because of the vacuum caused by orthodox medicine's nonparticipation in the market, the area of CAM has been a gold mine for charlatans and "snake oil" salesmen. Not a day goes by that some new miraculous substance does not appear (sold via a pyramid scheme or multilevel marketing), claiming to save the world and cure everything from warts to cancer. Nutritional supplements and herbal remedies have lead the way in the over-the-counter retail sector. In response to this billion dollar market, many large pharmaceutical companies have launched herbal and nutritional lines. Rexall has been in the homeopathic business for some time, while Bayer and Warner Lambert have just launched their branded herbal lines. By the time this book is completed, the list will have grown exponentially.

From the physician's point of view it is important to be knowledgeable about complementary and alternative modalities and therapeutics to ensure a level of comfort and trust when patients discuss these therapeutic alternatives and the herbs or supplements they may be taking. The appropriateness of remedies for different medical complaints and the interaction of herbs with regular drugs are important therapeutic issues. A recent review by Lucinda G. Miller, PharmD., focuses on the most popular herbs and their toxic and interactive side effects.[14] A recent CD-ROM release from Integrative Medical Arts in Beaverton, Oregon entitled *Interactions* has an excellent database of drug–herb, drug–nutritional, and herb–nutritional interactions. The list of problems includes: hepatotoxicity, nausea and vomiting, diarrhea, anticoagulant properties, nervousness, agitation, insomnia, depression, confusion and hallucinations, cholinergic toxicity, seizures, pulmonary hypertension, contact dermatitis, SLE, gynecomastia, menorrhagia, hypoglycemia, hypertension, diuresis, hypotension, palpitations, and tachycardia. These effects are not unexpected as many regular drugs are derived from herbal origins and consequently have physiological activity, both good and bad. The specifics will be dealt with under the section on Western and Eastern herbs.

A number of *ethical issues* that must be addressed by the practitioner of CAM, including:

## PATIENT ISSUES

Patients have the right to choose their modality of treatment and their practitioner. The freedom of medical choice is a fundamental freedom issue to many people selecting CAM as a first or complementary choice in medical care. Legislation regarding freedom of choice is being enacted in Washington state and other states are looking at similar laws. However, freedom of access to the treatment of choice also implies some real dangers in these choices based on emotional decision making and erroneous information or conclusions. Many times patients have no information as to the appropriateness and efficacy of their medical choices, other than anecdotal information or marketing information provided by a health food store or unsolicited pamphlets in the mail. None of these sources is a substitute for an informed medical assessment of the treatment and the patient's problems. Informed consent regarding patient expectations in an integrated medical practice is paramount. Some patients come with the idea that you are only going to utilize CAM even if allopathic medicine is appropriate. These ideas should be dispelled and the integrated approach of using whatever is needed in any particular clinical situation explained. Some patients will tell you how you are going to treat them in no uncertain terms, because they have read about a treatment or it worked in a friend's disease. You have to look at their directives with scientific and clinical impunity and, if the therapy does not fit, you must state that you do not think that this approach is indicated and explain your objections and alternative traditional approaches. If the patient insists on their approach, it is time to end your relationship with the patient. Many of these patients can be quite aggressive and developing a productive patient–doctor relationship is not possible. However, if anything were to go amiss, they may be the first to sue you.

Some patients believe that you will come up with the alternative magic bullet for their cancer, lupus, or multiple sclerosis. The outcome data, if any exists, regarding their disease and alternative medicine treatment together with your clinical experience must be carefully reviewed and compared with allopathic medical treatment. The patient and the doctor should come to a mutually acceptable course of treatment with objective time constraints and clear therapeutic objectives. A case that comes to mind is a very spiritual lady who felt strongly that the Archangel Gabriel was going to cure her hypothyroidism. Her thyroid stimulating hormone (TSH) at the time was 168 micrograms per milliliter with the normal being 1.5 to 5.0. I did not bring her belief system into doubt, I just gave the Archangel two weeks to reduce her TSH to a normal level. At the end of two weeks her TSH level had not changed and she happily went onto supplemental thyroid hormone. Everybody was a winner in this situation and good medical treatment was not compromised. Of course, if her TSH had normalized by itself in two weeks, I would have given Gabriel his due and been equally happy. The pathways to health are varied and many.

Patients are ethically obliged to inform their traditional practitioners what CAM modalities they are using and what supplements and herbs they are taking. Many of the herbs and herbal mixtures interact with regular drugs and some herbs are absolutely contraindicated in some diseases.

Informing one's doctor is important from two perspectives: (1) he or she needs to know what one's being taken as a therapeutic alternative which may augment, supplement, or even antagonize the drugs he or she is prescribing, and (2) the doctor needs to know that at some level the patient has lost partial faith in regular medicine and is now open to possibly unproved and inappropriate therapies, for which the doctor, if he or she is still treating the patient, will ultimately be held responsible for the clinical outcome. Playing games with one's practitioner and being less than honest is no way to establish a good healing rapport. A particularly CAM-adherent patient came to see me with complaints of palpitations and syncope of two days duration. On examination she had a pulse rate of 180 beats per minute and a blood pressure of 160/100 mm Hg. She had never had any cardiac pathology and her historic blood pressure was 110/70. On questioning she admitted to taking a Chinese patent medicine for a viral prodrome that she felt was coming on. I inquired into the name of the medicine and asked her what dosage she was employing. The patent medicine was Yin Chiao (Lonicera-Forsythia Dispel Heat Tablets), which is commonly used for viral infections in the first 48 hours of symptoms. The normal dose is 5 to 6 pills every 2 to 3 hours for the first day, then decreasing to every 4 to 5 hours the next day. She had been taking 8 pills every 2 hours for two days. In spite of the increased dosage, her symptoms did not make any sense, as the action of the formula does not cause palpitations and raised blood pressure, even in an increased dosage. Inspection of the bottle revealed the cause of her symptoms. Many of the newer Chinese patent formulas, as a reflection of the renewed interest of the Chinese in Western culture and medicine, include Western pharmaceuticals. Some of the formulas for arthritis will, for example, include some cortisone, and in this case the medication included rather large amounts of paracetamol, caffeine, and chlorpheniramine. She was virtually on a therapeutic dose of "speed" due to the Western pharmaceuticals included in her Yin Chiao. All her symptoms disappeared within 8 hours of stopping the patent formula.

## PRACTITIONER ISSUES

Every practitioner is ethically obliged to know as much as he or she can regarding their field of medicine. This is the reason for continuing medical education requirements for state licensure, board recertification, and medical staff privileges. Not knowing any CAM is akin to neglecting to learn the cardiovascular system in medical school. Yet, the great majority of U.S. practitioners has little knowledge of CAM and has little opportunity to acquire that knowledge. This defect in our medical knowledge is so important because CAM refers not only to different modalities of treatment, but a whole new way of looking at the patient, disease, and treatment. This recent appreciation of the "whole" rather than "components" leads to real healing and well-being far in excess of any expectations currently placed on traditional therapy.

Many practitioners of CAM are amiss in their approaches to their patients. Some MDs, chiropractors, and acupuncturists expound unrealistic expectations and results and a few practice far beyond their scope of practice. Many treat traditional medicine as an enemy to be fought against at all times and counsel patients not to go back to their traditional physicians. All of these attitudes are abhorrent and are to be deplored. The terms *alternative* and *complementary* are divisive and nonproductive. They indicate an "either/or" approach and should be discarded in favor of the term *integrated* or *integrative* which reflects the true nature of medicine and biology.

## REGULATORY ISSUES

The medical boards of different states seem to view CAM in many differing ways. In California, you can practice homeopathy with impunity if you are not a medical doctor, but with legal risk if you are a licensed physician. States such as Arizona, Alaska, Washington, Connecticut, and Nevada have specific legislation allowing the practice of CAM. Each state has adopted a slightly different approach to the "problem." These boards are now forced to deal with these licensing and practice issues because of pressure from their constituents. Most of these boards are poorly prepared to deal with these questions because they have steadfastly refused to acknowledge the existence of CAM. The most important issue relates to the prosecution of doctors solely because they choose to use CAM in their practices instead of, or together with, traditional medicine. The decisions regarding the appropriate use of CAM are difficult because of the lack of scientific outcome data utilizing CAM in different clinical situations. It should not be an issue unless CAM is used inappropriately in place of traditional medicine. When in doubt as to the efficacy of a CAM approach, the practitioner should monitor the patient closely, have a traditional backup approach documented, and be ready to medically defend his or her choices to the licensing board. In Nevada, the Nevada State Board of Medical Examiners has taken the pragmatic approach of stating that any modality and instrumentality may be used by a practitioner in treatment of his patient, provided that the practitioner can demonstrate adequate training in the modality, that the patient was informed, and that the treatment was not grossly inappropriate or fanciful. The use of homeopathy, medical acupuncture, Chinese and Western herbology, therapeutic nutrition, and neural therapy are all regarded as "the practice of medicine."[15] The issue of "customary and usual treatment" as a discriminatory tool against CAM will fall by the wayside as CAM becomes more customary and usual. The major problem for the boards is documenting practitioner competence in CAM modalities. A specialty board in CAM as is customary in all other medical specialties is needed.

Notwithstanding all the ethical issues that are arising as a result of CAM activity, most of the issues are really plain old medical ethics that have been addressed for eons, but now raise different questions.

# 3 A Brief History of Medical Thought and Politics

The concept of vitalism, that man is more than just the sum of his physical or mechanistic parts, reappeared within the elitist Western universities of Europe during the late 18th and early 19th centuries in a response to the new science of mechanics and rational thought. This concept of a vivifying force that made man alive and was the essence of his being had been the fundamental basis of most early medical philosophies and still has its expression in Ayurvedic medicine as "prana," in homeopathy as the "vital force," and in acupuncture as "Qi." Medieval biology, taking its roots from Aristotle and his concepts of natural laws and the theological dictates of the day, could not separate the mind from the body or the psyche from the soma. Thus, when reductionism, the concept that the body and its diseases can be totally described in terms of their parts and subparts, began to surface, the intellectual elites of the time began to resist this new science with a vitalistic attack. The vitalistic promise, however, could not survive the many discoveries and newer concepts that began to appear, including Descartes' separation of the body and the mind and the mathematical explanation of all things, the classification of disease by Thomas Sydenham, Morgagni's pathophysiological approach, and Virchow's discovery of cellular pathology. The vital energy tradition was carried on as a footnote in medicine by the Viennese physician Anton Mesmer (1734–1815), who conceived the notion of "animal magnetism" as the source and cure of all disease. This concept has matured over time and has been called "psychic force" by Robert Hare (1781–1858), "parapsychology" by Joseph Bank Rhine (1885–1980), "psionic energy" by Robert Thouless (1894–1984), and "auric or astral force," a term coined by the Theosophists (Madame Blavatsky 1831–1891), while modern teachers prefer the phrase "subtle energy." Others who developed this idea in a more spiritual manner were Phineas P. Quimby (1802–1866), who developed the concept of "Mind Cure," and his more famous patient, Mary Baker Eddy (1821–1919), the founder of the Christian Science Church. Modern day laying on of hands, prayer, and spiritual healing still carry on the vitalistic nature of our spiritual being.

However, the real battle between the vitalistic forces and the new medical sciences took place between the practitioners of homeopathy (the Eclectic or New School) and the practitioners of drug therapy and surgery (the Allopathic or Old School).[16] The war was somewhat subdued in Europe, but was vicious and heated in the United States. In the early 1880s medicine was in shambles. The drugs used and the techniques employed were crude, harsh, and ineffectual. Homeopathy had been imported from Germany to the Americas by Constantine Hering, MD. He published the *Domestic Physician*, the first homeopathic materia medica, in two volumes in 1835 and 1838. In 1844, due to the popularity of homeopathy and its numerous converts to the "new school," the American Institute of Homeopathy (AIH) was formed with Hering as its first president. This august body is still in existence. Although the aim of the institute was to be an accrediting organization for homeopathic qualifications and to discover new medications, it soon turned into a political body to face the growing counterattack from the apothecaries and the allopathic doctors of the old school. In 1846 the American Medical Association (AMA) was formed to counter the influence of the homeopaths and the AIH. By the turn of the century, 15% of the medical doctors in the U.S. used homeopathy and were supported by 1000 pharmacies and 22 medical schools in most major cities. Boston University, New York University, Hahnemann Medical College of Philadelphia, and the University of Michigan were all homeopathic medical schools. The University of California at San Francisco still has an unendowed Professorial Chair of Homeopathy. The University of Michigan has one of best homeopathic libraries in the world in its lower stacks. When I visited my college-going sons there, they had to drag me out of the bowels of that literary cornucopia with its 200 years of exquisite clinical information. The original printed sixth edition of Hahnemann's *The Organon of Medicine*, including his handwritten ink comments, is available for examination in the rare book section of the University of California at San Francisco medical school library.

During the great cholera epidemics in England in 1830 and 1854, Naples in 1854–55, Vienna in 1836, and New York in the 1850s, the average mortality rate of those using regular old school medicine was 60% to 70%. In the hands of homeopathy, the death rate across Europe was 9% and in New York 4% to 5%. The success of homeopathy during the epidemics led the AMA in 1855 to adopt a "consultation clause" in which it forbade consultation with homeopaths on the threat of expulsion from the AMA.

The AMA went so far as to expel a physician from his state medical society for talking to his homeopathic doctor wife about a patient. This AMA action brings to mind similar activities practiced by the AMA against chiropractors in the 1980s, a practice that was judged illegal and immediately dropped. After fifty golden years in the U.S., homeopathy went into decline due to newer medical techniques, more effective drug therapies, the economics of homeopathy, and internecine infighting. The final death blow to homeopathy in the U.S. was the publication of the Flexner Report in 1910. The AMA commissioned the Carnegie Endowment to examine the educational structure and curricula of all the medical schools in the country and to either give them a stamp of approval or discredit them. Abraham Flexner, accompanied by Nathan Colwell of the AMA, took the criteria for the allopathic medical schools (Johns Hopkins Medical School being the model of the new physical and laboratory approach) and used those criteria to discredit and thus close down all the homeopathic medical schools of the day. The last diploma in homeopathy was issued by the Hahnemann Medical School in 1950.

Homeopathy, and indeed all holistically based medicine, went undercover and was carried on by a few older doctors who had been taught homeopathy and by many lay practitioners. It was the lay practitioners who kept the art alive in the U.S. In Britain, doctors were still allowed to practice due to the insistence of the royal family and the establishment of the London Royal Homeopathic Hospital just around the corner from the Great Ormond Street Children's Hospital. In Europe homeopathy continues to be practiced by both doctors and naturopaths in conjunction with allopathic medicine without any problems. The German government just recently reintroduced homeopathy and natural medicine into the medical school curricula.

The United States Food and Drug Administration has had an ambivalent relationship with natural and homeopathic medicine. On one hand it has tried to stamp out practice of these modalities by targeting specific high-profile physicians and putting them out of business, while on the other hand it has to allow homeopathic medications because they are covered by the homoeopathic pharmacopoeia of the United States, which had its first edition printed in 1897 under the auspices of the Pharmacopoeia Convention of the American Institute of Homeopathy. The FDA has recently had a serious legal setback with the herb industry regarding the classification of herbs not as a drug but as a food. Its recent legal loss to Pharmanex for the herbal preparation Cholistin (a natural lipid-lowering substance) has finally put the FDA on notice that it better get seriously into or stay out of herbal and natural pharmacy jurisdiction. Pressures from organized medicine and counter-pressures from the lay public will eventually rule in this regard.

The medical schools, long the whipping boys of the drug cartel, have had to make their own changes as managed care and reduced reimbursement and consumer pressures have caused them to reassess their opposition to complementary and alternative medicine. There are now 63 medical schools that offer either an elective or some formal teaching in CAM.

We have come one giant circle in terms of the acceptability of a vitalistic medical philosophy and the wheel continues to turn even as I write this sentence. What the eventual politicoeconomic and medical outcome will be, no one yet knows, but it will certainly be different from the status quo.

# 4 Integrated Medical Biology

The doctor of the future will give no medicine, but will interest his patients in the care of the human frame, in diet, and in the cause and prevention of disease. —Thomas Edison.

## INTRODUCTION

Before we delve into the concepts of integrated medicine and its predecessors, we need to have a basic understanding of the underpinnings on which all physical form on this earth is based. This explanation is necessary because in medicine we never go far beyond the obviously apparent. The human manifestation is supported at all levels by the natural laws of physics that govern the cosmos, universes, galaxies, planet systems, and, indeed, our own existence as an energy–mass–information being. We need to understand that it is these laws of thermodynamics, entropy, and homeodynamic nonlinear equilibrium that we are dealing with when we try to cure a diseased patient, who really represents nothing more than a thermodynamically unstable system. This human system can, like the electron, be considered at any one time as a particle (mass) or as a waveform (energy), the yin and the yang as the Chinese describe it. The physics that relates to these issues in the universe includes the laws of thermodynamics, nonlinear dynamics, fractal geometry, and chaos theory.

## THERMODYNAMICS IN BIOLOGY

For the purpose of thermodynamics, the human body is a *local system*. This local system, however, is *open* because it can exchange matter and energy with its surroundings. Those surroundings consist of nonbiological and biological entities, such as heat or perhaps a virus. The human body and its surroundings constitute a *miniuniverse* in which we operate and exchange energy with our surroundings. However, because our bodies operate as an integrated whole, the body itself, while exchanging energy and matter with the outside, operates as a *closed universe*. All information–energy–matter changes within the body will, by necessity, have an impact on the form and integrity of all other parts. The Chinese were well aware of all these issues as evidenced by their recognition of the effect of the weather and seasons on the balance of the body. They also described the bodily organs without ever having performed an autopsy, not as physical tissues, but as interrelated functional–emotional–energetic concepts. For example, the kidney, which regulated some of the bodily fluids, was described as the seat of fear and the source of all energy within the body. The organ concepts were all connected on the outside and inside of the body by the energetic principal meridians and related functionally by the Ko and Sheng cycles. Changes in one area produced changes in all areas.

Because we are part of the total universe, however, we have to obey the universal laws that pertain to our particular manifestation, that is, as physicoenergetic beings. This leads to the *first principle of thermodynamics*: energy is conserved in the universe, but may change its form. Thus, the conversion of adenosine triphosphate (ATP) to running muscles represents a conversion of chemical energy to thermal and mechanical energy. This ability of the body to utilize energy to do useful work is termed *utility*. These concepts are more or less common sense and are part of our everyday experience.

The *second principle of thermodynamics* is a lot more important and a lot more subtle. The second principle states that the universe acts spontaneously to become more disorderly. This is the natural direction of change, to one of disorder. The measure of this disorder is called *entropy*. Thus, the second principle can be reworded to state that any spontaneous process increases the entropy of the universe. The second principle exhibits some general features. For example, entropy is not conserved but is always increasing, as spontaneous events are always happening. In a local system, for example, our bodies, entropy may decrease as long as there is an equal increase in the entropy of its surroundings; that is, another part of the body becomes more disordered or more entropic. So, in the human body, which is part of this universe, entropy is increasing unless we add some energy to reverse that process. This is the battle from birth and growth, which is highly neg-entropic, to death, which for us is the ultimate and maximum entropic state.

In the body itself, for example, the act of glycolysis and aerobic respiration causes the energy liberated by glucose metabolism to bond inorganic phosphate to adenosine diphosphate (ADP) to form adenosine triphosphate (ATP), which is the unit or quanta of energy utilized in the body. This decreases entropy by covalently fixing these atoms in place. However, the entropy in the region surrounding the ATP is increased by conversion of glucose into $CO_2$ gas and by the release of heat into the surrounding mitochondrial matrix. The increased heat causes an increase in molecular motion and entropy of the mitochondrion. Thus, the positive interplay of the external environment (the source of the glucose as food from photosynthesis) and the conversion of energy into a utilitarian neg-entropic currency allow the human body to retain its integrity and purposefulness rather than collapsing into a random collection of nitrogen, carbon, and oxygen atoms. The negative interaction of the surrounding environment in the form of radiation, trauma, or even harsh words causes further induced external sources of entropy that must be countered in order to maintain a suitable neg-entropic state. This purposeful movement towards a state of acceptable biological neg-entropy is a semi-steady state called the *homeodynamic equilibrium*. This is not the more commonly recognized "homeostasis," which is a more immobile fixed steady state that has some very negative physiological attributes, as we will see later.

As humans we are stuck in a double bind. We need to create energy to keep our integrity (neg-entropic organization), but its very creation causes increased entropy within us. This battle of entropy production and reduction is exemplified in free radical production by oxidation, the source of our neg-entropic energy. These free radicals, by their further interaction with membranes, lipids, enzymes, and nucleic acids, cause increases in entropy in these structures, which we term *inflammation*, *degeneration*, and finally *necrosis* or *aging*. We have internal mechanisms that dampen the activity of the free radicals, and we also ingest antioxidants, which help in reducing the entropic activity of these chemical reactions.

There is another fundamental issue that needs to be discussed in connection with the second principle. The change of energy from glucose to $CO_2$ causes an increase in the energy of the $CO_2$ bonds, thus increasing the kinetic molecular energy of translation, vibration, and rotation. This increases the *degrees of freedom* and movement of the $CO_2$. The increase in freedom of movement, however, is balanced by a loss of stability. We, as humans, are constantly in this precarious balance between freedom of movement (adaptability, biological choices) and stability (neg-entropy), and it is the interplay between these metaphorical thermodynamic poles that will determine the state of health or dis-ease that we experience. Choice, by reason of changing the status quo, makes us momentarily unstable, but if the choice is wise, it will create greater stability in the long run. We can also look at this phenomenon as a definition of evolution. Positive changes cause enhanced development of the being. Negative changes cause greater entropy with reduced permanent stability. As we shall see, it is this interaction with our external and internal being that will determine the eventual balance of our being at all levels, even our thermodynamic balance, and hence our final evolutionary form. Freedom of will, with the ability to choose, produces changes that represent the poles that vivify our very existence, just like good and bad, dark and light, and hot and cold. This polarity of being with the interjection of movement, unpredictable behavior, and circadian cycles appears to be the bedrock of existence as we know it.

If we start just before the "big bang," the most organized and neg-entropic time of the universe, the universe has been spontaneously expanding and becoming more disorganized ever since. In Stephen Hawking's book, *A Brief History of Time*, he relates time to entropy.[17] If there was no change in entropy, you could not possibly observe the passage of time, because the unwinding of a spring or the discharge of a battery all involve a change in entropy. In fact, in the human, entropy (degeneration) and aging (the passage of time) are intimately linked. One can think back to childhood when one hour seemed an eternity and now, when one day seems to go by in an instant. Our perception of time seems to be connected to our state of neg-entropy — the more neg-entropic we are (young, whole, and growing), the slower we perceive time to be; the more entropic we become (old, chaotic, and degenerating), the faster time seems to pass. Thus, we have now injected time into the evolutionary and thermodynamic equation.

Now let us get back to the ideal human state — *homeodynamic equilibrium*. In the cell, with its thousands of simultaneous and somewhat compartmentalized reactions, a state of *chemical equilibrium* (maximized entropy) is never attained as reactants and products are continually entering and leaving the system. The best we can hope for is a *semi-steady state*, in which reactants and products remain in somewhat constant concentrations, but there is no equilibrium in the system. In fact, if equilibrium is reached, it usually means the death of the organism.

We have to ask a question at this point: How does the human biology maintain its low entropy in a universe whose entropy (disorderliness) is always increasing? This orderliness is obtained by input from an external free energy source, namely, the sun. Thermonuclear reactions in the sun liberate orderliness as sunlight; the green plant incorporates some of the sun's orderliness in $CO_2$ fixation by photosynthesis; herbivores eat the plant, thereby incorporating some of the green plant's orderliness into their own structure; the herbivore dies and the remaining orderliness is lost as it decomposes. Thus, mammalian biology is a temporary blip of low entropy and orderliness in the continual expansion and chaos of the universe. In fact, the concept of the "flow" of orderliness through biological systems was first put forward by the famous physicist E. Schrodinger, in his book entitled *What Is Life?*[18] This specific order in biological systems is the reason we need to look to the patient's biology for the meaning and treatment of disease and not to the double-blind study, which is far removed from the discrete biology in front of us. Morowitz has restated this concept by saying that, "Living organisms, because of their low entropy, are improbable and their condition of existence is maintained by a constant inflow of free external energy from the sun, thus increasing the entropy in the rest of the universe."[19] The very reality of our existence then, is truly against all energetic odds and can lead some of us to believe that the human was ordained to be manifested, and with this ordination come certain responsibilities and tasks in relationship to the rest of the cosmos, because our existence causes a countercurrent perturbation in the rest of the universe. It is the disconnection from this path that causes poor choices, and hence positive biological entropy and the resulting premature aging and death — physical, energetic, and spiritual.

There are some interesting and practical consequences from these laws of thermodynamics. Suppose a herbivore was eaten by a carnivore, and that carnivore was eaten by another carnivore, etc. By the time the energy and orderliness of the original plant reaches the last carnivore, the amount of the original plant orderliness is extremely small. Thus, a large quantity of plant orderliness is needed to support the orderliness of carnivores down the food chain. This thermodynamic fact gives some credence to John Robbin's *Diet for a New America*, which emphasizes a plant source diet.[20] One can explain these concepts in considering a very simple food chain. The chain consists of grass, grasshoppers, frogs, trout, and humans. As each part of the food chain is devoured by the organism above it in the food chain, there is an 80% to 90% loss of energy as heat. Only between 10% and 20% of the energy devoured is available in the body of the predator to the next member of the food chain. It turns out that 300 salmon are needed to keep one human alive for one year;

90,000 frogs keep the salmon alive; 27,000,000 grasshoppers keep the frogs alive, and 1000 tons of grass keeps the grasshoppers alive. Therefore, a vegetarian is cheaper to feed than a carnivore. A low entropy protein diet can be very expensive if it is obtained metabolically far from the sun. It is better to eat the plant than the animal that ate the plant, in terms of thermodynamic efficiency and cost. Vegetables and fruits are cheaper sources of orderliness than equivalent amounts of meat. In the same vein, it is more efficient, more global, and less costly to treat the disease closer to the internal source and to work with the biology and encourage the energetic flow system instead of trying to change disease from outside the system, causing a loss of energy in the system and more entropy and disorganization. We will deal with the practical issues that these constructs present to medicine in the section dealing with the energetic and functional biological model.

## THE CURRENT MEDICAL BIOLOGICAL MODEL

The current medical model owes its origins to the machine age, which was championed by five great thinkers: Francis Bacon (representing the pragmatic practical approach), Rene Descartes (representing a mathematical approach), Isaac Newton (representing a physics approach), John Locke (representing government and society), and Adam Smith (representing the economic approach). The only two worldview philosophies that had preceded the mechanical worldview were those of the Greek and the medieval church. The Greeks had a view that although the world was created by deities, it was not immortal but had in it the seeds of its own destruction. Therefore, the idea that history was a decaying cyclical process made the Greeks believe that less change conserved order and energy. Growth did not signal greater value and order in the world, in fact, it indicated the opposite. Thus, the Greek worldview was somewhat congruent with the laws of thermodynamics. The worldview of the church and the Middle Ages was somewhat different. In those times, life was perceived as a mere stopover in preparation for the next life. The Greek view of cycles had been dropped in favor of history as a linear decaying process that had a beginning (creation), a middle (redemption), and an end (salvation or the "last judgment"). All of life's tasks were performed to this end of eventual salvation and the will of God. To add insult to injury, the doctrine of original sin precluded humanity improving its lot in its lifetime.

However, a single individual, in a single lecture given at the Sorbonne in 1750, changed all of that. Jacques Turgot single-handedly took the history of the world and turned it upside down in announcing that the cyclical and degrading view of the world was incorrect and that history proceeded in a straight line with each succeeding era an improvement on the era that came before it. He proclaimed that change and progress were the only true realities and virtues in the world. It did not take much for our five great thinkers to delineate and categorize progress and change, which all had to do with a more and more minute examination of the parts so as to understand the whole. One could then devise ways of manipulating these parts and have jurisdiction over change and the future. Thus, our modern worldview has been transposed to our modern medical view, which follows a similar edict.

These great thinkers gave birth to a number of fateful assumptions that have steered the course of modern medicine. These assumptions include, but are not limited to:

1. the separation of the mind from the body;
2. understanding of the whole from investigation of the parts;
3. imposing treatment upon the organism from the outside;
4. removal of symptoms or disease representing a cure.

We shall examine these constructs in more practical detail. Our minute understanding and dissection of physiology, biochemistry, and the physical, anatomical, human body has led to a conclusion that life is no more than a composite of these particular elements. *Disease*, then, is a departure from the normal framework of these elements, which can, through external manipulation by drugs or surgical or physical means, that is, medical therapy, be put back into its appropriate place of reference and be normalized. The prime arbiter and initiator of these normalizing or curing activities is the *medical diagnosis*. This logical mental manifest is the prime medical event around which all other medical activities relating to the patient take place. Without diagnosis there can be no therapy — they are inexorably linked. Diagnosis itself is of some practical use: it categorizes the disease by pathophysiology and organ system; it gives some idea of historical treatments and prognosis; and it puts a value on the frivolous or serious nature of the process occurring in the patient. All of this information is of practical value and must be factored into the integrated medical approach.

Diagnosis has some serious drawbacks, however, especially in multiorgan, multifactoral, and complicated chronic disease. Diagnosis is based on a listing of signs and symptoms that are seen as a repetitive coherent whole in the general population, and as such, through medical history, have assumed a clinicopathological identity that can be extrapolated to any one patient in particular. Many times this extension of the general case suffices to characterize the patient and his or her disease, but many times it falls short of the clinical needs of both patient and doctor. Problems occur when the patient's symptoms do not fall into a clean definition of any one diagnosis. Perhaps the patient has a disease that just can't be treated as so many single disease processes, or worse still, if the symptoms don't even qualify as "real," they are viewed as being "in the patient's head." The patient's reality and appreciation of their dis-ease may not be congruent with, or even part of, your understanding of disease. Nevertheless, the patient is presenting with an odd problem and to him or her it is real and it is causing dis-ease and you are expected to deal with it, even if you can't put a name on it. The patient with chronic disease represents a special case of difficulty, with each successive therapeutic intervention, based on a discrete medical diagnosis, causing a more complicated, muddled, and deeper pathology to appear. Another problem with diagnosis is that patients with the same diagnosis often do not respond to the appropriate therapy for that diagnosis. What is wrong? Is it an incorrect diagnosis or is the patient noncompliant or refractory to therapy? It is difficult to assess. One of the options is that some cases of a particular diagnosis arrive at their disease through a different etiologic mechanism than is usually the case, and hence a more defined alternate treatment is necessary. The concept of diagnosis and the associated therapeutic menu does not quite make the grade in every patient. Clearly, there are many instances in which the current biomedical diagnostic model does not quite fit.

The most important part of the diagnosis is the patient's symptom or symptoms. *Symptoms* are any manifestation of a deviation from a previous or generally recognized pattern of health perceptible by the patient, individuals around him or her, or by a physician. The collection of symptoms will often suggest a clinicopathological diagnosis. Often the symptom is the diagnosis, e.g., headache. Although the medical model can subdivide headaches into some pathophysiological subtypes such as cluster headaches or tension headaches or migraines, the real thrust of the treatment is to extinguish the symptom. Any subtyping is pursued only because it may have some therapeutic and prognostic subtlety. This is true of the approach of most of modern medicine. There certainly is no shame in ridding the patient of pain and suffering, and we would be remiss in not aspiring to that end. However, let us go back to that second law of thermodynamics and see where this superficial approach gets us.

If a symptom represents a departure from the normal steady state of energy flow, then it also represents a state of disorder with respect to the rest of the body. You now extinguish this disorder and make it more orderly by applying some directing or informational free energy from the outside, a drug, for instance, and the symptom is suppressed and order is restored to the body. You will remember that every time you create order in the system, you do so to the detriment of another part of the system that becomes more disordered. So, the acute outer symptom will be replaced by a more chronic internalized symptom whose disorderliness will be far greater than the disorder you corrected, because the body's own choice of disorder, i.e., symptom, is always the best and least destructive choice. When the system is barraged by multiple, acute, suppressive, and superficial therapeutic inputs of this type, it results in a system that is so disordered that it cannot be made orderly again by any amount of suppressive therapy and the end result is "chronic disease." So we end up curing the symptom and shifting the patient closer to an equilibrium state (total disorder), because we have suppressed the body's ability to respond to the internal disorder that was the problem in the first place (remember the discussion on the implicate and the explicate of David Bohm).

There are, however, instances in which such superficial and suppressive therapeutic endeavors are entirely appropriate. If the patient is tending toward death (the ultimate equilibrium state of disorderliness), it is quite appropriate to suppress the symptom and reinstate some orderliness to reverse this process. A good example of this special case would be an acute asthma attack treated with steroids or terbutaline. Modern medicine is extremely talented at this kind of diversional suppressive therapy as evidenced by spending a night in an emergency room or trauma unit. This kind of energetic thinking certainly does not go on in your head as you see patients in your office, but it should. The majority of our ambulatory patients do not fall into the acute suppressive category in spite of the fact that we treat them as if they do, with antibiotic, antidepressant, antipsychotic, antihypertensive, anticonvulsive therapies.

While I am being controversial and provocative, let us discuss disease. *Disease* can be defined as a state of ill health or discomfort experienced by the patient. The job of the modern medical doctor is to intervene and eradicate this polysymptomatic manifestation — or is it? Let's go back to thermodynamics. If the externally manifested disease constitutes a state of less order, blocked flow-through, or available energy, then it is being formed in response to an associated state of more necessary order or neg-entropy or balance somewhere else in the system. If this state of increased order in the inner system is more critical to the biological steady state than rectification of the peripheral disease, then by suppressing the symptoms of the peripheral disease we have done a biological and thermodynamic disservice to the body (that is, if the disease is not tending towards death as discussed above).

This discussion brings up the topic of *medical cures*. To most doctors *cure* means eradication or disappearance of the symptoms of disease. Thermodynamically, this process can be translated into changing the superficial disorderliness (disease) of the system to a more ordered state (cure), and thus the disorder (disease or symptoms) disappear. But remember the corollary of order on the surface is an associated deeper disorder, so the "cure" is but "skin deep" and the disease has been driven deeper into the system. Let me give you a commonly encountered example of this phenomenon. In atopic families it is common for young babies to present with eczema. This superficial disorder is commonly rectified by the suppressive action of a topically applied cortisone preparation. So the skin is made more orderly, but this new orderliness has now blunted the expression of superficial disorder (eczema) that the body was expressing for its own thermodynamic ends. Now the body must express that disorderliness in a new format or disease at a somewhat deeper level in order to satisfy the laws of thermodynamics. This new disease presentation will usually occur at a time of increased change and disorder in the body (stress), where the flow-through energetic resources fail the total energetic economy and a new compensatory disorder is forced to present to keep energetic balance. Examples could be starting school, parent's divorce, infectious mono-nucleosis, or even the occurrence of puberty. In the case of infantile eczema that has been suppressed, the new disease that invariably arises is asthma. This disorder is deeper in the organism, affects a more crucial organ, and is vastly more energetically disordered and threatening to the host's biology and survival than the original disease. If this disease is then similarly suppressed with sympathomimetics, steroids, and anticytokine treatment, the disorder once again submerges and will reappear many years later as an autoimmune disease or worse. So, it seems we have to be a little hesitant and less cavalier in removing symptoms right and left — the thermodynamics of the biological state have to be explored and understood to effect a deeper cure.

*Susceptibility* is a very poorly taught medical concept. It means to be open, submit to, or be unresistant to an external stimulus or agency. It is the ability to experience a state. In the more

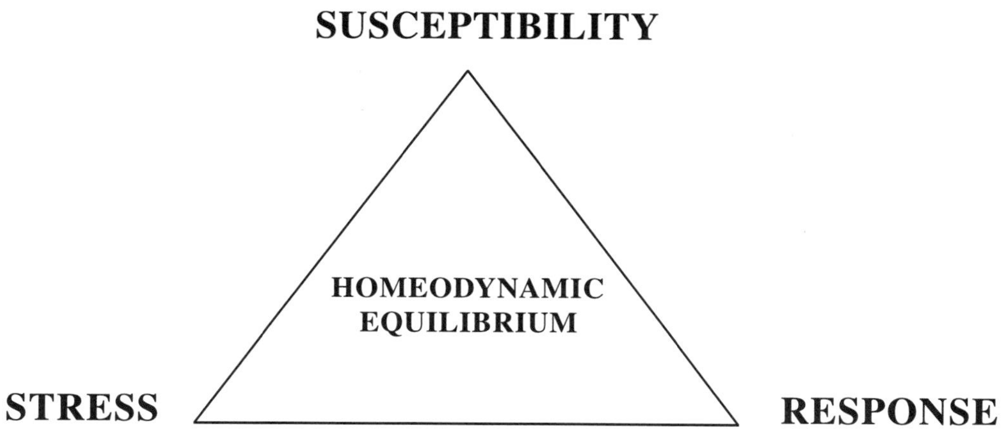

# SUSCEPTIBILITY

**HOMEODYNAMIC
EQUILIBRIUM**

# STRESS                                                          RESPONSE

**FIGURE 4.1** The Triangle of Homeodynamic Equilibrium.

specific medical sense, it implies your state of resistance or acceptance of an extraneous factor such as infectious disease.

Susceptibility forms the apex of the *triangle of homeodynamic equilibrium*. (Figure 4.1). If we look at this figure we see the three components that make up the potential of homeostasis or the steady state of thermodynamics: *external stressors*, *internal reaction or response*, and *susceptibility* that modifies both of these opposite forces. The thermodynamic relationship between the arms of this triangle is quite integrated. The external stressor is trying to induce disorder for its own acquisition of orderliness (the invading organism or your boss shouting at you); the response is to attempt to maintain homeodynamic equilibrium by matching the disorderliness of the stressor with a cybernetic reaction that stabilizes the internal milieu and is equal to or greater in energy than the offending outer disturbing force. The amount of susceptibility to the offending stressor will govern the impact of the stressor and how much response will have to be mounted. The less susceptibility, the less damage the stressor does, and the less energy needed to expend to offset its action.

Susceptibility then, acts as a modulator of any outer thermodynamic attack. The greater the constitution of the individual, the less the susceptibility to any stressor and the greater ease with which any stressor is countered. Modern medical therapeutics have focused on either trying to kill or offset the stressor or suppressing the reaction of the patient to the stressor, if this reaction is deemed unpleasant, e.g., fever in an infective processes. Very little has ever been done to decrease the susceptibility of the host. Both homeopathy and Chinese herbology are important therapeutic tools in this regard.

Another characteristic of modern medical thought is the compartmentalization of disease into organ systems which are handled by medical specialists. Scarce attention is paid to the relationship between organs and the body as a whole. Everybody is looking after an organ system, but who is looking after the patient?

The concept of *cure* has been dealt with to some extent; however, *wellness and health* have never been adequately defined in modern medicine. The absence of disease does not mean wellness or health. There are many people walking around who have no disease but are certainly not well. Growing numbers of people lack vitality and suffer from a host of "normal" complaints such as allergies, headaches, lack of energy or excessive fatigue, indigestion, heartburn, constipation, restless sleep, or dysmenorrhea and PMS, along with a variety of emotional states ranging from mild depression to mood swings and anxiety. They are in a state of "vertical ill health." They are not sick enough to lie down ("horizontal ill health") and yet consider themselves normal because most of the people they know are equally unhealthy. They rely on a barrage of antihistamines, antiinflammatories, analgesics, H1-blockers, antacids, soporifics, laxatives, antidepressants, and tranquilizers to maintain adequate daily homeodynamic balance. The side effects that they develop from these mostly over-the-counter drugs only add to their problems.

## THE CONCEPT OF AN ENERGETIC AND FUNCTIONAL BIOLOGICAL MODEL

I have used the physical domain of thermodynamics to anchor my energetic understanding of what is happening in biology and medicine. One of the tenants of the laws of thermodynamics is that they only apply to the physical activity of the world. These laws govern the horizontal world of time and space. However, when it comes to the vertical world of spiritual transcendence, all worldly laws are powerless. The spirit is a nonmaterial dimension and so does not obey the laws of fixed boundaries and limits. There is a relationship between the spirit world and the physical world. The physical world is a small manifestation of its greater whole and is eventually governed by the spirit force that gave it form and life. In medicine, we pay scant attention to the spiritual and ethereal origins and manifestations of disease. However, on pure clinical grounds, we cannot ignore this connection to the template of our physical being. In my experience there are too many instances of diseases that are connected to, and respond to, a discussion of spiritual issues concerning the patient to ignore this vast source of positive and negative manifestation and inspiration. We have discussed the concept of entropy, the state of disorganization and chaos toward which the universe and our bodies are heading. It turns out that if we take a look at the evolving entropic state, there seems to be some underlying order. This underlying order (the implicate order of Bohm) has recently been expanded upon with the defining and new understanding of *Chaos Theory* and its physical concepts of *strange attractors*, *nonlinear paradoxes*, and *fractal geometry*.[21,22] It seems that variability, unpredictability, and discontinuous irregular biological behavior has some vitality and purpose to it that can only be explained at this time by a higher purpose and connection. Some physical law is governing the body's organizing response to entropy and the eventual physical and emotional forms that this response manifests. These responses seem to be characteristic of, and common to, all living forms on this planet. Let us examine these theories and see how they might fit into our evolving understanding of disease and health.

### Chaos Theory, Nonlinear Dynamics, and Fractals

The reductionistic mind-set is ruled by the logical order of a linear systems theory. The magnitude of a linear response is proportional to the strength of the input stimulus. These linear systems can be fully understood and predictions made by examining their component parts. The subunits of a linear system add up — there are no anomalies or surprises. However, as we have postulated, the human biology is interconnected, and its components obey a different set of system dynamics that interrelate all the components, as if they all operated as a single integrated unit. This kind of anomalous holistic and collective deterministic behavior is governed by another system: the *laws of nonlinear dynamics*. By contrast, in nonlinear dynamics, system proportionality does not hold because the output is not proportional to the input, and nonlinear systems cannot be understood by analyzing their parts (is this starting to sound familiar?). These systems are characterized by a "chaotic" behavior inasmuch as small changes introduced into control of the system cause it to abruptly change from one type of behavior to another. This enables our bodies to respond to large insults with small defined inputs to effect balance. This abrupt, nonlinear behavioral transition in chaos theory is called a *bifurcation*. A more understandable term that could be used is a *step-down* or *step-up modulation*. *Deterministic chaos* relates to an aperiodic, seemingly random behavior that can arise from the operation (internal feedback loops) of even the most simple nonlinear system. *Chaos*, in its new meaning, is seen as a form of underlying order disguised as disorder. These nonlinear, emergent, collective, biological properties are the result of the summed and integrated activities of seemingly independent single parts that have come together to operate as a unified whole, and in doing so now have new collective properties not possessed by the sum of the individual components. Such a dynamic collection is seen, for example, in an ant colony, a flock of birds, or a school of fish. The ability of these integrated biological systems to react to a wide range of complex biological situations is governed by the components of the system and the degree of interaction between the individual units. These qualities augment the system's ability to react to any stressor more efficiently and with greater adaptivity. This self-organization and plasticity is seen in complex adaptive systems, such as the brain (neuronal cooperation) and the heart (myocytes contracting together), and in acupuncture as the *Law of Five Elements*. It has been suggested by Langton that evolutionary natural selection has spawned complex systems that adapted toward the boundary between order and chaos. Living systems seem to evolve toward this boundary and Kauffman has proposed that in these systems the maximum fitness occurs at the interface of order and chaos — being on the leading edge without being on the bleeding edge.[26]

These systems, however, are not allowed to go to chaotic extinction but, because of the underlying order, are limited in their randomness by a mathematical value called the *attractor* (the implicate order of Bohm). The attractor stabilizes the new state until it is no longer biologically tenable and the system is forced to move to a new chaotic state and a new attractor and so on. In some instances the attractor is so strong that it prohibits movement to any other state, the biology is then stuck, and its plasticity and its reactive abilities are compromised. The attractor seems to represent any agent with an organizing ability and so, perhaps we should refer to it as a *phase or level organizing stabilizer (PLOS)*. Anything altering the deterministic chaotic nature of the collective features of a self-organizing biological system will cause disease. This is classically seen in chronic heart failure and epileptic seizures.

If one then graphically plots the coordinates of a chaotic system, the underlying orderliness of the system is revealed by a geometric shape called a *fractal*. A fractal is a geometric shape composed of subunits upon subunits, all with the same shape, that gets smaller and smaller as you look deeper and deeper into the structure, a property known as *self-similarity* (Figure 4.2). Many common forms in nature are nonlinear and obey fractal dimensions, e.g., coastlines, clouds, snowflakes. In the

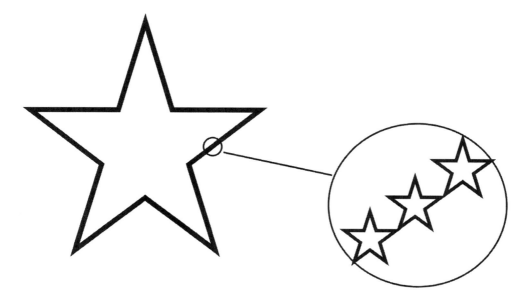

**FIGURE 4.2** Fractal self-similarity.

human anatomy we can point to the tracheobronchial tree with its ever-narrowing but similarly patterned bronchi, bronchioles, and alveoli. We can also consider the arterial and venous trees, the His-Purkinje network, and the collecting system of the kidney and calyces. These self-similar anatomic structures all serve a common physiological function: rapid and efficient transport over a complex, spatially distributed system. Other distributive features are seen involving information (nervous system), nutrient absorption (bowel), and collection and transport (biliary ducts and renal calyces). The fractal concept can also be used to graph physiological numbers, say, heart beats per minute, or the timed space between beats, or beat-to-beat variations. The jagged line of peaks and valleys on the graph represents the physiological data. If you then magnify any one part of the line, you see a similar line of jagged peaks and valleys and this picture continues at any higher magnification (Figure 4.3). This self-similarity is indicative of a fractal and hence indicative of a chaotic process and will follow nonlinear dynamics. Because this information is chaotic, it is by definition more healthy than data without fractal values. Complex fluctuations with the statistical properties of fractals have been described not only for heart-rate variability, but also for fluctuations in respiration, systemic blood pressure, human gait, and white blood counts as well as certain ion-channel kinetics. These fractal properties seem to be associated with most central organizing principals of biology and the absence of such a fractal scale is associated with disease.

The antithesis of a fractal scalar system is one that is dominated by one frequency or scale. A system that has only one frequency or dominant scale is especially easy to recognize or characterize, because it is by definition periodic and repeats its pattern in a highly predictable pattern. The paradoxical appearance of highly periodic dynamics in many disease states is one of the most compelling examples of the notion of complexity loss in disease, e.g., Kussmaul breathing. *Complexity* here refers specifically to a multiscale, fractal-type variability in structure or function. Many disease states are marked by dynamics less complex than those seen under healthy conditions. This decomplexification of systems seems a common feature of many diseases, including aging.[23] When physiological systems become less complex, their information content is degraded. As a result, they are less adaptable and less able to cope with the exigencies of a constantly changing environment.

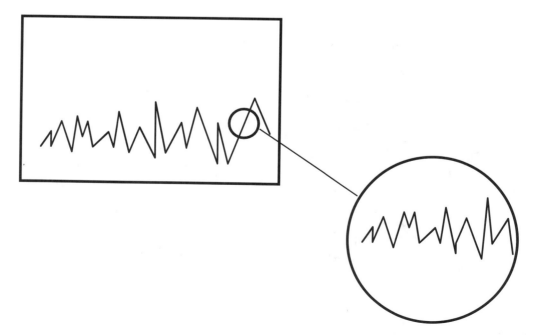

**FIGURE 4.3** Physiological fractals.

Generally, the practice of bedside diagnosis would be impossible without the loss of complexity and the emergence of such pathological periodicity. These periodicities and highly structured patterns — the breakdown of multiscale fractal complexity under perturbed conditions — allow clinicians to identify and classify many pathological features of their patients, i.e., a stable observable symptom.

Another important finding about nonlinear dynamics and chaos theory is that the outcome is very *sensitive to initial conditions* and that *very small inputs can cause very large changes*. The classical example is that a butterfly flapping its wings in Bejing could cause a tornado in Kansas if the initial conditions were unstable enough. In medicine this theory can be used in any disease state in which a key physiological parameter (e.g., blood pressure, hormone levels, immunological responses) is shown to be chaotic and is potentially amenable to control by introducing small, critically timed perturbations into the system with appropriate initial conditions.

Findings from nonlinear dynamics have also challenged conventional mechanisms of physiological control based on classical homeostasis, which indicates that healthy systems seek to attain a constant steady state. By contrast, nonlinear self-organizing systems with fractal dynamics are described as dynamic, far from equilibrium, and absorbing energy from their surroundings to maintain their state. This kind of complex variability, rather than a single homeostatic steady state, seems to define the free-running function of many biological systems.

In summary, it would seem from chaos theory, that disease represents a static, steady state of narrowed response, less complexity, and perhaps a dominant attractor. Our task, as caretakers of this biology, is to reinfuse information and energy that will broaden bodily responses and complexity, facilitate appropriate attractor adherence, and stimulate the physiology and cybernetic systems to be mobile and responsive once again.

In this discussion on thermodynamics, chaos theory, nonlinear dynamics, and fractals I have had made liberal use of, and extensively quoted from References 24–26.

These concepts were extremely hard to comprehend in a practical way and it took numerous repeat readings of the material for the concepts to crystalize. You may need to read the above section many times for its significance to become apparent and of some practical purpose. I have outlined these issues in a previous book.[27]

## COMPONENTS OF DISEASE

I think it would useful at this time to review an approach to the components of disease. The task of the doctor is to empower the patient at all levels of his or her being, knowing that one's state of health is the ability of the body–mind to balance the stresses that confront one everyday, and to strive to maintain connection to one's spiritual path. If the stresses and our body's response are evenly balanced, then we are in a state of homeodynamic equilibrium and good health. If the stresses are too strong and our response is too weak, then we are in an imbalance that can lead to ill health and disease. This concept of health as a balance will be repeated many times in the section on Traditional Chinese Medicine. Biological imbalance, seen as disease, has four major components, and each has to be treated to attain complete rebalancing of the human body. Treatment of only one or two components will result in either no change in symptoms, new symptoms, or reappearance of the disease at a later date. The four components of disease are:

1. **Emotional-Mental (Spiritual)** — probably the most important component, and the least addressed by modern medicine. The influence of genetics is included in this component, as it reflects the fixed spiritual information with which we come into this life. The expanding knowledge of psychoneuroimmunology (PNI) is the framework around which the biological reality of this component revolves. This will be dealt with in detail in the next section entitled Disease as a Chronological Continuum.

2. **Biochemical** — we are more familiar with the biochemical components of disease, but I will take a slightly different approach, focusing not so much on the biochemical laboratory diagnosis of disease. Rather, I will explain how the biochemistry of the body can be viewed from a functional point of view, both in health and disease. The concepts of detoxification, metabolic modulation, immune system regulation, hormonal supplementation, and therapeutic nutrition will be discussed.

3. **Structural** — the structural component includes the influence of the autonomic nervous system, which governs the activity and reactivity of the organs, circulation, muscles, fascia, and dermatomes. The relationship between these integrated entities and the bony skeleton will be elucidated and techniques and treatment discussed.

4. **Energetic** — the energetic component is foreign to the medical mind, and the most difficult to conceive. It relates to the flow of electrical and electromagnetic energies within and around the body. We are all familiar with EKGs, EEGs, and similar electrical measurements. The energetic parameters we are talking about are an extension of these gross electrical parameters. The internal electrical milieu of the body and its biological activities of regulation, embryogenesis, limb regeneration, and nonunion bone fracture healing have been well documented by Robert O. Becker, M.D. in multiple publications[28,29] and by Bjorn Noodenstrom, M.D. of the Karolinska Institute in Sweden, in his 1983 book *Biologically Closed Electrical Circuits*.[30]

As previously stated before, health or wellness is not the absence of disease. There are progressive quantum steps from the disease state to health. This progression represents a widening of the spectrum of biological reactivity, movement, or potential of the patient. If you follow the progression of the patient from disease to health you can see any of the following stages manifested:

1. *Suppression* — with disappearance of symptoms (what Western medicine usually accomplishes). The disease process is suppressed, the symptoms disappear, and the patient appears well. This wellness is only temporary as the symptoms have been driven deeper into the organism and will manifest at a later date in a more critical organ.

2. *Recovery* — return to a previous state of health with removal of major symptoms. This can be spontaneous (after treatment) or after the removal of a maintaining cause.

3. *Cure* — a much deeper and more significant process. This represents a return to a more complex and energetic nonlinear and chaotic state (to be discussed below) and can be defined in four ways:
   a. The whole process is cured (patient and disease).
   b. The patient is cured, not the disease, such as the patient who changes her conception of her reality after acquiring breast cancer, but goes on to die from the disease.
   c. There is complete restoration of health. The patient is cured, as is the disease, and the energetic state of the whole organism is advanced.
   d. The cure is permanent with no relapses. The patient's susceptibility is changed for the better.

4. *Change of susceptibility* — the patient's susceptibility is lowered. This often represents the removal of hereditary traits or miasmatic layers as described in homeopathy.

5. The physical changes may be seen as adhering to *Hering's Laws of Cure*. Hering was the most important American homeopath of the last century, and on pure clinical observations of disease, he postulated medicine's only laws of cure. Life is a centrifugal and organizing force, while disease is a centripetal and disorganizing force such that:
   a. disease disappears from the top downward.
   b. disease disappears from within, outward.
   c. disease disappears in reverse order of appearance — the last manifestation is the first to go.
   d. disease disappears from a more critical organ to a less critical organ.

Let me give a good example of these laws as they applied to a patient I saw in the sixth month of practice.

The young wife of a prominent professional in my town came to my office with fulminating ulcerative colitis. She had refused all regular medical treatment on emotional grounds and stated emphatically that she would rather die in my office than have regular medication. She had a fever of 103°F, a hemoglobin of 9.0 gm/dl and a white cell count of 16,000/ml with a left shift, a sedimentation rate of 46 mm in the first hour, and been having between 6 and 10 fluid bowel movements a day that exhibited blood and mucus. On examination she had diffuse abdominal tenderness and a thready pulse of 120 beats per minute, and she appeared dehydrated. This was not a good situation for me at all. Having a patient (the wife of a prominent official) expire in your office is not exactly a morale booster or a practice builder. She steadfastly refused to leave and so I had to biologically think my way through this serious clinical dilemma.

She agreed to have an intravenous drip as long as it contained no medication. So, she was rehydrated and started to pass urine for the first time in 24 hours. I then treated her with acupuncture (ST 25, ST 36; LV 2; LI 11; CV 4 and 12 and moxa to the umbilicus), homeopathy (Mercurius corrosivus 200c every 10 minutes), and hypnosis (to access the emotional trigger of the episode) as she lay on the acupuncture table. When she was examined two hours later, her fever had dropped to 100°F, her abdomen was decidedly less tender, and her pulse rate had dropped to 90 beats per minute. Her tongue was moist and her skin turgor was normal. She agreed to be driven home with instructions to keep her fluids up, eat only a bland diet, see me in the morning, and call if anything untoward happened during the night.

At 3:00 A.M. I got a call saying her bowel and abdomen were fine. She had had no further bowel movements at all, her temperature was normal, but she had excruciating leg pain and could not walk. I told her to come in at 7:30 A.M., which she did. On examination she exhibited the most amazing presentation of erythema nodosum of the lower legs I have ever seen. The swellings were of baseball size, glistening hot and fiery red in color. Another dilemma. She was quite upset in spite of her abdominal progress and demanded an explanation for the condition. I thought quickly on my feet and good old Hering came to my rescue.

I told her that this clinical presentation was a healing response, that it heralded the disappearance of her disease, and that it would defervesce in time with the homeopathic remedy that I would give her (Belladonna 200c every hour). How could I be so sure? In looking for elements of cure or worsening of disease, I noted that her legs were below her colon and her skin was more outside than her colon, which was, of course, internal. So, the disease had progressed from above, downward and from within, outward. The skin was a less critical organ than the gut and the legs were more centrifugal than centripetal. These carbuncular-looking swellings were more organized than the phlegmon of the inflamed gut mucosa. It turned out that Hering's Laws were correct! She was symptom free in three days and did not have another episode of colitis until eight years later when her husband divorced her.

6. *Total cure* — culminating in health, represents removal of all obstacles to cure and the full expression of the potential of the organism at all levels.

## DISEASE AS A CHRONOLOGICAL CONTINUUM

In Western medicine we are all aware that time plays a part in disease. Disease as diagnosed by the doctor, or related by the patient, has a beginning, a middle, and an end (if it is cured). We are aware of the pathological issues with regard to the intensity of disease as it relates to time — acute, subacute, and chronic disease. The length of suffering is short with acute and generally prolongs as the disease becomes more chronic.

We are also aware that there is a temporal precedence to disease. Smoking for a long time can lead to emphysema, menorrhagia for years leads to anemia, and high lipid levels for years can lead to atherosclerosis. What I wish to discuss has little to do with the pathophysiology of disease, but rather encompasses the concept that all disease that occurs in a patient, even from the time of preconception, is cumulative, interrelated, recorded, and logical. To explain what I am referring to, we need return to our discussion on the thermodynamics and chaos theories pertaining to biology.

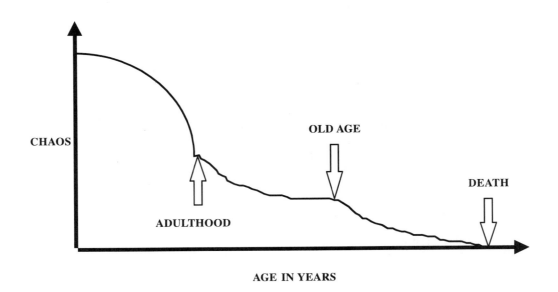

**FIGURE 4.4** Cycle of Life.

Let us look at the life history of a patient and try to understand the biology as it moves from two separate gametes, the sperm and the oocyte, to a single fused human zygote, from a morula to the blastocyst, from trilaminar germ disc to embryo, from fetus to newborn, from infant to toddler, from child to teenager, from adult to midlife, and from old age to death. If we look at these changes thermodynamically, we can see a left-shifted sine curve of early chaos and potential, gradually growing and becoming more mature, organized, and defined — the period from conception to adulthood. We then see a gradual flattening out of the curve from adulthood to middle age, and a downward drop of the curve with a decrease in organization and complexity and an increase in degeneration, the return of maximized entropy, and finally death. The cycle of life has been fulfilled (Figure 4.4). If the individual had perfect parents, a perfect birth, and a childhood, adulthood, and old age with no adverse effects on his or her life or biology, this is the curve we would see. However, because of the nature of life, this is rarely true, and what we see is a curve that has multiple points of negative and positive impact that influence and mold the curve to real-life dynamics (Figure 4.5). Now you will remember that one of the issues in nonlinear dynamics is that the system is exquisitely sensitive to initial conditions. In human biology the initial condition is genetic inheritance. This initial condition is probably the most important component of the biological nonlinear dynamic. It is also known that the phenotypic expression of this component may also be influenced by circumstances that occur throughout life — the classical nature versus nurture debate. Both have value and need to be considered in the final analysis.

Now back to the discussion on what is happening during these periods of change and development. What we are dealing with is a series of semistable, planned chaotic states, each with an attractor limiting the extent of the manifest chaos we call the human being. During the formation of the embryo, an extremely strong series of attractors called *morphogenic chemical organizers* and perhaps *morphogenetic fields* hold sway and cause the physical formation of the fetus. Problems in the initial condition, that is, the genetic information, or perhaps imposition of an external chaotic force, for instance, mother smoking or drinking alcohol, will cause a new chaotic condition in the embryo and force gravitation to a new stabilizing attractor that could be an inherited metabolic disease or the fetal alcohol syndrome. The effects of prolonged or obstructed labor, forceps delivery,

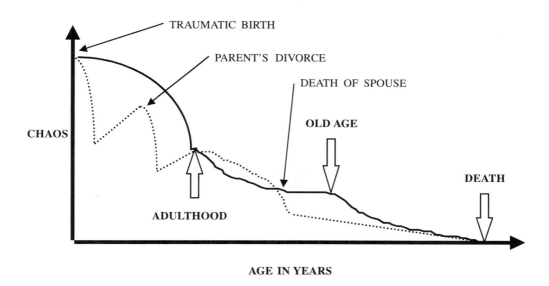

**FIGURE 4.5** Dynamics of Life.

meconium aspiration, or cephalhematoma all have their chaotic inputs, limiting attractors, and eventual response by the body to return to the ideal, most stable chaotic template. We could then go on and enumerate all the stressors of life — traumatic, metabolic, infective, and emotional — each of which has the potential to induce a new chaotic balance on top of the previous one with a new set of attractors and, hence, a new composite manifestation. Depending on our susceptibility and constitution — let's call this quality our *predominating anchoring attractor* — we are more or less influenced by these many inputs into our internal semistabilized chaotic milieu. Remember, as each new chaotic state develops, the underlying preceding chaotic state is the initial condition, and as we know, the chaotic state and its outcome are very sensitive to each new starting point, i.e., the previous underlying state. Multiple stressors that have similar characteristics will amplify their effects because the starting state is already a reflection of the new stressor. Repeat exposures to a similar stressor will increase sensitivity and susceptibility to that particular stressor (because of repetitive similar initial conditions), until the biology responds adequately to extinguish that stressor once and for all. If the biology does not extinguish that stressor, as happens for instance with a woman who keeps marrying abusive males, the biology accepts that chaotic state as being stable and will remain there until a larger perturbation of the system results in a quantum jump for survival into another more acceptable chaotic state. A large influence can knock us off balance and we jump into the next most appropriate chaotic state. Each time we do this, we change the underlying composite layering of chaotic states upon which we have built our present manifestation. That is, our present state of being is a composite history of our many previous chaotic states of being. So when recognizable disease strikes (an explicate manifestation that is strong and stable enough to be recognized as such), it is a result of, and the cumulative summation of all the chaotic history of the human that has come before. What does this actually mean in practical day-to-day medical clinic terms?

When a patient walks into your office with a medical complaint, this complaint did not have its origins the day before. This complaint is the final presenting accumulated, interrelated, and sequenced response of the body to everything that has happened before, and represents the best and least destructive pattern of chaotic and attractor response that the biology can muster at that time and place. It is conceivable that some recent acute episode was the final initiating trigger, such as the "Yuppie Flu" that hit Incline Village at Lake Tahoe where I was the attending pathologist, and spawned a whole new disease state — CFIDS. But it would not have manifested if the starting conditions (prior composite states) had not been present — a harsh, cold, and demanding climate in an isolated and close community, composed of overextended type-A personalities laced with alcoholism, drug addiction, and status symbol collection that exemplified "the Lake People." In integrated medicine we call these prior states the *biological load*. Some of us can withstand a large biological load without manifesting disease, because we have a strong constitution or anchoring attractor, while others have poor resistance and stamina and manifest one disease after another. The biological load can be composed of a number of stressors, some physiological: birth, puberty, and menopause; some biological and traumatic: the full spectrum of infectious disease and traumas, both physical and emotional; some deficiencies and excesses of nutrients: intoxications both internally and from the environment. The list could go on forever. In every individual there is, however, a time when the totality of the biological load exceeds the organism's capability to respond to another insult, and the patient hits the *biological wall*. Many older people have reached this state where their cybernetic response to stressors has been so compromised by suppressive therapy that they are no longer capable of mounting any type of response and are now on a slippery slope to accelerated chronic disease and eventual death. On pure clinical grounds I have found that it is relatively easy to return function on the left side of the biological wall, but it becomes increasingly more difficult to accomplish change of any kind the further you advance to the right of the wall (Figure 4.6). Here regular Western medications must be employed to support and control the fixed and unresponsive state that this represents.

We have dealt with the accumulation of insults and we should inquire how these insults are related and interrelated to each other, although they occur at different times in the organism's life. The most amazing biological "find" to me is that every single traumatic stressor in a patient has been recorded and is available to the subconscious for retrieval and comparison with the present situation. How do I know that? I know that this is true based on a number of clinical observations that are repetitive from patient to patient, and also within the same patient. I have seen Hering's Laws of Cure manifest clinically on homeopathic treatment, when old diseases return for a short period in the exact reverse sequence of when they first appeared.

It seems that every time we are faced with an overwhelming stressor, we compare the stressor with what has come before prior to jumping into the next chaotic state to accommodate the stressor. Some of this information is instinctual — what to do when cold, hungry, or in danger. Most of our stressors in modern life, however, do not pertain to survivalistic instinctual information. Many of them are circumstantial and emotional in nature rather than physical threats, although these still do exist. The brain accesses the stored instinctual centers for help (probably the Amygdala-Hippocampal Complex), but none match up. So, being survivalistic, the brain lays down a new memory that, if it is successful in resisting the stressor at hand, will become the new instinctual information specific for this current stressor and, paranthetically, the preferred attractor. These are called *learned memory responses* (LMRs) and have some interesting characteristics that lead to some surprising outcomes. We can see the origin of these learned memory responses in the early childhood history of all patients. We are all traumatized to a greater or lesser extent by our parents, siblings, and childhood circumstances. Each time we are traumatized, we lay down the traumatic memory and evolve a counterstrategy to stabilize ourselves, which becomes our modus operandi or anchoring attractor for that type of trauma. Repetitive, similar traumas eventuate into a more consolidated static counterresponse because of the enhancement and recruitment of the same response each time. These responses to stylized stressors mold, and may stifle our personalities, and in doing so, open us up to disease associated with the attractors we are continually calling forth for homeodynamic assistance. Large traumas such as incest, physical beating and neglect, witnessed or experienced violence, parents divorcing, or perceived abandonment have long-lasting effects on the quality of the anchoring attractor and cause the range and complexity of the stressor

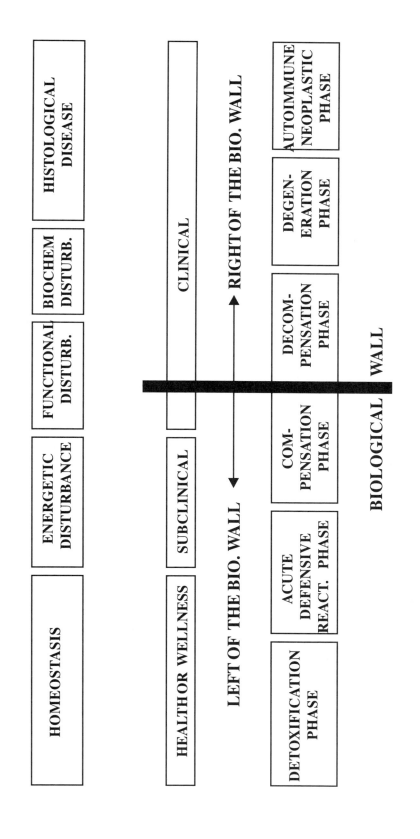

FIGURE 4.6 The Biological Wall.

response to be permanently narrowed down to a single response to all stressors, regardless of their type and quality. Such a biology is at permanent risk for abnormal behaviors and inappropriate biological responses, those physiological, emotional, and therapeutic. Thus, the cruel web of memorized childhood trauma reaches out to distort and truncate the natural history of the abused child.

Another interesting and somewhat bizarre finding of these acquired memorized responses is that they are often "state and scenario" dependent. This biological phenomenon has been described in the hypnosis literature as *state dependent learning*. Let me explain this phenomenon with two examples. If you were to be involved in a motor vehicle accident and were to be interrogated by a law officer immediately after the accident, with the adrenalin rushing through your veins, you could provide an account in great detail of exactly what had happened. If you were asked about the incident by your insurance company one month later, the general story would be the same, but some small details or nuances of fact would change. I have seen this personally when I was involved with testifying before a grand jury. As a case dragged on, the repeat testimony of the same witnesses seems to change in small increments over the course of questioning. In the motor vehicle case, however, one could jog the participant's memory to recall in exquisitely accurate detail by infusing the participant with adrenaline at the time of questioning. The brain has laid down the memory during a certain physiological state, in this case, of increased adrenaline, and the perfect recall of this memory is dependent on reproduction of the identical physiological state. This is also the reason why many postmenopausal females lose their memory and change their personality and sometimes their whole physiology, until they are put back into their state-dependent hormonal-memory state with an adequate estrogen level. In fact, it may turn out that hormonal activity is not only mediated at the target organ cellular level, but performs a portion of its general homeostatic activity by activating central nervous system pathways through hormonally state-dependent memorized physiological parameters set up in utero or at puberty.

The existence of these imprinted behavioral responses has been eloquently documented in homeopathy by Annanda Zaren in her two-volume *Core Elements of the Materia Medica of the Mind*.[31] I will quote from her summary in the introduction to her first volume with my energetic interpretations in brackets: "In summary, the *wound* [initiating external stressor], the *wall* [biological chaotic response — the implicate order] and the *mask* [external manifestation — the explicate order] are models that can provide a method for discerning and interpreting the symptoms in a case, such that the rubrics [patient's symptoms] used and the remedy selected will address the central disturbance or core pathology. The wound is a traumatic event that overwhelms the organism's ability to respond. Whether any specific event will cause a wound depends on several factors, including the sensitivity of the individual [susceptibility to the stressor, and initial condition], the constitutional vitality [anchoring attractor], miasmatic predisposition [strength or weakness of the anchoring attractor], and the safety and support of the individual's emotional and physical environment [initial conditions]. The memory of the wound is often 'suppressed or hidden.'" She continues: "The wall is either generated by miasmatic predisposition [hereditary weaknesses], or else it is created as an adaptation to protect the wound. The wall surrounds the entire organism, creating a barrier to both the outside world and the inner consciousness of the wound. Formation of the wall results in symptoms on the mental, emotional and physical planes. . . . The mask is the persona, a secondary layer over the wound. It represents a more superficial adaptation than the wall. . . . This model can provide a map to illuminate the deeper levels of a case and to permit the homeopath to determine the future clinical course and prognosis. . . . We have taken the inspiration from Samuel Hahnemann and become 'accurately observing physicians,' encouraging our patients to reveal their innermost pain and having the sensitivity to read, interpret, and comprehend the meaning of their suffering" (pp. 43–44).

One of the prime clues to disease etiology is the temporal association of important transitional or traumatic events in the patient's life with the onset of disease symptomatology. Any change in biological state, i.e., the appearance of a newly appreciated symptom, is de facto evidence of a bodily response to a recent stressor, internal or external. The body does not spontaneously develop symptoms — they are always in response to something. The appropriate biological treatment is always to understand the initiating event, what it means to the patient, and how and why the patient responded as he or she did, and to deal with that complex entity. Many times the initiating event is a recapitulating trigger of an old traumatic event, frozen in time and rehashed at every opportunity until it is expunged by psychotherapy or other therapeutic modality. This state of chronic poor adaptation or imprinting, utilizing a strong, paralyzing attractor, will potentially severely limit the full expression of this patient's innate capabilities unless this block is resolved. Let me give you an example.

A young man came into my office quite upset that his girl friend, also a patient, had made a terrible scene at a nearby restaurant where they had agreed to meet for lunch. He had arrived two minutes late and when he sat down at the table, she had started to cry uncontrollably, did not say a word, and proceeded to lock herself into the unisex bathroom at the restaurant. He had eventually persuaded her to come out, but she left in a huff without a word of explanation or apology.

Although it seemed to be simply a little lover's tiff, what really happened? The girlfriend had produced a very inappropriate and somewhat exaggerated response (symptom) to her boyfriend's arriving two minutes late to their appointment. One can only surmise that it was the small infraction of arriving two minutes late that initiated the response. The boyfriend knew that he was two minutes late because he was a punctuality freak and had been delayed at the office by his boss.

I then evaluated this infraction in light of what I knew about the lady's childhood history. She had been abandoned by her father at the age of 12, when he had left the family for another woman. She had been devastated by the ordeal and swore it would never happen to her. She had locked herself up in her room for weeks following the divorce and could be heard sobbing at night for months. So, an old childhood trauma, abandonment, had been retriggered by her perceived abandonment by another male authority figure, her boyfriend, who was not there for her at exactly the time he said he would be. Her response was exactly the same response she had used as a 12 year old. She cried and locked herself away in the only room available — the restaurant bathroom.

This story, and I could give you a hundred different ones, brings out two consistent, interesting biological observations:

1. Severe childhood traumas permanently imprint a delusionary state (the wound) on the child that forever colors the way he or she looks at that particular issue. Energetically this represents a marked narrowing of emotional response to almost any issue, because this attractor is so overriding. In the above case, all men are bound to abandon you, so watch out! The issue is always magnified, as it was in this case, and assumes a larger than life existence in the psyche of the patient. This patient had never been able to step up to, or down to, another chaotic phase of experience to stabilize this happening. She had been victim to the same delusionary chaotic state for 14 years.

   The particular issue or stressor will always elicit an inappropriately large response irrespective of the size of the infraction because it has an initial condition that needs only a small input for a maximal inappropriate response. The trigger or stressor may be covalently linked with other issues that occurred at the time of the initiating incident, to create a complicated woven picture of interrelated initiators and responses. When these large stressors occur, the body records the whole incident with every modality at its disposal — smells, sounds, tastes, sight, and thoughts. As it so happened, I learned later that her father's favorite Italian aria was being played as her boyfriend entered the restaurant. The initial conditions needed only a very small input to produce a large unexpected output. We will discuss these covalently linked biological states later in the book.

2. In very strong childhood imprinting, if the response is "successful," that is, the child survives, then that particular response (the wall) will be the modus operandi for all stressful situations, irrespective of the initiating stressor. This particular patient will

always cry and then retreat to a safe place in any stressful or confrontational situation. I had been privy to one such incident with this patient when she had arrived on the wrong day for her appointment. We had offered to work her in if she would just wait a while, but instead of sitting in the waiting room, she had run off to the bathroom and could be heard sobbing until she was seen.

The response or wall does not have to be an emotional response, and in fact, most often it is a physical manifestation or symptom, for example, headache or asthma or allergy. These surrogate physical responses replace an emotional response that is unable to be felt or expressed. Because the body has to respond in some way in order to maintain balance, it defaults to the next manifest level, the physical body. The only problem with this response is, although it creates a temporary stability, it is energetically the wrong response — emotional response must counter emotional stressor. The person is in the wrong responsive modality and this dysfunctional pattern or symptom complex will stay in place until he or she retraces his or her steps with the appropriate emotional response.

This last statement regarding the somatization of unresolved emotional stressors or conflicts as the major cause, if not the entire cause of all physical disease, will be met initially by most doctors with strong resistance and denials, if not ridicule. However, as you start to look to the initiators and triggers of disease, this truth becomes more and more real. Dr. John E. Sarno, Professor of Clinical Rehabilitation Medicine at New York University School of Medicine, in his two landmark books, *Healing Back Pain*[32] and *The Mind Body Prescription*,[33] developed the notion, which he gleaned from 30 years of observing his patients, that:

1. Emotions stimulate the brain to produce physical symptoms.
2. The Tension Myositis syndrome (TMS) is a major cause of back, neck, shoulder, and limb pain.
3. Repressed emotions lead to peptic ulcers, colitis, tension and migraine headaches, hay fever, and a host of other ailments.
4. Disabling painful conditions such as carpal tunnel syndrome, fibromyalgia, and post-polio syndrome are all part of TMS and can be treated successfully.

He encourages his patients to repudiate the structural diagnosis and the physical reason for the pain, acknowledge the psychological basis for the pain, and accept it and all its ramifications as normal for healthy people in our society. He makes the point that the body is able to produce symptoms in areas of weakness. So a bulging disc or a weak ligament is chosen as the place of manifestation and the body will initiate TMS pain where a structural abnormality exists. The tendency to attribute the pain to that structural abnormality is irresistible, and in some instances may be legitimate, but in most cases is clearly not, because the speed with which the person becomes free of pain tells us that the disc herniation was not responsible for the pain. Structural abnormalities are widespread and seldom symptomatic. A report in the *New England Journal of Medicine* in July 1994 from the Cleveland Clinic showed that there were lumbar disc bulges and protrusions on MRI in 64 of 98 men and women who had never had any back pain.[34] This finding is congruent with the findings in acupuncture where sometimes the worst backs respond with one treatment, while apparently normal backs on MRI are refractory to multiple treatments. The reason for this symptomatic subterfuge, he states, is: "to divert attention from what's going on emotionally and to keep you focused on the physical body. In essence it is a contest for conscious attention." I disagree with this statement, as I do not think it is a diversion. As I have discussed above, it is a purposeful strategy of sacrifice (the symptom) to balance the whole. We will develop this idea slowly with adequate scientific evidence to make you consider the issue with less doubt.

Issues will arise with this psychological theory of disease manifestation. By inference, these statements put the "blame" and causation of all disease at the patient's door. These are valid questions. If this is true, why then do babies contract cancer? The issue of young victims involves issues of a spiritual and religious nature, which I will answer if anyone wants to talk personally to me. The issue of responsibility for your disease is absolutely true. However, the conscious knowledge as to the whys and wherefores may not be at a conscious level in the patient, and to that extent, the patient is an "innocent" victim of his or her body's subconscious search for stability.

This concept of our subconscious being in control of our physical manifestation is certainly not new. We can trace this line of thought back to the late 1800s and the earlier part of this century. During that time, the Psychoanalytic Society of which Sigmund Freud, Sandor Firenczi, and Ernest Jones were members, spawned the father of psychosomatic medicine, Georg Groddeck (1866–1934). He was an entirely self-taught psychoanalyst who had been influenced in his young medical years by Ernst Schweninger who had been Bismark's personal physician. Schweninger's ideas clustered around the concept that the doctor was merely the catalyst that started off the therapeutic process. Groddeck took the concept much further and in his landmark work, *The Meaning of Illness*, he expounded his theory that there was no difference between organic and mental illness, that all organic disease was a conversion reaction mediated by an inner intelligence, which he called the "It."[35] This word was borrowed by his friend and contemporary Sigmund Freud as the "Id," but its entire meaning was lost in the Freudian interpretation. Groddeck did not differentiate between organic and mental illness or between health and illness. For him health was just another form of the "It" manifestation. The "It" decides on whether a person is ill, healthy, or recovering from an illness. The "It" also decides on what disease to utilize for tying a person down or causing him to rest. For example he maintained that headaches were one of the most widespread and well-known methods used by the "It" to immobilize thoughts and drives; that short-sightedness could serve to spare a person the sight of objects unbearable to him and, conversely, that the farsightedness of the elderly helps them symbolically make death appear far off. He was also aware of consciousness of the "It" in the bodily tissues and often used vigorous massage or hydrotherapy to change the "state" of the "It."

An article in the September 11, 1999 issue of *New England Journal of Medicine,* entitled "An International Study of the Relation Between Somatic Symptoms and Depression," brings into sharp focus the issues we are discussing.[36] Gregory Simon at the Center for Health Sudies, the Group Health Cooperative in Seattle looked at the presenting symptoms in 25,916 patients at 15 primary care centers in 14 countries on 5 continents. A total of 5,447 of the patients underwent a structured assessment of depressive and somatiform disorders. A total of 1,146 patients met the criteria for major depression, but between 45% and 90% reported only somatic symptoms and were unaware that they were depressed. A somatic presentation was more common where there was a poor patient–doctor relationship. Half the depressed patients reported multiple unexplained somatic symptoms. The conclusions were that somatic symptoms of depression are common in many countries, but their frequency varies depending on how somatization is defined. From this study we can see an example of the explicate (somatization) and implicate (depression) chaotic patterns that seem to be worldwide in distribution. We can also conclude, due to the general distribution of these phenomena, that somatization is widespread and is a normal biological manifestation and not an abnormal psychiatric disease.

In a recent review in *Lancet* entitled "Functional Somatic Syndromes: One or Many?" Professor S. Wessely and colleagues in the Department of Psychological Medicine, Guy's, King's and St. Thomas' School of Medicine in London have even more to say about the basis for functional somatic syndromes and their interrelationships.[37] They examined the literature regarding what is known in medical parlance as a functional syndrome — situations in which there are no objective medical findings to explain the patient's subjective complaints. In fact, it seems that each medical specialty has at least one functional syndrome. These are:

1. Gastroenterology — irritable bowel syndrome, nonulcer dyspepsia, esophageal spasm (Globus Hystericus), chronic cholecystitis without stones.

2. Gynecology — PMS, chronic pelvic pain.
3. Rheumatology — fibromyalgia.
4. Cardiology — atypical or noncardiac chest pain.
5. Respiratory — hyperventilation syndrome, panic attacks.
6. Infectious Disease — chronic (post viral) fatigue syndrome.
7. Neurology — tension headache.
8. Dentistry — temporo-mandibular joint (TMJ) dysfunction, atypical facial pain.
9. Allergy — multiple chemical sensitivity.

They believe, on examination of the overlapping criteria for diagnosis for each of the above syndromes, that the existence of specific somatic syndromes are largely an artifact of medical specialization and that similarities between them outweigh their differences. They come to this conclusion on the basis of the following observations in the literature:

1. Large overlap in case definitions of specific syndromes.
2. Patients with one functional syndrome frequently meet the criteria for other syndromes.
3. Patients with different functional syndromes share nonsymptom characteristics such as: most patients are female; functional complaints are all correlated with increased psychological distress especially to the number of current and past episodes of anxiety and depression; history of childhood maltreatment and abuse.
4. All functional syndromes respond to the same therapies such as antidepressives and cognitive behavioral therapy. There seems to be a clustering of the functional syndromes, for example, chronic fatigue and immune deficiency syndrome (CFIDS), fibromyalgia, and irritable bowel syndrome would form one cluster, while atypical chest pain, hyperventilation and panic attack would form another cluster. They believe, as do I, that all of these syndromes represent a specific somatic manifestation peculiar to each patient, but having very similar underlying mechanisms. (When you come to the section on patterns in Traditional Chinese Medicine, you will recognize that all of these syndromes have at their root only one pattern — restrained Liver Qi, the primary cause of which is repressed anger.) They also mention that these concepts are not new and have been brought up in the past as overlaps in what was then called "psychosomatic syndromes," and that these physicians also recognized the alternation or sequence of different syndromes in the same individual. They make the argument that reinstatement of these concepts is overdue.

## DISEASE AS A MEANINGFUL ENTITY

The next area that needs development in our search for an understanding of integrated medicine is the true meaning of disease. As we have seen, anything that the body does is in response to a stressor that knocks it out of balance at one level or another. We have discussed that symptoms are the body's response to balance the whole against the intruding stressor and that the body's response represents the most efficient response against that stressor at that time and place. Anything you do will not be as efficient, appropriate, or successful. The same stressor at a different time and place might induce an entirely different symptom response. These findings are based on having to listen to what your patient is telling you, even if it does not make sense, and to customize your treatment not only for each patient, but for every time that you see that patient, because the initial conditions are changing all the time. Symptoms are observable by the senses (no testing necessary) and, as such, are valid and constant over time from eon to eon. Diagnoses come and go as our understanding of disease progresses, but the symptom is absolute and real, needing no interpretation, classification, or fancy nomenclature.

*Symptoms* are the indications of the internal states of the patients (the explicit manifestation of the implicate order), indications of where they are in their evolution, and where they are "stuck." Symptoms are always a sacrifice or limitation on the organism as a whole, as they represent a narrowing of potential, less complexity, and reduced adaptability to all stressors. All symptoms occurring in a short time period are interrelated in spite of the fact that they occur in different organ systems or represent different pathophysiology. For example, take the case of a professor of engineering from South America who presented to me with a chronic history of migraines (right sided), fatigue, TMJ (right sided), and right-side hip pain. To the uninitiated, these disparate symptoms appear to be unrelated, but to the doctor educated in Traditional Chinese Medicine this case is a slam dunk. She was a foreign female operating in a male world of engineering at the university. She was treated with disdain and contempt in spite of the fact that she had more research grants than all of the males put together. She was very well brought up in the Hispanic old world fashion and never expressed her anger at being so poorly treated. Her body needed to balance this emotional stressor and defaulted to the organ and energy system relating to suppressed anger — the Liver/Gall Bladder system. The Gall Bladder energy line from its origin at the outer canthus of the eye, goes horizontally backwards to the temporomandibular joint, around the ear and then crisscrosses the temporalis muscle before extending into the posterior occiput, crossing the trapezius before coursing down the side of the trunk, passing through the gallbladder, downwards through the sciatic notch and hip joint before ending in the fourth toe (Figure 4.7). She had blocked off the flow of Qi through her right gallbladder meridian which explained all her pain — migraine, TMJ, and hip pain. The Liver, which distributes energy to the body, is the complementary energy line to the Gall Bladder (the Gall Bladder is the Yang line, liver the Yin line). The Liver Qi was also blocked and resulted in her low energy and fatigue. She was restored to a more appropriate state by her filing a complaint with the Dean of Engineering, receiving acupuncture to relieve the blocked Qi, and being treated with the homeopathic remedy Staphysagria for suppressed anger and humiliation.

What this all really means is that the body uses symptoms and the associated symptom complex called the "disease" to its own thermodynamic and evolutionary ends. All symptoms have their own logic and meaning and biology is goal oriented in its manifestations. In many instances the choice by the body–mind of symptoms does not seem to make much obvious sense, but deeper inquiry will always reveal the intelligence of the body at work. One way to elucidate the purpose of the presenting disease is to ask the following questions:

1.  What are the symptoms protecting in the patient, or what are the symptoms preventing them from doing?
2.  What is being sacrificed by having these symptoms?
3.  What could the patient do if these symptoms were not there?

A combination of these questions will often give you the clue to the source of the problem. Let me give you an example of such a case. A young lady presented to the office having been referred to me by a local neurologist who admitted to me that he did not know what was going on neurologically with the patient. She complained of double vision and bilateral wrist drop. Her MRI and CSF chemistry were negative, her EMG noncontributory, and her lab findings all normal. On examination she indeed did have bilateral wrist extensor weakness and assured me that her double vision was quite bad at times. She had no history of any toxic material or lead exposure. I treated her homeopathically with Plumbum metallicum for the wrist drop and Gelsemium for the double vision. She came back in two weeks without any change at all in her clinical presentation. I retook the case and inquired into her daily life and childhood. She related the following story: She was an only child of divorced parents and had always lived with her mother. She had become the surrogate husband and felt that her mother could not make it by herself without her support. At the time she presented, she had been looking after her mother for five years. Her mother took full

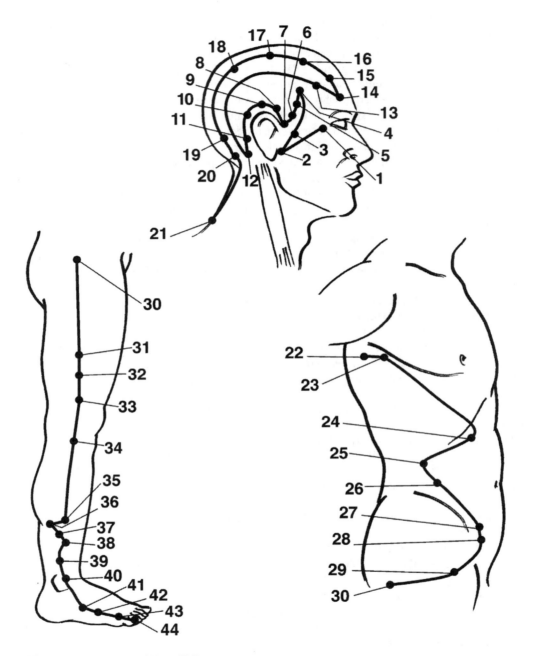

**FIGURE 4.7** Gallbladder Meridian (GM)

advantage of the situation and sat at home and watched television all day in spite of the fact she was quite capable of working and supporting herself. I asked her what she did for a living to support the two of them. She replied that she worked in a very busy travel agent's office where she sat in front of a computer all day booking vacations. I asked her if she liked her job and she said that she hated it! I asked why she could not leave and she said that it was not possible at that time, because she made such good money and she needed the extra money to buy things for her mother. That put me into a completely different thought pattern about the case. I turned to her with my prescription pad and gave her two weeks sick leave to stay at home and rest and to return in two weeks for assessment. She returned in two weeks with no wrist weakness or episodes of double vision. Quite simply she hated her job, but she could not leave it, and so her body had selectively removed the two key elements of the body necessary for utilizing a computer — her eyes and her typing hands. She left the job a month later and never had a return of those symptoms.

Some of you will say that's all well and good, but what about external trauma, heavy metal poisoning, being the victim of a drive-by shooting, or being burned or stung by an insect. Are these all self-induced? Maybe yes and maybe no. I was referring to the body's response to emotional issues, but I also believe that there are no accidents and whatever you need for your evolution you will draw to yourself. Borrowing from our local industry in Reno, Nevada — "life is no crap shoot!" We are always in control of our destinies. If it were any other way, life on this planet, for me, would have no meaning. We would all be just a jumble of chaotic random happenings in a more random universe, but our very existence speaks to the opposite view. I draw from my strong beliefs in a deterministic and purposeful life's being the bedrock of existence and the template for our physiology and reason for being.

*Disease is often symbolic or metaphorical.* In many cases the presenting disease is a metaphor for the emotional state of the patients. Some have chips on their shoulders (shoulder pain) or they cannot stomach a situation (peptic ulcer) or they have not the heart for the problem (angina or infarction). In some patients you will see symptoms that appear bizarre unless seen in the context of the patient's pain. Let me give you another example.

An elderly lady came to me with unilateral exophthalmos, which she had had for ten years. She had suffered from Graves' disease and had been adequately treated. However, her vision had remained poor in the right eye since the exophthalmos had started. Her left eye was unaffected and appeared quite normal to me. The unilateral nature of her ophthalmopathy was a little unusual, and as there was nothing else to go on with the case, I inquired of her why she thought that just one eye was affected. Her reply was astounding! It turned out that her husband had been unfaithful to her ten years before. She had been unable to deal adequately with this terrible situation and it was only after she developed Graves' disease and the exophthalmos that she was able to resume her life again. I again asked why the right eye? She smiled at me and said, "Because that was the eye I used to peer through the keyhole when I saw him making love to her in my bed." I was never able to cure that eye, it was such a powerful attractor. She had used the Graves disease to turn off the terrible vision of her husband's infidelity and had said nothing.

Another interesting issue with the thyroid is, that I have never seen any thyroid disease in a female that does not have to do with poor or suppressed communications within the family or at work. They shut down the fifth, throat chakra — the chakra of communication — and the body produces a physical manifestation at that anatomical spot.

# Section II

## Traditional Chinese Medicine (TCM)

# 5 Patterns of Diagnosis in Traditional Chinese Medicine

## INTRODUCTION

I am not going to rediscuss allopathic or Western medicine, as I think I have dealt with its basic elements in the foregoing chapters. When each integrated therapy is discussed for an individual disease, the appropriate issues of allopathic treatment will be raised, for and against. Let it suffice that allopathic or Western medicine is important in the quick acute rescue, the replacement of necessary nutritional, hormonal, or chemical elements, and the removal or reconstruction of physical deformity. Our time would be better spent trying to understand other paradigms of illness and how we can integrate them into allopathic medicine.

Traditional Chinese medicine (TCM) was introduced to the U.S. by James Reston's account of his acupuncture analgesia during an emergency appendectomy in Beijing, while he was covering the Sino-American ping-pong tournament in 1971. His account, on the front page of the *New York Times,* was the first popular account of Chinese medicine to reach the mass media in the U.S. There were Chinatowns and practicing acupuncturists and herbalists in many major American cities, especially on the West Coast, but there was little public awareness of Chinese medicine until that report. President Nixon's visit to China with his personal physician in 1972, and the earlier visit of three American physicians in 1971, added credence to Chinese medicine with a positive report in *JAMA* on several observed surgeries using acupuncture analagesia.[38]

The history of TCM in China goes much farther back. The roots are probably from the natural and folk medicine practiced during the Warring States period (475–221 B.C.) of the Zhou dynasty (1027–221 B.C.). The first classical book on traditional Chinese medicine was the *Huang Di Nei Jing* (The Yellow Emperor's Classic of Internal Medicine) and is ascribed to the Yellow Emperor, Huang Di, with its nucleus being written in the first century B.C. during the Han dynasty. It is presented as an 81 part dialogue between the Yellow Emperor and his private physician, Chi Po. The book is in two sections: the Su Wen (simple questions), which deals with preventative medicine and Chinese medical principles; and the Ling Shu, which deals with therapeutics. There are over 10,000 ancient Chinese medical treatises surviving from previous centuries and each has had its share of influence as Chinese medicine has evolved and matured over time. The introduction of Chinese medicine into Japan, Korea, and Southeast Asia, starting in the sixth century A.D., led to a regional and secular approach to Chinese medicine that was specific for each country that embraced the medical system. This development of Chinese medicine continues to this day in France and the United States.

Traditional Chinese medicine is composed of an array of therapeutics: *acupuncture, moxibustion, herbal medicine, diet, exercise,* and *spiritual approaches.* We will discuss herbal medicine, acupuncture, and moxibustion as useful therapeutic modalities in the Western medical office. The modalities of Chinese food therapy, Tai Qi, and Qi Gong are too impractical to be used in the office and will not be discussed in detail here.

# DIAGNOSIS IN TRADITIONAL CHINESE MEDICINE

TCM has at its basis the *maintenance of balance* in the body. Illness or disease always represents a state of imbalance. We could consider this concept the need to find the most appropriate and stable chaotic state, with a strong attractor. Over time, TCM has elucidated methods of restoring balance to the body, thus curing disease. The two most important methods are herbal therapy and acupuncture. Although many imbalances can be treated by either method, herbal medicine is excellent at tonification, that is, increasing the energy of a particular organ or the whole body, while acupuncture is more successful at removing energy blockages or stagnations of energy, and balancing the energy when there is excess in one part of the body and deficiency in another. Of course, in integrated medicine we often end up using acupuncture and herbal medicines together — acupuncture for the acute problem, and herbs to shore up the underlying deficiency that allowed the acute disease to manifest.

## THE LANGUAGE OF CHINESE MEDICINE

Chinese medicine is somewhat simplistic in the language it uses for diagnosis. The diagnosis is not the name of a disease, but the description of a pattern that seems to be preeminent in the whole person. The pattern is elucidated by the *Chinese physical exam*, which includes:

1. Looking — examination of the eyes, tongue, lips, nose, and ears (five senses); examination with special reference to color (the five colors).
2. Listening — to the breathing and the voice (five vocal expressions).
3. Smelling — the skin, sweat, breath, and urine.
4. Palpating — the abdomen (the Hara), the Channels or Meridians (Alarm Points and Ah-Shi points).
5. Asking — relevant questions as to the nature of the imbalance.
6. Pulse diagnosis — taking the radial pulses.
7. Tongue diagnosis — inspecting the color, shape, coating, and quality of the tongue tissue.

(All these diagnostic issues will be discussed in practical detail in the section: The Integrated Physical Exam).

The Chinese physical exam is able to show a predominant pattern of imbalance in the patient, which, in the Chinese physician's eyes, *is* the disease to be treated. Many dissimilar Western diagnoses will have similar Chinese patterns of disharmony, and many similar Western diagnoses will have different Chinese patterns of disharmony. In Chinese medicine there have been periods in which one theory of harmony and disharmony dominated over another. Thus, during one period, the Five Element Theory of disharmony reigned supreme and during another period, the Yin–Yang and Eight Principles Theory of disharmony reigned supreme. In this paradigm of healing, the Western diagnosis is unimportant, as we are treating the patient's explicit response to his or her inner disturbance, which is going to be different for each patient according to his or her initial condition.

The language and concepts of Chinese medicine describe the ways we get out of balance. The most important issue in the Chinese way of thinking about disease is not, is X causing Y, but what is the relationship of X to Y? In order to differentiate these patterns we have to learn the language of these patterns under the headings: *The Eight Diagnostic Principles*, *The Six Evils*, and *The Five Fundamental Substances*. These headings relate more to a herbal therapeutic diagnosis than to an acupunctural imbalance. The Five Element Theory, the Channels, the Six Stages, the Four Levels, and the Three Burners will be considered under the section dealing specifically with acupuncture as they specifically explain disharmonies and movements of Qi or energy. The Six Evils act as stressors on the body and produce a reactive change in the Chinese Zang-Fu organs and the Five

Fundamental Substances, to produce a bodily response called "The Pattern of Disharmony" — the illness or imbalance, represented as a mixture of the Eight Diagnostic Principals.

# IDENTIFICATION OF PATTERNS OF DYSHARMONY

The identification of patterns underlying the basic imbalance or disharmony in the patient is the most important "diagnostic" activity in Chinese medicine. This activity is consistent with Chinese philosophy where relationships rather than causes are of paramount importance. There are several methods used to define these patterns. Each method is more applicable in certain disease processes, and this distinction will become more apparent in the next pages, and with clinical experience.

The methods of pattern identification are according to

1. The Eight Diagnostic Principles.
2. Qi, Blood, and Body Fluids.
3. Pathogenic factors (the Six Evils).
4. Internal organs.
5. The five elements.
6. The Channels (Meridians).
7. The Six Stages.
8. The Four Levels.
9. The Three Burners or Heaters.

## THE EIGHT DIAGNOSTIC PRINCIPLES

The Eight Diagnostic Principles are:

1. Yin and Yang
2. Cold and Heat (Wet and Dry)
3. Interior or Exterior
4. Deficiency and Excess

When we look at a patient in TCM we need to define the patient in reference to each of the paired four diagnostic principals. We will address the clinical presentations of these paired concepts and then go on to understand the concepts of the external factors that cause disharmony — the six evils — and the constituents of the body — the five fundamental substances and the Zang-Fu organs.

**Yin and Yang** — Yin/Yang is a symbolic representation of the universe that embodies the concept of change, relationships, patterns, process, or flow from one concept into the other, at all levels of existence. Yin and Yang can only be defined in relationship to each other. This relationship is seen graphically in the Yin/Yang symbol (Figure 5.1), where Yin gradually turns into Yang, but even when Yang is full, it still has a small dot of Yin contained within it. The same is true of a full Yin. Another way of looking at it is that a part can only be understood in relationship to the whole. Yin and Yang are two convenient polar opposites that are used to explain how things function in relation to one another and to the universe. No entity can be seen in isolation; everything is connected and related in some fashion — so are Yin and Yang. Everything in the universe has two aspects to its nature — a Yin and a Yang aspect. Any Yin or Yang aspect can be further subdivided into another level of Yin and Yang and so on until infinity. This aspect of self-similarity on every level should remind you of the concept of fractal geometry, which relates to nonlinear dynamics and chaos theory that was discussed under the energetics of the body. Yin and Yang mutually create each other and they depend on each other for definition. Yin and Yang also control each other; when one is weak, the other is strong and vice versa. If the imbalance between the two occurs for a

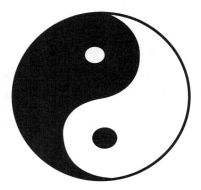

**FIGURE 5.1** Yin/Yang.

prolonged period, without the possibility of rebalancing, then the extreme disharmony means that the deficiency of one cannot support the excess of the other and they will transform into the opposite pole, or existence will cease. This is reminiscent of the concepts of chaos theory where, unless there is unimpeded change and unrestricted flow, the attractor will cause maladaption and reduced reactivity and adaptability of the organism, and cause a quantum jump to another chaotic level, or result in permanent stability, which means death of the organism. A good clinical example of this collapsing concept is seen in the diabetic patient who has a superficial skin infection with streptococcus, seen as a boil. The lesion is on the surface, is red and hot, and, therefore, qualifies as being a Yang presentation (see below). The patient neglects the problem and the streptococcus invades the body and becomes systemic in nature. The body responds with fever (excessive Yang) and finally cannot hold off the invading organism and goes into septic shock, a cold, inert, collapsed Yin state.

The qualities of Yin and Yang are polar opposites. Yin has all the feminine attributes and is quiescent, yielding, static, and contracting, while Yang is masculine and dynamic, active, and expansive. Yin is at the core, sinking, condensed, and internal; Yang is at the surface, rising, dispersed, and external. Clinically, Yin and Yang are related mostly to the two elements, which in combination, permit life to exist on this planet, that is, sunlight or heat, and water. Yin is cold, wet, and dark; Yang is hot, dry, and light. If we consider Hering's Laws of Cure, it is then apparent that Yang symptoms are more on the surface, acute, and less dangerous than Yin symptoms, which are internal, chronic, and more at the core of the patient. The Yin aspects of the human body are then internal and, because we can curl up into a fetal position and bury our chest and abdomen under our arms and legs, at the front of the body. The upper body closest to heaven tends to be Yang, while the lower body closest to the earth tends to be Yin. The exposed back of the body and skin are considered to be Yang. The internal organs, while having both Yin and Yang elements, are usually considered to be predominantly one or the other. When I refer to organs, it will be in the Chinese sense, that is, not just meaning the physical organ, but the whole emotional, energetic, and functional attributes of that "organ." The Chinese were not allowed to vivisect and had no concept of the organ anatomy. Some "organs" have similar or overlapping Western attributes such as the Lung, but the Spleen, for instance, is seen in TCM to be the center of the digestive function in the body. All the parenchymal, solid, or dense organs (Zang organs) are considered to be Yin and more essential for life and include the Liver, Heart, Spleen, Lung, and Kidneys. The hollow organs (Fu organs), which have to do with movement, are all Yang and include the Gall Bladder, Small Intestine, Stomach, Large Intestine, and Bladder. When discussing the Chinese organ or bodily status or fluid as a spiritual, emotional, and functional concept, the organ etc. will begin with an upper case letter, .g., Liver, Heat, Phlegm. The Yang organs are really an internalization of the exterior surface and, therefore, still represent the exterior Yang. Because they are Yang, their energy lines or meridians,

---

**TABLE 5.1**
**Yin/Yang**

| Yin Signs | Yang Signs |
| --- | --- |
| Feels Cold | Feels hot |
| Quiet manner | Agitated active manner |
| Low voice/without strength | Coarse strong voice |
| Reduced appetite | Strong appetite |
| Lies in a curled position | Lies in stretched position |
| Desires warmth | Dislikes Heat |
| Clear urine | Dark urine |
| Thin white tongue coating | Thick, yellow tongue coating |
| Thin, empty, weak pulse | Full, rapid, strong pulse |
| Tired and weak | False strength |
| Cold, diarrhea | Constipation |

---

tend to manifest as the primary imbalances on the surface of the body and are associated with muscular skeletal symptomatology and pain.

It follows from our discussion of the implicate and explicate orders of Bohm that every acute, superficial, excess Yang presentation is a manifestation of lack of control by the underlying deeper Yin deficiency. The Chinese teach that, to eradicate a recurring acute disease, for example, seasonal hayfever, it is necessary to tonify the underlying internal deficiency that is allowing the acute disease to appear. So, Yang symptoms are acute, easily seen or appreciated by both patient and doctor, and manifest more on the back or sides and upper body of the patient. Yin symptoms are more chronic, covert, internal, and degenerative.

Practically speaking, Yin and Yang are not all that important when trying to establish a pattern of disharmony in a particular patient. The deficiency or excess of Yin or Yang in relationship to each other will place the patient's biology into a particular pathological state (Table 5.1). It is therapeutically more important to address the patterns of Heat versus Cold, Wetness versus Dryness, and Excess versus Deficiency. The concepts of interior versus exterior are not all that important as part of the pattern, but tend to fall into place as the pattern of disharmony is defined. That is, it is easily apparent whether a pattern is Interior or Exterior. Since most diseases are rooted in Deficiency, most disease is Interior. The importance of Exterior versus Interior is mostly related to the depth of invasion of the pathogenic principle in the patient. Exterior disease is less harmful than Interior disease.

**Heat and Cold** — The concepts of Heat and Cold define two important states of bodily imbalance. Most diseases or symptoms may be hot or cold. For example, acute rheumatoid arthritis is Hot because the joints feel hot and look red, while osteoarthritis is Cold, because it has none of the Heat symptoms. A headache can be either a Cold or a Hot pattern, usually differentiated by the general pattern of the patient as well as the observation that the pain is better after application of ice in the case of a Heat-pattern headache or heat in the case of a Cold-pattern headache. A leucorrhea that is abundant, watery, and pale or white has a Cold pattern, while a thick, yellow, smelly leucorrhea is a Heat pattern. Some patients will have mixed patterns that are difficult to treat, for example, the patient may have an overall Cold pattern, feeling chilled and wanting warm drinks, but have pneumonia and be coughing up thick yellow spectum, which is a Heat pattern. In general, dryness is usually associated with, and is a major symptom of Heat, but may be caused by other factors, such as Blood deficiency. Heat patterns tend to be easier to treat because they represent a vigorous reaction on the part of the patient's immune system. These patterns are seen classically in children who have a high fever and look heated in the face, with rosy cheeks, in no time at all. This represents a good response to the invading principle and should not be suppressed with antipyretics. In the last five years I have noticed that this pattern of response has become less and less apparent especially in adults, and the relationship to most viruses, for example, has been

**TABLE 5.2**
**Cold/Heat — Wet/Dry**

| Cold/Wet | Heat/Dry |
|---|---|
| Pale face | Red face |
| Cold limbs | High fever |
| Slow movement | Rapid movement |
| Fear of Cold | Dislikes Heat |
| No thirst | Thirsty |
| Clear urine | Dark urine |
| Pale, white mucus/discharge | Dark, yellow, brown, green, or Bloody discharge |
| Watery stool | Constipation |
| Desire for warm drinks | Desire for Cold drinks |
| Lesions that are cold, pale, wet, and waterlogged | Lesions that are hot, red, dry, scaly, and cracked |

a Cold response. This indicates either a fundamental virulent change in the viruses we see or a decrease in the general immunity of the populace or both, Table 5.2, delineates the clinical differences between Cold and Heat patterns.

Wetness or Dampness is a condition where the Body Fluids congest and accumulate in the body. Dryness is the opposite condition, where body fluids are lessened. Dryness is often a symptom of Heat, as Heat will dry up the body fluids. Dryness is readily apparent if we look at the skin and mucous membranes, which have little moisture. Wetness, however, also relates to not so obvious wet conditions, such as sinus congestion and peripheral edema. Table 5.2 also relates to the important clinical signs and symptoms of Wetness and Dryness.

**Excess and Deficiency** — One can consider Excess and Deficient conditions either as a general state of the patient or as an excess or deficiency of a particular bodily substance such as Qi, Blood, or Phlegm (see below). In Deficiency conditions the bodily functions are weak or underactive. In Excess conditions, the bodily functions are overactive, or there may be obstructions, stagnations, or excessive accumulations of substances in the body.

Let us look at the more general concept with a clinical example. Two men telephone into the clinic on a Friday afternoon during the flu season with a report of low-grade fever, myalgia, and sore throats. Neither can come in at that time so both elect to be seen on Monday. On Monday morning both have become more invaded by the pathogen and present with bronchopneumonia with cough and copious sticky yellow sputum — a Heat condition with dryness. Neither wants to be treated with Chinese herbs and both are given an appropriate antibiotic, a cooling substance. They are asked to come in for a check on the following Monday. The first patient has cleared the cough, has no sputum, fever, or lung sounds, while the second patient has developed a chronic dry cough, with fatigue and shortness of breath. The first patient had an Excess condition that was easier to treat and cleared up with the antibiotic; the second patient had a Deficient condition for which the antibiotic was not sufficient, as it did nothing to tonify his weak lung Qi (cough and shortness of breath) and his overall low Qi as seen by his fatigue. The issue in these two patients is the strength of the invading pathogen versus the susceptibility and response of the patient. When they are mismatched and the invading pathogen is too strong, or the response is too weak and the patient is super susceptible, then the disease will not be cleared and become chronic as evidence of the patient's underlying deficient condition.

The most important indicator of Deficient conditions or patterns is that they are chronic and the symptoms do not clear within 7 to 10 days. Table 5.3 delineates the most important Deficiency and Excess patterns.

**Combinations of the Eight Principles** — One of the most confusing issues for medical doctors when considering the Eight Principles is the concept that when any two principles are out of balance and not controlling one another, then one will see symptoms of Excess or Deficiency in one of the

**TABLE 5.3**
**Deficiency/Excess**

| Deficiency | Excess |
|---|---|
| Weak movement | Heavy movement |
| Shortness of breath | Coarse respiration |
| Pressure relieves discomfort | Pressure increases discomfort |
| Weak or frail pulse | Full pulse |
| Low voice, fatigue | Loud voice |
| Dizziness, little appetite | Increased appetite |
| Little tongue coating | Thick tongue coating |

pairs. That seems rather straightforward and self-explanatory, but the difficulty arises when one tries to understand what exactly is producing the pattern that is seen clinically. For example: when a patient utilizes all of his Yin, his Yang, which is neither in Excess or Deficiency, but is out of balance in relationship to his Yin, appears to be increased or in excess. An excess Heat condition shows up clinically, despite the fact that the problem is actually a Deficient Cold, Yin condition and has to be treated by increasing the Yin. This is called an *Empty Heat* condition as it derives from a Deficiency. One may see an almost identical Heat Excess pattern when the Yin is unchanged but the Yang is in actual Excess, and there is not an increase in Yin to balance it. This is called a *Full Heat* pattern as it comes from a true Excess. Figure 5.2 compares the symptoms of an Empty Heat and Full Heat presentation. In this case the treatment is to decrease the Yang. An Excess Cold condition usually arises when there is an actual decrease in Yang that is not sufficient to balance the normal Cold Yin component. The treatment here is to increase the Yang to balance the Yin and Heat up the patient. These relationships are shown graphically in Figure 5.2.

## THE FIVE FUNDAMENTAL SUBSTANCES

The five substances are Qi, Blood, Body Fluids, Jing (Essence), and Shen (Spirit). Chinese medicine sees the working of the body–mind as the interaction of these substances. All of the other substances are seen as manifestations of the most important substance, Qi, varying from the very substantial Blood and Body Fluids, to the more ethereal Jing and Shen.

Harriet Beinfield and Efrem Korngold said it best: "Qi, Moisture, Blood, Essence and Shen are interdependent, cogenerating and mutually regulating constituents and processes. Moisture cannot be separated from the function of moisturizing, Blood from nourishing and Qi from moving. Without proper Moisture, Qi becomes Hot and agitated and Blood dries up and congeals. Without Blood, Moisture is dispersed and Qi is scattered. Without Qi, both Moisture and Blood stagnate, coagulate and stop circulating. Without Essence, the body has no material source; without Shen the body lacks presence, having neither spirit nor mind. Thus, Chinese medicine identifies disease as a disorder of relationships, not a singular, unvarying entity."[39]

Associated with the Five Fundamental Substances and related to their primary activities are the *Five Fundamental Processes*. These processes, which go on in all living organisms, are generation, transformation, movement and circulation (transport), storage, and regulation. These Western physiological concepts apply to the Chinese substances, each one being subject to specific combinations of the Fundamental Processes as its nature demands.

## Qi

The concept of Qi or energy indicates that it is something that is at the same time material and immaterial. It lies between the atomic particle and the waveform. In man, it represents the source

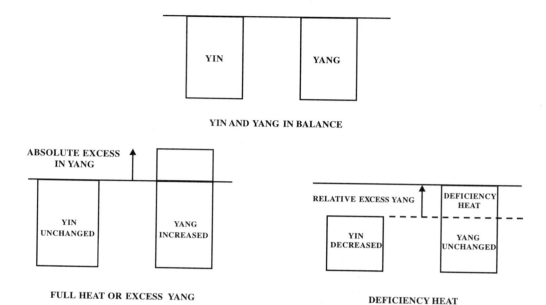

**YIN AND YANG IN BALANCE**

**FULL HEAT OR EXCESS YANG**          **DEFICIENCY HEAT**

FIGURE 5.2 Full and empty Heat.

of all things, being the interaction of the Qi of the heavens and the Qi of the Earth that came together to create man.

Where does Qi come from? We all inherit a certain amount of Qi from our parents, which is termed *prenatal Qi*. However, the main way we obtain Qi is by eating and breathing. This involves digestion, so we are talking about the Spleen, which processes the food to form *pure Qi*, which is moved upward to the Lungs, and *impure Qi*, which is discarded through the Large Intestine. It is the Stomach's job to separate out the pure from the impure Qi and to move the impure Qi downward into the Intestines. When the Stomach becomes rebellious, the impure Qi will move upward instead of downward, and that is when we experience belching and vomiting. In the Lung, the *air Qi* is mixed with the pure Qi from the Spleen to create *essential Qi (Zheng Qi)*. The essential Qi, if not immediately used, is moved downward in the body and stored in the Kidneys, the root of all energy, where the prenatal Qi and Jing are stored.

Last, we have the regulation of Qi which is the work of the Liver. The Liver is responsible for the smooth regulation of both Qi and Blood and, indeed, is the "Great Regulator" of the body. The Liver is very sensitive to emotions, especially anger, and constrained emotions will cause a decrease in regulation and a decrease of Qi in the body.

In summary, Qi is:

- Created and raised upward in the Spleen,
- Energized (transformed) and moved downward by the Lungs,
- Stored in the Kidneys,
- Regulated by the Liver.

Practically, this cycle of energy production is important to appreciate, because it focuses your attention on the areas of energy production in those patients who are weak, fatigued, or chronically ill. These patients must have a breakdown in the Qi cycle at one or multiple points. Clinical experience reveals the following patterns of Qi production breakdown:

1. The number one problem of energy access in patients is *constrained Liver Qi* regulation of smooth energy flow to the rest of the body. This syndrome occurs in patients who are angry, resentful, frustrated, and feel trapped. It is made worse by dietary indiscretions of sugar, fats, and alcohol that further congest the liver, and by decreased detoxification ability of the liver because of the unavailability of detoxification cofactors, vitamins, and minerals for Phase I and Phase II hepatic detoxification. Increased intestinal toxicity, due to constipation, food allergy, or intestinal dysbiosis, with increased enterohepatic toxin circulation, taxes the liver's ability still further. Female hormones also have a negative effect on the liver's ability to distribute Qi, and this is seen predominantly during the premenstrual period and also in some patients on certain birth control pills. **Treatment:** Address the emotional issues; Chinese herbs to move stagnant Liver Qi and Blood; acupuncture to move constrained Qi; nutritional counseling and addition of appropriate supplementation.

2. The second problem encountered is the *low level of Qi storage in the Kidney*. These patients have undergone chronic stress for a prolonged length of time and have no reserves left. First, the Yin is used up and they get a brief respite of false energy due to Deficiency Fire (relative excess Yang and all its Heat symptoms), and then they use up all the Yang and collapse. This syndrome is seen mainly in Type-A workaholic men, or in females who have to keep up the family as well as work for a living. They will demonstrate symptoms of both Qi and Kidney Deficiency, such as fatigue, low back pain, sore knees, nocturia, sleep disturbances, tinnitus, and dizziness. They will also become fearful and may display more severe symptoms such as panic attacks, agoraphobia, and idiopathic chest pain of a severe nature. **Treatment:** Lifestyle counseling; restoration of Kidney Yin and Yang with Chinese herbs.

3. The third syndrome seen is the *inability to derive pure Qi from the food that is ingested*. These patients have a multitude of gastrointestinal problems, such as indigestion, bloating, heartburn, constipation, or diarrhea, and many suffer from food allergies and intolerances. Many of them have had a previous Liver syndrome that went away and transformed into this Spleen problem. **Treatment:** Restore Spleen Qi with Chinese herbs; acupuncture allergy desensitization for food allergies; restoration of normal bowel flora and possible Chinese herbs for food stagnation together with digestive enzyme supplementation.

4. *Problems with Kidney grasping the Essential Qi from the Lungs* is one cause of asthma (Kidney Deficient asthma) and rarely seen as an isolated energy problem. Seen in exercise-induced asthma and nonspecific shortness of breath in stressed-out patients. **Treatment:** Specific Chinese herbal formula.

5. *Problems with provision of air Qi by the Lungs* is seen in typical Western diseases, such as emphysema, asthma, chronic obstructive airways disease, and all diseases causing poor oxygen transfer across the alveoli, or a mismatched aeration–perfusion ratio in the lung. **Treatment:** Chinese herbs for Lung Qi deficiency, viral and bacterial infections, and allergy and respiratory tract smooth muscle spasm.

6. Not included in this discussion is the effect of poor circulation or the movement of Blood, which is inseparable from the availability of Qi, as they move together, and will be discussed in the next section.

Two other forms of Qi that fall under the Zheng or essential Qi are the Wei Qi and Ying Qi. They are both of paramount clinical importance. *Wei Qi* is the surface circulation of Qi in the skin and the muscles and is the body's outer defense against invading pathogens. This Qi can be tonified using certain herbal combinations. These combinations are used as a prophylaxis against viruses and other infections and they are the "immune stimulants" of Chinese medicine. The *Ying Qi* is the Qi that is partly the meridian Qi circulating in the Chinese acupuncture meridians and is also part of the nutritive Qi in the Blood. It is the energy that is moved when administering acupuncture. It is the Qi that is augmented with the use of moxabustion and electrical stimulation of acupuncture points.

**TABLE 5.4**
**Rebellious Qi and Symptoms.**

| Organs | Normal Qi Direction | Pathological Qi Direction | Symptoms |
|---|---|---|---|
| Lung | Downward | Upward | Facial swelling, cough, asthma |
| Heart | Downward | Upward | Mental restlessness, insomnia |
| Spleen | Upward | Downward | Prolapse, diarrhea |
| Stomach | Downward | Upward | Belching, hiccup, nausea, vomiting |
| Liver | Upward | Excessive Upward Downward Horizontally To the stomach To the spleen To the intestines | Headache, dizziness, irritability, burning sensation, pain, belching, nausea, distention, diarrhea, constipation |

Qi is subject to conditions of congestion and depletion called *Qi pathology. Congestion of Qi* results from the pathogenic influences of *Heat, Cold, Wind, Dampness,* and *Phlegm* as well as from trauma, shock, emotional inhibition, and overeating. *Depletion of Qi* occurs with overwork, excessive sex, undernutrition, overexposure to environmental, mental or emotional stress, and prolonged or difficult illness.

1. **Deficient Qi** — characterized by weakness, lethargy, fatigue, chills, sweating, anorexia, loose stools, and organ dysfunction. **Treatment:** Tonify the Qi with herbs, e.g., mushrooms and ginsengs.
2. **Collapsed Qi** — an extreme case of Deficient Qi. Usually manifests as the inability to hold organs in their anatomical positions. Therefore, all syndromes with organ prolapse, hemorrhoids, feeling of bearing down (see Sepia in homeopathy) and the accumulation of Dampness in the lower body fall into this category. **Treatment:** Tonify the Spleen with herbs and acupuncture, e.g., Astragalus. The Spleen is responsible for holding the organs in their place and the Blood within the vessels.
3. **Rebellious Qi** — the Qi of each organ has a particular orientation of flow and if the flow is disturbed or reversed, then symptomatic disease occurs. See chart of Rebellious Qi and associated symptoms (Table 5.4). The common syndromes encountered are Rebellious Stomach Qi, which moves upwards and causes vomiting, belching, or hiccups; and Rebellious Liver Qi (Liver Fire) which either invades the Stomach and causes GERD (gastroesophageal reflux disease), gastritis, or gastric ulcers, or invades the Spleen and causes diarrhea and nausea. **Treatment:** Treat the underlying cause and tonify the invaded organ.
4. **Stagnant or Blocked Qi** — this is when the Qi does not flow and is related closely to Blood Stagnation. The organ involved is invariably the Liver, since it is responsible for the smooth distributed flow of Qi to the organs. Any situation causing anger, irritability, stress, anxiety, or depression will lead to Liver Qi and Blood Stagnation. Stagnation of Liver Qi and Liver Blood results in low energy, a feeling of distention and stiffness of the subchondral abdomen and the rib area, tight shoulders, breast soreness, and distention. Stagnation of Lung Qi results in cough and weak voice. Stagnation in the Stomach Qi results in belching and Stagnation of Qi in the acupuncture meridians results in shifting pain and numbness along the path of the meridian and is better for firm palpation. **Treatment:** Disperse or purge Liver Qi and Liver Blood; Lung Qi and Stomach Qi. Deal with the anger issues.

**TABLE 5.5**
**Chinese Organ Clock**

| Organ | Most Active Time of Energy Flow |
|---|---|
| Lung | 0300–0500 Hours |
| Large Intestine | 0500–0700 Hours |
| Stomach | 0700–0900 Hours |
| Spleen | 0900–1100 Hours |
| Heart | 1100–1300 Hours |
| Small Intestine | 1300–1500 Hours |
| Bladder | 1500–1700 Hours |
| Kidney | 1700–1900 Hours |
| Pericardium | 1900–2100 Hours |
| Triple Heater | 2100–2300 Hours |
| Gall Bladder | 2300–0100 Hours |
| Liver | 0100–0300 Hours |

The Qi circulates through each organ in two-hour segments at certain times of the day and night. This is known as the *Chinese organ clock*. Each organ has a two-hour maxima of Qi energy flow in the day or night and a corresponding minima or nadir at the same time twelve hours in the opposite diurnal segment (Table 5.5). For instance, the Liver Qi maxima is at 1:00 A.M. to 3:00 A.M., while its minima is at 1:00 P.M. to 3:00 P.M. These energy–time flows often explain the occurrence of certain symptoms at different times of the day and night.

The clock also indicates that it is better to eat breakfast than dinner, as all the digestive and assimilating organs are active in the morning and none in the evening. It also offers advice as to the best time to take your Chinese herbs for various organs as they are usually taken at the time of maximum activity if the therapeutic aim is to strengthen the organ, or they can be taken in the previous two hours or at the nadir of activity if the therapeutic aim is to calm or decongest a particular organ. Herbs may also be taken when the problem is manifest such as in the morning for morning sickness or in the afternoon for afternoon fatigue.

## Blood — Xue

Blood circulates through the body, nourishing and moistening the organs, sinews, muscles, mucous membranes, and skin, and is under the domain of Yin. The concept of Blood in Chinese medicine is somewhat different from that of Western medicine. In TCM, Blood is a form of very condensed and materialized Qi. Blood and Qi are inseparable. Blood gives Qi form and movement and Qi creates Blood. We could look at this concept as the relationship between oxygen (Qi) and the blood (Blood) in which it is flowing within the hemoglobin of the red cells. Blood is made in the Spleen from the Body Fluids that are distilled from food in the Stomach and combined with Zheng Qi from the Lung and Kidney Jing (marrow). In Western medicine anemia is connected to deficiencies of iron, $B_{12}$, or folic acid absorption. In TCM, anemia (Blood Deficiency) is associated with a weak Spleen and Lung and poor digestive function. The Blood is circulated by the Heart Qi. One of the difficulties in learning TCM is that there is just enough similarity with Western physiology to lull us into thinking in Western terms. The Blood is stored in the Liver. This is especially true when we go to sleep. The Blood moving into the Liver sedates consciousness. The Liver also regulates the Blood, for example, the Liver regulates menstruation, and the whole way Blood is released from the body.

In summary, Blood is:

- created by the Spleen, Lung, and Kidney Jing (marrow),
- moved and circulated by the heart,

- stored in the Liver,
- regulated by the Liver.

Blood is subject to conditions of depletion and congestion, called *Blood pathology. Congestion of Blood* occurs as a result of trauma, emotional distress, and the development of other pathogenic conditions such as *Heat, Cold,* and *Phlegm* which disrupt, retard, or obstruct its circulation. *Depletion of Blood* arises from overwork, undernutrition, excessive bleeding, exhaustion from difficult or prolonged illness, difficult pregnancy or childbirth, excessive thinking, and chronic sleep deprivation.

1. **Blood Deficiency** — causes a pale complexion and tongue, dry hair and skin, alopecia, infertility, dizziness, poor vision, scanty menses and amenorrhea, vitiligo, livido reticularis, and psorrhiasis (with Blood Heat). The deficiency in Yin of Deficient Blood causes insomnia and vivid dreaming. At night the Blood embraces and calms the mind, but if the Blood is deficient the mind "floats" and cannot sleep. Blood anchors the mind and if it is deficient, the person will have vague anxiety, irritability, and a feeling of dissatisfaction. **Treatment:** Tonify Blood by tonifying Spleen, Liver, and Heart. Tonify Qi as well.
2. **Blood Heat** — this is mostly due to Liver Heat. This causes red, hot, and itchy rashes, feeling of heat, and dry mouth. Heart Blood Heat can cause anxiety, manic depression, and mouth ulcers. Blood Heat can cause excessive menstrual bleeding especially in young women. **Treatment:** Acupuncture and herbs to purge Heat and tonify Blood.
3. **Blood Stagnation** — this means just what it implies, the Blood is not moving or circulating and is congested in one area or in one organ. This causes local muscle cramping and fixed local pain. The tongue appears dark or purple in color. Firm pressure on the area causes increased pain. Stagnant Blood is commonly seen in gynecology where it causes menstrual cramping, PMS, dark and clotted menstrual blood, or heavy bleeding. Blood stagnation is, not surprisingly, often a component of chronic illness. **Treatment:** Move and disperse the Blood. Exercise is important in this regard.
4. **Congealed Blood** — the Blood has stopped flowing at all in an area and, as in Western medicine, will cause a swelling or tumor with associated sharp pain. This is seen with traumatic injury, surgery, or long-term stagnation. **Treatment:** Purge the Blood.

Inasmuch as Blood and Qi are so much a part of each other, as blood and oxygenated hemoglobin are, problems of Blood are also problems of Qi and vice versa. So, treatment of one also requires treatment of the other. At all times, for example, we will be moving the Blood and moving the Qi at the same time in stagnations of either. However, acupuncture is much more successful in dealing with blocked or stagnant Qi problems, while herbs are much more effective in purging and moving Blood, especially in gynecology.

## Body Fluids — Jin-Ye

Chinese medicine distinguishes two types of Body Fluids. *Jin* is translated as Fluid and refers to the light, clear, watery fluid of sweat, tears, mucus, urine, and saliva. These Fluids circulate with the Wei Qi just under the skin and are controlled by the Lungs. The function of Jin is to moisten the hair, skin, and muscles. The most refined portion of these Fluids forms part of the Blood and keeps it thin and prevents blood stasis (plasma). *Ye* is a more dense and turbid substance translated as Liquids. These liquids circulate with the nutritive Qi and are controlled by the Spleen and Kidneys. Their function is to moisten the joints, bones, and spine while lubricating the orifices and sense organs. When Heat congeals the fluids, *Phlegm* manifests. There are two types of Phlegm:

Substantial (having form) and Nonsubstantial (without form). *Substantial Phlegm* is similar to the Western concept of phlegm or mucus and is seen in the Lungs or the Stomach. *Nonsubstantial Phlegm* has no correlation in Western thought, cannot be seen, but can "obstruct" the Heart, channels, and joints. *Dampness* is a term for a more watery substance than Phlegm. Dampness and Heat together will produce *Damp-Heat*, often seen in the pelvic area or Lower Burner and, manifesting as a UTI or as a vaginal infection.

In summary, Body Fluids are:

- Generated and raised by the Spleen,
- Further transformed and sent down by the Lungs,
- Further transformed and sent up by the Kidneys.

Moisture (the consequence of Bodily Fluids) is subject to conditions of congestion and depletioncalled *body fluid pathologies*. *Congestion of Moisture* occurs due to the pathogenic influences of wind, Heat, and Cold resulting in the accumulation of Body Fluids under the skin; in the channels and vessels that transport Qi, moisture, and Blood; inside the joints; within the body cavities; and even within the organs themselves. *Depletion of Moisture* occurs due to the presence of Heat, external dryness, loss of fluids due to sweating, vomiting, diarrhea, coughing, nasal discharge, and excessive bleeding.

1. **Deficiency of Body Fluids** — The typical symptoms of dehydration as well as some atypical symptoms are seen in a deficiency of Body Fluids. Dry skin, mouth, nose, lips, and tongue as well as cough are caused by a deficiency of Body Fluids. Body fluids are a part of Yin and, when they become deficient, they always cause Dryness. This pattern looks very much like, and may precede or be caused by, a Yin deficiency. Another cause of Body Fluid deficiency may be the loss of body fluids through excessive or *prolonged* sweating, vomiting, or diarrhea. Similar changes will be seen in Blood loss or chronic Blood Deficiency. The Lungs (cough), Stomach (epigastric burning), Kidneys (dark, scanty urine), and Large Intestine (constipation) are most affected by a deficiency of Body Fluids. **Treatment:** Replace fluids and tonify Yin.

2. **Accumulation of Body Fluids (Edema)** — Edema is caused by a weakness in the Spleen, Lungs, or Kidney, and sometimes in all three. These three organs are responsible for the transformation and movement of Fluids, and if any one is dysfunctional, Fluid is not transformed, overflows out of the channels, and causes subcutaneous edema. Each organ produces a specific area of edematous presentation:
Lung — edema of face and hands.
Spleen — edema of the middle (ascites).
Kidney — edema of legs and ankles.

3. **Accumulation of Phlegm (Substantial Phlegm)** — Substantial or gross physical phlegm (mucus) accumulates in pathologies of the Lungs, Stomach, and Large Intestines.
    1. *Wind Phlegm* — dizziness, nausea, vomiting, numbness of the limbs, phlegmy cough, rattling in the chest and throat, aphasia, and stroke.
    2. *Phlegm Heat* — yellow thick phlegm, red face, dry mouth and lips, restlessness, and red tongue.
    3. *Cold Phlegm* — white, watery phlegm, cold limbs and back, nausea, and pale tongue.
    4. *Damp Phlegm* — very profuse, white phlegm, no appetite, no thirst, sticky white tongue coating.
    5. *In the Kidney and Gall Bladder* — stones and gravel.

4. **Accumulation of Phlegm (Nonsubstantial Phlegm)**
   1. *Under the skin* — takes the form of lumps, nerve ganglia swellings, swelling of lymph nodes, or thyroid swellings and can be a component of fibroids and lipomas.
   2. *In the channels* — swellings that cause numbness.
   3. *Misting the Heart* — can obstruct the Heart orifices giving rise to mental illness and epilepsy.
   4. *In the joints* — chronic rheumatoid arthritis and bone deformities.
   5. *Qi Phlegm* — feeling of swelling in the throat with difficulty swallowing, stuffiness of the chest and diaphragm — the "plum pit syndrome" (globus hystericus).

Clinically speaking, Phlegm represents the end stage of the body's ability to react to its hostile environment — on the physical plane with tumors and cancer and on the mental plane with psychosis (see Heart patterns).

## Essence — Jing

Jing is the source of life — the unfolding etheric template through time that governs our growth, reproduction, and decline. It is a mostly Yin substance but has characteristics between that of Yin and Yang, is stored in the Kidneys, and is fluid in nature. Jing has two sources:

1. *Prenatal (Pre-Heaven) Jing* is inherited from our parents at conception and defines the strength of our constitutions. A lot of Essence equals a strong constitution. This is a fixed amount and, when it is used up and no more is produced, death results.
2. *Postnatal (Post-Heaven) Jing* is maintained and replenished in life from the food that we eat in conjunction with the activity of the Spleen and Stomach.

Jing circulates through the body and most particularly through the "Eight Curious Meridians" or "Eight Extraordinary Vessels," especially the Governing and the Conception Vessels. It vivifies the body and, with Original Qi, determines how long we will live. Therapeutics aimed at longevity need to focus on replenishing and maintaining Jing. Jing is naturally depleted as we age and is used up with excessive sex (mostly ejaculation in men, hence the many nonejaculatory techniques in China), and when we go against our nature (in denial of ourselves or our role in life).

### Functions of Jing

1. Growth, reproduction, and development;
2. As the basis of Kidney Qi;
3. Producing marrow, the common matrix of the bone marrow, spinal cord, and brain;
4. As the basis of constitutional strength.

In summary, Jing is:
- Partly inherited from birth,
- Partly sustained and nourished by the same process that makes Qi,
- Stored in the Kidneys.

*Essence* can be eroded (Jing pathology) as a consequence of injury, overwork, abuse of drugs and medicines, inadequate nutrition, difficult or prolonged illness, abortions or miscarriages, multiple births, and excessive or frequent loss of Blood and Body Fluids. Essence deteriorates as a natural consequence of aging and this decline is responsible for many of the observable changes in our bodies with aging. The clinical features of decreased Essence are:

1. Stunted growth, poor bone development, and mental retardation in children;
2. Infertility and habitual miscarriage;
3. Bone deterioration, loose teeth, balding, and premature graying in adults;
4. Poor sexual function, impotence, weakness of the knees, nocturnal emissions, and tinnitus and deafness;
5. Susceptibility to colds and flus, and chronic allergy.

Treatment of Jing pathology includes lifestyle accommodations, healthy diet, restrained sexual activity, and Chinese herbal therapy.

It could be forecast that Viagra use in patients with decreased Jing, and hence decreased libido and impotence, would cause death as the Jing that they were conserving was used up with inappropriate sexual emissions. The use of Viagra in these Jing deficient patients should be supported with Jing tonics.

Many of the modern disease plagues are a consequence of behaviors that deplete Essence or Jing and include degenerative and autoimmune diseases such as arthritis, diabetes, cancer, lupus, multiple sclerosis, CFIDS, and AIDS.

## Spirit — Shen

*Shen* can be thought of as the vibrancy or aliveness of consciousness. It is really more than just consciousness and mental functioning. It is the vitality behind Qi and Jing in the human body. It is the integrative, animating quality we think of as mind, spirit, and intelligence. Shen is not created by an organ, but is part of the vitality of the organism that connects it to the greater universe. It is stored in the Heart, nurtured by the Blood, and supported by Yin. The quality of the Shen can be seen in the clearness and luster of the eyes. It has to do with the willingness to be fully in the "here and now" and to be grounded in reality. Shen is associated with the dynamics of the personality and the ability to think, discriminate, and make appropriate choices. It enables the mind to form ideas. The spirit is anchored to the Heart. When the Shen starts to wander, we see disturbances of consciousness and sleep.

In summary Shen is:

- Obtained from both parents,
- Nourished by the environment after birth,
- Nurtured by the Blood and supported by Yin,
- Stored in the Heart,
- The primary integrative element of the body–mind,
- The overriding "chaotic" state in bodily nonlinear dynamics.

Shen is subject to conditions of disturbance and detachment called *Shen pathology.* Shen becomes *disturbed* by traumatic or shocking events internally or externally, both physical and emotional. Shen becomes *detached* from the body–mind by severe emotional and physical shock or severe weakness due to extreme depletion of other body constituents, especially Blood and Qi. Without adequate Blood and Qi, the Shen does not have a well-knit matrix to contain it. Because Shen is also the capacity of the mind to form ideas and make appropriate responses to the environment, a *Shen disturbance* causes muddled thinking and forgetfulness, insomnia (because the Heart is not anchored), and incoherent speech, madness, and unconsciousness.

With the concept of Shen the Chinese were able to articulate the concept of body–mind as a substance that was ingrained in the body — the Blood and Qi — yet was the vivifying quality of the mind and embraced the concept of consciousness and creative intelligence.

We can now go on to discuss the Six Evils as contributors or instigators of the pathology of the Five Substances.

## THE PATHOGENIC FACTORS OR SIX EVILS

The six evils are pathogenic factors that cause imbalance within the patient and lead to a specific pattern of disharmony. The six evils are Wind, Cold, Heat/Fire, Wetness or Dampness, Dryness, and Summer-Heat. The presence of activity of the evil is determined by the manifestation of symptoms and signs specific to that particular evil. The evils can appear alone or in combination. If the defensive system is strong, it repels the invasion or adjusts to the sudden changes. If the body Qi is weak or the evil is particularly strong, an illness develops which, if not stopped, goes progressively deeper into the body. The evils are natural environmental phenomena that stress the body and tend to occur as a predominant cause or aggravation of disease in their related seasons. We have dealt with Cold, Heat, Wetness, and Dryness in the Eight Principles as states of disharmony. These states of disharmony, however, can also be considered as pathogenic principles, that is, Cold can invade the body and produce a Cold state of imbalance. We will complete the topic with the discussion of Wind, Cold, and Summer-Heat, as they are the more important invading pathogenic principles.

### Wind

Wind is the "Spearhead of a Hundred Diseases." It is the invading evil that Western medicine calls virus or bacteria. It is related mostly to the Liver–Gall Bladder channel as wind is said to enter into the human via the Gall Bladder points in the occipital region at the back of the head. Wind can appear at any season and is usually combined with another evil such as Heat or Cold. It changes rapidly, is light, and rises to the upper part of the body. Wind may enter from outside the body, as in an invading virus, *External Wind*, or come from within (Liver Wind), *Internal Wind*. The origin of the Wind leads to two very different clinical manifestations.

**External Wind** — is characterized by a rapid onset of chills and fever, headache, and muscular tension — colds and flus. External Wind can also cause acute migrating skin eruptions (rashes and itching skin such as hives and urticaria), as well as acute and migrating arthralgia and early stage arthritis. External wind may also invade the Lung and nose and cause allergic rhinitis. External Wind is usually classified as being either Hot or Cold. Hot External Wind would have a red face, fever, and thick yellow mucus and be treated with cool surface relieving herbs, while Cold External Wind would be pale with abundant clear watery mucus and be treated with warming surface relieving herbs.

**Internal Wind** — frequently, though not exclusively, accompanies a chronic disorder of the Liver. Liver Wind is usually classified as being deficient (deficiency of Liver Yin or Blood) or in excess (excess of Liver Yang). Wind can manifest in symptoms of tinnitus, chronic headaches, numbness of limbs, tremors, spasms, convulsions, epilepsy, and hypertension. Substances that extinguish Wind and herbs that tonify Blood are beneficial in subduing deficient Liver Wind, while herbs that clear Heat and extinguish Wind, address excess Liver Wind.

### Cold

Cold is a Yin pathogenic factor and will damage Yang. Cold can be brought in by Wind to form Wind–Cold or can itself invade the channels and cause obstructed Cold pain such as arthritis, worsened by cold and better for heat. Apart from invading muscles, channels, and joints, Cold can invade organs directly. The organs most susceptible to Cold invasion are the Stomach (causing epigastric pain and vomiting), the intestines (causing abdominal pain and diarrhea), and the uterus (causing acute dysmenorrhea).

The case of Cold invasion of the uterus is quite interesting. This is often seen as the complaint of sudden development of acute dysmenorrhea in young school girls who are sportswomen or cheerleaders. The reason for this is inappropriate clothing during times of outside activity when it is Cold or frigid. The Cold can enter directly through the vagina into the cervix and hence into the uterus where the Cold causes Blood stagnation, pain, and spasm. This also happens postpartum, after sexual intercourse, or during menses when the uterus is open and exposed to any invading pathogen, Cold and Heat included. In these cases, symptoms would be accompanied by chilliness and pain and relieved by heat.

## Summer-Heat

Summer-Heat occurs in the summer, is a Yang excess factor, and injures the Yin. It is associated with prolonged exposure to the heat of the sun, or being in a hot room or situation without adequate ventilation, or working in a hot environment. It is close to a Western diagnosis of heat stroke. It is characterized by aversion to heat, sweating, headache, scanty dark urine, dry lips, thirst, a rapid pulse, and red tongue. It can be mild or go on to damage the Pericardium causing clouding of the mind, delirium, slurred speech, and unconsciousness. This is very similar to extreme heat stroke.

## THE SEVEN INTERNAL EMOTIONS AS DISEASE ETIOLOGY

The degree of balance within an individual and his or her harmony is eloquently discussed by Giovanni Maciocia in his book entitled *The Foundations of Chinese Medicine*.[40] This balance within the environment is dependent on physical health, a balanced flow of emotions, and proper development of intellect.

Emotion is not in and of itself pathological, but is reflective of the inner balance of the being — the implicate order of Bohm. Emotions become pathological when their flow becomes obstructed or irregular, when they become deficient or excessive, or when one or more becomes predominant.

Emotional imbalance gives rise to organ pathology, and organ pathology can give rise to emotional imbalance. In some cases the two origins form a vicious circle. For example, the harried housewife becomes angry at her situation, congests her Liver, which in turn makes her Liver emotion predominant (anger), and the cycle is established. All pathology of the liver causes an increase in irritability, resentment, and anger. I had a very interesting case of an extremely intense, perfectionistic Type-A patient who had had the misfortune to ingest carbon tetrachloride as a child. She eventually, after many years of high potency homeopathic treatment, went on to liver transplantation. When she came back in after the transplant, I did not recognize her! She was so sweet and relaxed, it was quite amazing. Her new liver was no longer part of the vicious organ-emotional cycle of anger, irritability, and impatience that were marks of her previous personality. Another example would be when chronic stress and anxiety, a regular presentation in the doctor's office, causes Kidney Deficiency because it is using up an inordinate amount of stored Qi and Essence. On the other hand, the Kidneys may become Deficient because of too many pregnancies too close together, which may cause an emotional state of anxiety and fear.

Each of the Zang-Fu organs has an emotional attribute and the emotions are integrally entwined in organ imbalance and pathology. *The Seven Emotions* are (1) joy (Heart), (2) anger (Liver), (3) pensiveness or worry (Spleen) (too much thinking), (4) grief (Lung), (5) anxiety or sadness (Lung), (6) fear (Kidney), and (7) fright or shock (Heart-Kidney). Each of the emotions has a particular effect on Qi and affects a particular organ.

- Anger makes Qi rise and affects the Liver.
- Joy slows Qi down and affects the Heart.
- Pensiveness and worry knot Qi and affect the Spleen (worry also affects the Lungs).
- Sadness and grief dissolves Qi and affects the Lungs.
- Fear makes Qi descend and affects the Kidneys.
- Shock scatters Qi and affects the Kidneys and Heart.

Most of the emotions over a period of time will eventually be seen as Heat or give rise to Fire in one or another of the organs. Clinically, *The Five Feelings* and the *Five Zang Organs* are the most important.

### Fear — Kidneys

Fear depletes Kidney Qi and makes it descend. In children, the descending Qi causes enuresis, while in adults it results in deficient Kidney Yin with low back pain, and the rising of Empty Heat (Kidney Yin not able to control Kidney Yang, which rises in the body and causes Heat or Fire symptoms in the upper half of the body) within the Heart. This is the same energy line as the Kidney, the Shao Yin energy axis, where the Kidney water is unable to put out the Heart Fire and includes associated atypical noncardiac chest pain, heat in the face, night sweating and hot flashes, palpitations, and dry mouth and throat with unquenchable thirst.

The deficiency in Kidney Yin, if left untreated, will eventually cause the Kidney Yang to be used up and the patient will go from the agitated, sleepless Kidney Yin false Heat to a collapsed Cold state of deficient Yang as well.

### Anger — Liver

Anger can be represented by resentment, repressed anger (the most commonly seen), irritability, frustration, rage, indignation, animosity, or bitterness. Anger causes Liver Qi and Blood stagnation with the resulting Heating up of the Liver and causing the rising of Liver Yang or Fire. Anger makes Qi rise and most of the symptoms will be seen in the region of the chest, neck, and head. The most common presentations are headaches and migraines, tinnitus, dizziness, red blotches on the neck, red face, thirst, red tongue, and a bitter taste in the mouth. Liver Qi will commonly invade the Spleen and cause diarrhea, while Liver Fire will invade the Stomach and cause nonulcer dyspepsia and GERD. If anger is repressed for a long time, then again the patient tends to collapse as in Kidney Yang deficiency and what one sees is the picture of depression. Depression is usually due to long standing, unresolvable resentment towards family members or situations.

### Joy — Heart

Joy should be interpreted in a very broad sense. Joy in itself is not pathological, but when the whole aim of life is to work hard at pleasure and enjoyment, then the Heart Qi is squandered and the excessive stimulation of the Heart leads to Heart–Fire or Heart–Empty–Heat. The Heart is the last affected organ and is always eventually injured in any general disturbance in the body of Yin and Yang balance.

### Sadness — Lung

The Lungs govern Qi and sadness depletes Qi. The Heart is usually involved together with the Lungs. The symptoms seen are extensive sighing, breathlessness, depression, and crying. In women, sadness with Deficient Lung Qi leads to Blood Deficiency with irregular periods and amenorrhea.

### Worry/Pensiveness — Spleen

Pensiveness means excessive thinking, excessive mental work, or studying. This weakens the Spleen causing tiredness, loss of appetite, and loose stools. Splenic deficiency is very common in our overworked and mentalized society and is the main deficiency seen in HIV infected individuals. Worry depletes Spleen Qi much in the same way that excessive mental work does. Worry also knots Lung Qi leading to anxiety, breathlessness, and stiffness of the shoulders and neck, a scenario we see everyday in the office.

## OTHER CAUSES OF DISEASE

### Weak Constitution

Every individual is born with a certain constitution dependent upon the parent's general health (genetics and lifestyle), state of parent's health at conception, and the mother's health during the pregnancy. The fetus is nourished by the prenatal Qi and we replace our Essence and Qi throughout life according to the way we eat and conduct our lives. The state of the mother during pregnancy is extremely important and any physical, toxic, or emotional trauma to the mother during the pregnancy will cause a similar effect on the fetus and its eventual development. It is important to gauge a patient's constitution, as it will largely determine treatment success and will help you determine agressiveness of treatment. Patients with weak constitutions should be counseled regarding lifestyle changes that will conserve their Qi and Essence.

### Overexertion

Overexertion of some type is an important pathological cause of disease in the West. Patients are overdoing everything. They work too hard, play too hard, get no exercise, usually get too much exercise, etc. What is needed, of course, is a balance between work, play, and rest. The relationship between Qi and activity and Qi and rest is quite simple. Activity uses up Qi and rest allows time for restoration of Qi. When we are talking about Qi we are first talking about short-term energy storage (probably Aderosine Triphosphate, ATP), which we term Postnatal Qi. This Qi is readily utilized and restored from food by the Stomach and Spleen, on a day-to-day basis for our daily lives. Essence, on the other hand, is our fundamental inner energy and vitality and has a long seven-year cycle, and so is only slowly affected by our daily activity. However, if we are continually in a daily Qi deficit because of out-of-control overactivity, the body starts to draw on the Essence energy and slowly starts to deplete it. This depletion will eventually show up as a Yin deficiency, usually of the Kidneys. This energy cannot be quickly replaced and needs slow herbal tonification together with a more balanced lifestyle for replenishment.

There are three types of overexertion to be considered:

1. **Mental Overwork:** This is very common in our fast, competitive, materialistic, and industrialized society. The Qi of the Stomach, Spleen, and Kidneys becomes exhausted, especially if poor and erratic diets are followed.
2. **Physical Overwork:** This tends to deplete Spleen Qi, as the Spleen dominates the muscles. Excessive use of one part of the body will cause Qi Stagnation and associated pain. This is seen in repetitive motion injuries such as carpal tunnel or tennis or golf elbow. Excessive lifting or standing causes Kidney weakness with low back and knee pain.
3. **Excessive Physical Exercise:** Excessive exercise will deplete Qi. This is particularly so if carried out during puberty and especially so in young girls, who may later develop menstrual problems. Weightlifting affects the lower back, jogging the knees, and tennis the elbows. Lack of exercise is also a cause of disease. Regular exercise is important for the circulation of Qi and the prevention of Blood and Qi stagnation and Phlegm (tumor, blood clot) formation.

### Excessive Sexual Activity

Excessive sexual activity tends to deplete the Kidney Essence. Because it is difficult to replenish Essence, one must conserve it by restricting sexual activity. By "excessive sexual activity" the Chinese mean ejaculation in men and perhaps orgasm in females, although this does not seem to be much of a problem in females. Sexual energy in females is not so much related to Kidney Essence, but is more related to Blood. With the stoppage of blood loss after menopause, the sexual energy of the female may, in fact, increase from its low point of multiple births and menstruation with blood loss. The use of Hormone Replacement Therapy with extension of menses, and hence blood loss, may lead to Blood deficiency and decreased sexual energy. Sexual activity without ejaculation is not thought to be harmful, which is why many sexual techniques without ejaculation are seen in Chinese texts. Normal sexual activity relates to the status of the Kidney Essence at any one time, the age of the male, his state of general health, and the season. Increased sexual activity is allowed in the spring, but should be curtailed in the winter.

Sexual desire and libido are related to Kidney energy, especially Kidney Yang. Low libido and erectile performance are best treated with herbal mixtures restoring Kidney Essence and Yang. Viagra causes a False Heat and usage of Essence with immediate sexual stimulation and injures the Heart. Deficient Kidney Yin with the rising of empty Fire will cause an insatiable demand for sex with vivid lascivious and wet dreams and can only be dampened by restoring the Kidney Yin.

## Diet

This chapter will not discuss the quality of food and all the issues of contamination, nutritional values, and processing. In TCM, dietary habits can be a cause of disease if the diet is unbalanced in terms of quality or quantity. Malnutrition is seen in both third world and first world countries, as a deprivation of nutrition in the former and as poor eating habits and inappropriate dietary interventions in the latter. I was amazed to see two cases of pellagra in well-to-do young females, one a nurse. Both of them had dementia, a persistent dermatitis, and diarrhea, all of which cleared up with oral B-complex.

Starving causes a weakened Spleen, which in turn stops producing Qi and does not burn food that is stored, and so the weight increases. Therefore, a steady eating pattern throughout the day causes more weight loss than starving or missing meals.

Overeating causes Stomach and Spleen weakness and leads to stagnation, a feeling of distention, nausea, and mucus accumulation. Excessive consumption of cold foods such as ice cream, raw foods (salads), and iced drinks causes damage to the Spleen, in particular the Spleen Yang.

Excessive consumption of sugar, sweets, and candy blocks the Spleen's function of food transformation and leads to Dampness with upper respiratory catarrh, abdominal distention, and fullness, mucus in the stools, and vaginal discharges (yeast infections).

Excessive consumption of hot and spicy foods such as curry, chili, alcohol, lamb, beef, or spices gives rise to Heat symptoms. The Heat usually affects the Stomach and the Liver, with symptoms of heartburn, GERD, and thirst.

Excessive consumption of greasy and fried foods, milk, cheese, and butters gives rise to the formation of Phlegm (mucus) and obstructs the Spleen function, which in turn causes more Dampness and Phlegm formation and leads to symptoms of sinusitis, allergic rhinitis, head fog, dull headaches, and bronchitis.

It is also important to eat in the correct surroundings and the correct frame of mind. Eating on the run in a hurried manner or in a state of emotional tension will lead to poor nutrition, poor digestion, and Stomach Yin deficiency.

## Trauma

Trauma refers to physical trauma, which causes local stagnation of Blood and Qi. This gives rise to the familiar pain, swelling, and bruising. Minor trauma causes Stagnation of Qi, major trauma stagnation of Blood. Old unresolved traumas represent an area of weakness where exterior pathogenic forces can produce symptomatic manifestations, such as where headaches or knee pain will manifest.

## Zang-Fu Organ Pattern Identification

### Lungs (LU)

The Lungs are the most delicate and most exterior of all the organs. They control the skin and are the most susceptible to exterior stressors. The Lung Qi plays a major role in supporting the immune system through the Wei Qi or surface protective Qi. Deficient Lung patterns stem from Lung Qi deficiencies, while excess patterns derive from exterior pathogenic factors.

*Lung Patterns*

The Lungs are most affected by exterior factors such as Wind, Heat, Cold, Dampness, and Dryness. The Lungs influence the strength of the Wei Qi or surface immune barrier.

External wind impairs the Lung's function of descending and dispersing, creating the excess conditions that are seen at the onset of a viral cold or flu. Dampness also affects the descending and dispersing function the Lungs, allowing the External Wind to invade the body. This is evidenced by catching a cold after getting wet or chilled.

A diet of cold and raw foods and dairy products will affect the Lungs via the Spleen. Excessive consumption of these foods will weaken the Spleen, creating phlegm that is stored in the Lungs. This is the reason children, who have undeveloped Spleen function and hence are more prone to Spleen weakness, produce a lot of phlegm with the ingestion of dairy products.

Emotions of sadness and grief strongly affect Lung function. Prolonged sadness will disperse Qi and cause Lung Qi Deficiency, while grief knots the Qi and causes stagnant Qi in the chest.

Excessive cigarette smoking causes drying up of the Lung Yin and stagnant Lung Qi. After many years of smoking, the Lung Qi becomes chronically stagnant and gives way to Dampness and Heat.

The state of the external skin and body hair will reflect the state of the Lung. The nails and head hair are a reflection of the Liver, Blood, and Kidney Yin. The nose and the sinuses are regarded as being part of the Lung.

The main Lung patterns include Deficiency and Excess patterns.

1. **Lung-Qi Deficiency** — Caused by hereditary weakness, an invasion of Exterior Wind (virus or bacteria) not treated properly, bending over a desk all day long, or chronic sadness. The Lungs govern Qi and respiration. When Qi is deficient, shortness of breath occurs especially during exertion. When the Lung Qi is weak and does not descend, a deficient cough results. With decreased Lung Qi the voice is weak. Because Lung Qi controls Wei Qi, it will not be able to protect the body from wind invasion and the patient will be susceptible to viruses.

   Lung Qi deficiency is seen with pertussis, viral croups, asthma (exercise-induced type), common colds, allergies, bronchitis, and emphysema. Lung Qi deficiency is most often described together with Wind Invasion and Phlegm in the Lung. **Treatments:** with herbs by tonifying Lung Qi and warming the Yang; with acupuncture: LU-9, LU-7, Ren-6, BL-13, Du-12, ST-36. Tonify with moxa.

2. **Lung Yin Deficiency** — Caused by chronic Lung Qi deficiency, Kidney and Stomach Yin Deficiencies, External Dryness invading Lungs, and cigarette smoking. A lack of body fluids leads to Dryness and eventually to Heat symptoms. The patient exhibits dry cough, sticky thick sputum, night sweats, dry mouth and throat, and hoarse voice. This picture is seen in chronic bronchitis, bronchiectasis, asthma, and emphysema and is worse in the dry Southwestern climates of Nevada, Arizona, and New Mexico. **Treatment:** with herbs by tonifying Lung Yin, nourishing Body Fluids, and clearing Empty Heat; with acupuncture: LU-9, Ren-17, BL-43, BL-13, Du-12, Ren-4, KI-6, Ren-12, LU-10.

3. **Lung Dryness, Lack of Moisture** — Caused by long periods of dry weather or surroundings or by Stomach Yin Deficiency. This state precedes Yin Deficiency with dryness

without Deficient Heat symptoms. Symptoms include dry cough, dry skin, dry throat, thirst and hoarseness, and dry constipation. **Treatment:** with herbs by nourishing Bodily Fluids and moistening Lungs; with acupuncture: LU-9, Ren-4, KI-6, Ren-12.

4. **Invasion of Lungs by Wind–Cold, Excess Pattern** — Caused by exposure to wind and cold in a patient with weak Qi or deficient Wei Qi. This can happen in air conditioning or refrigerated store rooms. Fever results from the battle between the Wei Qi and the invading Wind–Cold. The Cold obstructs the descending function of the Lungs, such that the Qi in the nose is obstructed with stuffiness. Cold also obstructs the circulation of the Wei Qi, causing head and body aches and aversion to Cold. This represents the Tai Yang stage (most superficial and external) of disease invasion.

   This picture is seen in viral invasion especially influenza, rhino virus, and some enteroviruses. This pattern represents a hyporesponsive immune response and is termed a "cold viral" pattern, which is more dangerous than a "hot viral" pattern (seen as fever and sweating). **Treatment:** with herbs by purging the External Wind and Cold; with acupuncture: LU-7, BL-12, Du-16, (Cupping BL-12).

5. **Invasion of Lungs by Wind–Heat, Excess Pattern** — Caused by exposure to external Wind (virus or bacteria) and Heat, artificial sources of heat such as central heating, weakened Wei Qi, and constitutional heat intolerance. External Heat dries up the Bodily Fluids and causes fever, dry sore throat, thirst, head and body aches, stuffy nose, yellow mucus, slight sweating, and cough. This is seen in most productive bronchopneumonias of "hot viral" or bacterial origin. **Treatment:** with herbs by purging External Wind and Heat; with acupuncture: LI-4, LI-11, LU-11, Du-14, BL-12, Du-16, GB-20. Needle in dispersion.

6. **Invasion of Lungs by Wind–Water, Excess Pattern** — Due to exposure to External Wind and Dampness. This impairs the Lung's ability to control the waterways of the body and results in facial edema or swelling around the eyes. The descending function of Qi is also weakened leading to scanty urination, cough, and breathlessness. This is seen in nephrosis, angioedema, and congestive cardiac failure. **Treatment:** with herbs by purging External Wind and Cold and resolving Dampness and edema; with acupuncture: LU-7, LI-6, LI-7, LI-4, BL-12, BL-13, Ren-9.

7. **Damp-Phlegm Obstruction of Lungs, Excess Pattern** — Due to an underlying Spleen Qi and Yang Deficiency caused by recurrent attacks of Exterior Pathogens or excessive consumption of cold, raw, or dairy foods. This is an Excess pattern caused by a Deficiency — the impaired Spleen function of transforming and transporting leads to the formation of Phlegm which is stored in the Lungs. The pale complexion is a sign of Spleen Yang Deficiency. This causes chronic bouts of coughing with profuse white sputum, congested lungs, pale complexion, and shortness of breath that is worse when lying down. This is seen in bronchiectasis and chronic bronchitis. **Treatment:** with herbs by resolving Phlegm, tonifying Spleen, and restoring Lung descending function; with acupuncture: LU-5, LU-7, LU-1, Ren-17, ST-40, PC-6, Ren-22, Ren-12, Ren-9, BL-20, BL-13. All in dispersion except BL-20 and Ren-12.

8. **Phlegm–Heat Obstructing the Lungs, Excess Pattern** — This is a chronic condition similar to Damp Phlegm, but accompanied by Heat. An underlying weak Spleen Qi is transformed into Heat by Wind–Heat invasion by long-term excessive smoking and excessive consumption of greasy hot foods. Symptoms include a barking cough with thick yellow-green mucus, wheezing and shortness of breath, and lung congestion. This is seen in chronic bronchitis and some infective asthmatic cases. **Treatment:** with herbs by resolving Phlegm, clearing Heat, and stimulating the Lung's descending function; with acupuncture: LU-5, LU-7, LU-10, LU-1, LI-11, BL-13, Ren-12, ST-40. All in dispersion except Ren-12.

9. **Phlegm–Fluids Obstructing the Lungs, Excess Pattern** — This is caused by chronic Spleen and Lung Yang deficiency from overexertion and poor diet or overconsumption of raw, cold foods. This is a condition of chronic Phlegm in the Lungs, characterized by its watery quality and profuse amounts, and is seen mostly in older individuals. Symptoms include cough and breathlessness with splashing, bubbling sounds in the chest and the bringing up of copious watery sputum. The patients are cold. This is seen in congestive cardiac failure and chronic bronchitis. **Treatment:** with herbs by resolving Phlegm, tonifying Spleen Yang and Qi and Lung Qi; with acupuncture: LU-9, LU-5, Ren-9, Ren-12, Ren-17, BL-13, BL-43, ST-36, ST-40. Use moxa.

## Large Intestine (LI)

The main function of the Large Intestine is to receive food from the Small Intestine, absorb fluids, and excrete feces, making all the Large Intestine patterns having to do with the dysfunction of bowel movements.

### Large Intestine Patterns

The Large Intestine can be invaded by External Cold as a result of prolonged exposure to cold or to normal seasonal cold without proper clothing. Cold and Dampness can penetrate the Lower Burner resulting in abdominal pain and diarrhea.

The emotions of sadness and worry can also effect the Large Intestine, depleting the Lung Qi, which inhibits its ability to descend. This results in Qi stagnation in the Large Intestine causing spasmodic abdominal pain with alternating constipation and diarrhea. Anger stagnates Liver Qi which in turn will stagnate Large Intestine Qi creating irritable bowel syndrome (IBS).

Dietary issues include the intake of too much cold food, which will cause Cold in the Large Intestine resulting in diarrhea. The overconsumption of greasy hot foods will also create Damp Heat in the Large Intestine.

Large Intestine patterns are closely related to the Spleen, Stomach, and Small Intestine. The main Large Intestine patterns include:

1. **Damp–Heat in the Large Intestine** — Caused by overeating hot, greasy foods, which results in the Large Intestine's not absorbing fluids with resultant diarrhea and mucus (Phlegm from Dampness). If blood or anal burning is present it is a sign of associated Internal Heat. Symptoms include diarrhea with mucus and blood. The tongue will be red with a sticky yellow coating. These symptoms are seen in most bloody diarrheas including ulcerative colitis, Crohn's disease, or severe infective diarrheas or food poisoning. **Treatment:** with herbs by clearing Heat and resolving Dampness; with acupuncture: LI-11, ST-37, BL-17, BL-20, BL-25, Ren-12.

2. **Heat In, and Heat Obstructing the Large Intestine** — Caused by eating hot foods and in the more severe obstructive stage by febrile diseases heating up the intestine and drying it out, causing constipation with dry hard stool or even acute fecal obstruction. The Heat extends to the Stomach which in turn becomes heated and the rebellious Stomach Qi moves upward causing vomiting. This is seen in fecal impaction with reflex vomiting and in acute appendicitis. **Treatment:** with herbs by clearing the Large Intestine and Stomach Heat and promoting moisture in the bowel; with acupuncture: LI-2, LI-4, LI-11, SP-6, SP-15, ST-25, ST-44, TH-6, KI-6, Ren-4 and 12.

3. **Large intestine Dryness** — Caused by drying up of the moisture and fluids, including Blood and Yin, in the Large Intestine, due to a hot climate or in elderly people who are thin. It can also be seen postpartum if there was extensive blood loss. Symptoms include constipation with dry stool and dry mucus membranes with dry mouth. **Treatment:** with

herbs by promoting fluids in Large Intestine and Stomach; with acupuncture: ST-36, SP-6, KI-6, Ren-4.

4. **Large Intestine Cold and Collapse** — Caused by excessive amounts of cold and raw foods, exposure to cold on the abdomen, or associated with a chronic Qi and Yang deficiency of the Stomach, Spleen, and Large Intestine. Symptoms include chronic loose stool, cold limbs, dull abdominal pain, and rectal prolapse in extreme cases. Yang Deficiency leads to loss of appetite, coldness, and fatigue. Seen in elderly and fatigued, lifeless patients. **Treatment:** with herbs by tonifying Large Intestine and Spleen and raising Qi; with acupuncture: ST-25, ST-36, ST-37, SP-3, BL-20, BL-21, BL-25, Ren-6, and Du-20 with moxa.

## Spleen (SP)

The Spleen belongs to the Earth element and represents the late summer. It is the primary source of nourishment of the body because it governs digestion and the production of Qi. The Spleen also governs the transformation, separation, and transportation of fluids in the body. If this process is deficient then Phlegm and Dampness occur. Spleen Deficiencies cause diarrhea, fatigue, and bloating.

The Spleen is responsible for keeping the Blood within the vessels and is also responsible for generating Blood. Hemorrhages, anemia, and Blood Deficiencies require Spleen tonification. The musculoskeletal system is ruled by the Spleen. Weak muscles, poor tone, myopathy, and myalgias all require Spleen Qi tonification. The Spleen is responsible for the raising of Qi and holding the organs in their place within the abdomen. Any organ prolapse is a Spleen Deficiency.

The Spleen is the residence of thought. Our capacity to think, study, concentrate, focus, and memorize relies on our Spleen Qi.

### Spleen Patterns

The Spleen is most susceptible to the evil of Dampness. The Spleen needs to be warm and dry to perform properly. Damp may invade from the environment in the form of wet clothes, Damp weather, swimming, etc. Women are more susceptible to Dampness during menses and postpartum.

A diet of cold or raw foods with an abundance of dairy foods is also important in the generation of Dampness and Phlegm. This is the origin of excess mucus in the sinuses and lungs especially in children, who have a poorly developed Spleen Qi.

Patients who worry, brood, study excessively, or are continually in their heads will weaken their Spleens.

The main Spleen patterns include:

1. **Spleen Qi and Yang Deficiency** — Caused by irregular and poor dietary habits together with excessive mental work and chronic disease. This is a very important and fundamental deficiency that has ramifications to almost every other organ in the body, with Liver Qi Stagnation, Lung Qi Deficiency, and Kidney Yin Deficiency. The Yang deficiency is from a primary Kidney Yang Deficiency that does not provide the Heat to transform the fluids in the Spleen.

   Symptoms relate to the digestive system with associated bloating, indigestion, Heat in the Stomach, fatigue, loss of appetite, weakness in the limbs, memory problems, loose stools, and edema. This is one of the scenerios from which CFIDS develops. A deficient damp Spleen and simultaneous Stomach Heat is a common combined pattern seen in overweight and obese patients. This is also seen in chronic diarrhea and chronic gastritis. The tongue is pale and swollen with teeth marks. **Treatment:** with herbs by tonifying Spleen Qi and warming Spleen Yang; with acupuncture: SP-3, SP-6, SP-9, ST-36, ST-28, BL-20, BL-21, B-l22, Ren-12. Use moxa for Yang Deficiency.

2. **Spleen Qi Sinking** — Caused by Spleen Qi Deficiency, but the focus of the problem is that the raising of Spleen Qi is impaired with consequent organ prolapse. This is often the result of poor muscle tone and standing for many hours a day.

   Symptoms include a bearing down sensation in the pelvis and perineum with rectal, uterine, or bladder prolapse. Additional symptoms include urinary stress incontinence and frequency, hemorrhoids, and varicose veins. In homeopathy this picture is an exact replica of the remedy Sepia. Liver Blood and Qi Stagnation should be treated along with varicose veins and hemorrhoids, reflecting the role of liver portal vein congestion with backflow into the hemorrhoidal plexus and down incompetent venous perforators. **Treatment:** with herbs by tonifying Spleen and general Qi; with acupuncture: Du-20, Ren-6, ST-21, Du-1.

3. **Spleen Not Controlling Blood** — This is caused by a Spleen Qi Deficiency with the focus on the extravasation of Blood out of its holding vessels — blood vessels or uterus. This is a deficient bleeding pattern in contrast to, for example, epistaxis which is an Excess Heat pattern.

   Symptoms include petechiae, hemorrhage, ecchymoses, bruising, hematuria, breakthrough bleeding, dysfunctional uterine bleeding, menorrhagia, and any Spleen Qi Deficient symptoms. Also seen with bleeding hemorrhoids and hemophilia. This is seen in ITP, TTP, and all anemias as well. **Treatment:** with herbs by tonifying Spleen Qi and herbs to stop bleeding (often the same that induce bleeding!); with acupuncture: same as Spleen Qi Deficiency and add SP-1, SP-10 and BL-17.

## Combined Patterns

Because it is so central to Qi, Blood, and fluid formation and control, the Spleen is often seen in combined pictures with other related organs of the same endodermal embryonic derivation — the Lung and the Liver.

**Spleen and Lung Qi Deficiency** — this patient is extremely weak and needs slow, long tonification. This patient is burned out and is probably Jing Deficient as well.

**Spleen Qi and Liver Blood Deficiency** — the Spleen does not make Blood, so the Liver is Blood Deficient with the consequent symptoms of fatigue, dizziness, pale tongue, and blurred vision.

**Damp Spleen and Liver Qi Stagnation** — anger stagnates Liver Qi, and Dampness stops the flow of Liver Qi in the Middle Burner. Over time the Spleen Dampness turns into Heat and aggravates the Heat produced from the Liver Qi Stagnation. The tongue is swollen with red edges and a thin white-yellow coating. There is a bitter taste in the mouth with hypochondriac pain, nausea, and fatigue. This pattern can be seen with splenomegally due to immunological dysfunction, malignant cellular infiltration, or cirrhosis.

## Stomach (ST)

The Stomach is responsible for "rotting and ripening" food, that is, digesting and transforming food to make it available to the Spleen. The Stomach and Spleen are closely linked and are sometimes treated as a unit, although pathologically, the Spleen tends to Cold and Dampness, while the Stomach tends to Dryness and Heat. Stomach Qi descends while Spleen Qi ascends to the Lungs.

## Stomach Patterns

The state of the Stomach is governed by the Hot–Cold nature of ingested food in relationship to the patient's constitution and the environment. If the patient is a type-A hot reactor, he or she is at risk for heating up the Stomach if hot, greasy, and spicy foods including alcohol, sugar, and coffee are consumed. Raw salads should be eaten in the summer to balance the Hot and Cold aspects of the body and environment. If, on the other hand, the patient is a weak, cold-bodied individual, he or she can't afford to eat raw and cold foods in winter without the risk of inducing a Cold Invasion of Stomach and Spleen with stagnation, indigestion, and nausea.

One should eat at regular times and at the best time for assimilation and digestion of food. The Chinese organ clock peak two-hour period for Stomach Qi is between 7:00 A.M. and 9:00 A.M. Overeating causes food stagnation and prevents Stomach Qi from descending, hence that feeling of fullness and nausea. Undereating and starvation diets cause Stomach and Spleen Qi Deficiency. Eating late at night causes Stomach Yin Deficiency and, if it is after 11:00 P.M. it causes the Liver Yin to be unsettled, obstructs the Heart Qi, and insomnia results.

Eating during emotional situations of worry or arguing or eating on the run will cause Qi and food stagnation. Eating while reading causes Stomach Qi Deficiency.

The main Stomach patterns include:

1. **Stomach Qi Deficiency** — Caused by a poor diet or chronic debilitating disease and often accompanied by Spleen Qi Deficiency. The deficient Stomach Qi fails to descend and causes discomfort in the abdomen.

   Symptoms include lack of appetite and taste, early morning fatigue, loose stools, and indigestion with epigastric discomfort. This pattern is seen as nonulcer dyspepsia or nonspecific indigestion. **Treatment:** with herbs by tonifying Stomach Qi; with acupuncture: ST-36, Ren-12, BL-21.

2. **Stomach Yin Deficiency** — Caused by an irregular diet, chronic vomiting, or eating late at night with a background of Yin Deficiency. Symptoms include thirst without desire to drink (Yin Deficiency), dry mouth and throat, and constipation. This is seen in bulemic and chemotherapy emesis. **Treatment:** with herbs by tonifying Stomach Yin; with acupuncture: Ren-12, PC-6, ST-36, SP-3, SP-6.

3. **Stomach Deficiency and Cold** — Very similar to Spleen Yang and Qi Deficiency. Feels better after eating and worse after a bowel movement.

4. **Liver Qi Invading Stomach** — A very important and commonly found presentation, especially in men. This pattern is caused by a combination of Stomach Qi Deficiency and Liver Qi Stagnation. This is always caused by repressed emotions, usually anger, resentment, or frustration. The Liver Qi is stagnant and causes the Liver to heat up and overcontrol the Stomach–Spleen causing the Stomach Qi to ascend causing belching, sighing, and bloating. The Stomach heats up and causes burning abdominal pain. The constrained Liver Qi also causes Liver Yang to rise, and headaches and migraine may be part of the picture.

   Symptoms are epigastric pain (burning) with repressed emotions, belching, sighing, irritability, and bloating. This is classically seen in GERD, which is primarily a Liver problem, not a Stomach problem. It also connects the emotional component of gastric ulcer to its angry origins. **Treatment:** with herbs by soothing the Liver, regulating Qi, and purging Heat; with acupuncture: LR-2, LR-3, LV-14, PC-6, ST-21, ST-36, Ren-12, GB-34.

5. **Stomach Fire or Phlegm Fire** — Caused by eating bad food or excessive hot, greasy, or spicy foods. The Full Heat burns up all the fluids and causes thirst, constant hunger, and a burning sensation in the stomach. The heat causes the Stomach Qi to ascend causing sour regurgitation, vomiting, and nausea. The Full Heat in the Stomach channel causes Blood Heat resulting in bleeding gums or epistaxis. Symptoms include a burning sensation in the epigastrium, constant hunger, bleeding gums, sour regurgitation, vomiting, and nausea. This pattern is seen commonly in advanced GERD and peptic ulcer. **Treatment:** with herbs by clearing Stomach Heat; with acupuncture: ST-21, ST-44, ST-45, SP-6, PC-6, Ren-12, Ren-13.

6. **Retention of Food in the Stomach** — Caused by overeating or eating too quickly. Food stasis obstructs the Stomach Qi from descending. This obstructs the Middle Burner and prevents Heart Qi from descending, causing insomnia.

Symptoms include satiety, fullness, nausea, and distention relieved by vomiting; foul breath from food fermenting in the stomach; belching; and insomnia.

This is a typical picture in Reno, Nevada where happy casino patrons stuff themselves at the cheap buffets, end up uncomfortable and unable to sleep, and hence go back to the gambling tables for more action. There seems to be some wisdom in supplying cheap food in this instance. One Saturday night, while on autopsy call, I had to minister to one unfortunate casino patron. His stomach exploded and he terminated rather quickly with a diffuse chemical peritonitis. An extreme case of ascending, or rather exploding, Stomach Qi. **Treatment:** with herbs by resolving food stasis and stimulating the descent of Stomach Qi; with acupuncture: ST-21, ST-44, ST-45, SP-4, PC-6, Ren-13.

7. **Stasis of Blood in the Stomach** — Caused by chronic Stomach Fire, food retention of Liver Qi invading Stomach. The stagnant Qi turns into stagnant Blood. Symptoms include stabbing stomach pain made worse with pressure and after eating, vomiting of dark blood, or blood in the stools. This pattern is seen in bleeding ulcer with hematemesis and malena. **Treatment:** with herbs by resolving Blood Stasis and stimulating the descent of Stomach Qi; with acupuncture: ST-21, ST-36, SP-10, Ren-10, BL-17, BL-18.

# Heart (HT)

The Heart is the "monarch" of all the organs, controls the blood vessels, and regulates and controls the flow of blood in the body. The Heart is also the residence of the Shen, the source of "mind" and the transformation of Essence and Qi. When the Shen is healthy, by reason of a flowing and adequate Blood and Yin, then the person is happy and vital. The Shen enables us to live in the present and to make appropriate responses to our environment. The Shen is susceptible to emotional upset.

*Heart Patterns*

TCM is similar to Western medicine in its concept of the Heart as being responsible for the circulation of blood around the body. The Heart also takes part in the formation of Blood by transforming the grain Qi into Blood. If the Blood is adequate and the Heart function strong, the patient will have a strong constitution and vitality.

In controlling the blood vessels, the vitality of the Heart can be felt in the pulse, which should be full and regular. It is necessary to have both Heart Qi and Heart Blood for a strong pulse.

The state of the Heart Blood is reflected in the complexion of the individual:

- Heart Blood abundant — rosy, healthy complexion.
- Heart Blood deficient — pale complexion.
- Heart Blood stagnating — bluish or purple complexion.
- Heart Blood heated — red or flushed complexion.

The *Shen* resides in the Heart. When the Heart is strong and the Heart Blood abundant, the individual will have adequate Shen, seen as balanced emotions, clear consciousness, good memory, keen thinking, and sound sleep. The Shen needs to be rooted in the Heart Blood or mental restlessness, depression, anxiety, palpitations, and insomnia will result. The Shen has influence on the spiritual aspects of the Kidney, Liver, Spleen, and Lungs. When the Heart and Shen are healthy, the individual is happy and healthy. When Shen is in excess, the individual is manic and may have symptoms of mental illness. Our Heart and Shen status determines our interrelationships with people and our environment.

The tip of the tongue indicates the status of the Heart. If the tip is red, the Heart has Heat. With severe Heat, oral ulcers will form or there will be glossitis. Stuttering and aphasia are due to Heart Deficiencies. Inappropriate laughter and babbling reflect a Heart imbalance.

By governing the Blood, the Heart controls bodily sweating. With Heart Qi Deficiency there will be spontaneous sweating, while Heart Yin and Kidney Yin Deficiency will give rise to night sweats.

Pathology in the Heart is usually due to emotional issues, and it is said that all disease has its origins in a lack of love and joy, the two emotions connected to the Heart. Joy in excess can damage the Heart Yin by providing to too much stimulation and input, much as is seen in patients who are exclusively self-indulgent. Sadness, an emotion primarily of the Lung, can also damage the Heart by causing Heart Qi Deficiency, which chronically causes Qi Stagnation and Heat, with resulting Heart Fire. Anger from the Liver causes Liver Heat and Yang to rise and attack the Heart with resultant Heart Fire.

The dysfunctional Heart patterns follow a progression of severity from Heart Qi Deficiency to Heart Blood Deficiency to Heart Yin Deficiency to Heart Yang Deficiency to Heart Fire blazing to eventual Phlegm–Fire in the Heart. *Each pattern generates the following more serious pattern* in a predictable sequence such that you can clinically estimate just how severe a Heart problem your patient has.

The main Heart patterns include:

1. **Heart Qi Deficiency** — Caused by excessive or chronic blood loss or chronic sadness. Symptoms are palpitations, fatigue, sweating, pallor, shortness of breath on exertion, and any other sign of general Qi Deficiency. These symptoms are seen post-hemorrhage, in significant anemia, or in patients following a death of spouse or loved one, with excessive sighing, depression, and listlessness. Heart Qi Stagnation, together with Heart Phlegm, may be seen in the depressive aspects of a bipolar disorder. **Treatment:** with herbs by tonifying Heart Qi; with acupuncture: HT-5, PC-6, BL-15, Ren-6, and Ren-17 with tonification.

2. **Heart Blood Deficiency** — Caused by associated Spleen Qi (important in Blood formation) and Heart Blood Deficiency. A diet composed of cold or raw foods will initiate or exaggerate this condition. The Shen becomes unrooted because of the lack of Heart Blood and Shen Deficient symptoms occur. The Heart Blood does not nourish the brain, which causes dizziness and poor memory.

   Symptoms include palpitations, insomnia (cannot fall asleep), dizziness, poor memory, anxiety, dream-disturbed sleep, and pale complexion and lips. This pattern is seen in emotionally disturbed patients who have a rootless Shen and so deplete their Heart Blood and Qi. They are fearful and anxious and worry about everything. They appear drawn and tired from not sleeping because their minds race at night stopping them from falling asleep. These symptoms also occur in postnatal depression where there has been an excess loss of Blood. **Treatment:** with herbs by tonifying Heart Blood, Blood in general, and Spleen Qi; with acupuncture: HT-7, PC-6, BL-17, BL-20 tonify, Ren-4, Ren-14, Ren-15.

3. **Heart Yin Deficiency** — Caused by an excessive and overactive lifestyle associated with high stress and poor coping mechanisms. The first sign is Kidney Yin Deficiency, which then leads to Heart Yin Deficiency. Because Blood is a Yin substance, there is often an associated Heart Blood Deficiency, which leads into or precedes this pattern.

   Symptoms include chronic anxiety, palpitations, chest pain, poor memory, insomnia (cannot fall asleep = Heart Yin Deficiency; cannot stay asleep = Kidney Yin Deficiency), mental restlessness, dry mouth, and night sweats. These patients also demonstrate 5 Palm Heat. This a reflection of the deficiency in Kidney Yin allowing the Yang (hot) to be out of control and produce a False Heat of the palms of the hands, soles of the feet, and a feeling of Heat in the chest, hence "5 Palm Heat."

   This is a very common pattern seen in extremely busy professionals who work 60+ hours per week with no downtime. The most common presentation in males is night sweats and inability to stay asleep (Kidney Yin Deficiency), fatigue, 5 Palm Heat (relative excessive Yang), and very often idiopathic chest pain, usually associated with Coxsackie

B virus infection. The most common presentation in females, which is becoming more common with both parents working, is palpitations, headaches, extreme fatigue, emotional outbursts, and menstrual irregularities due to Blood (first two weeks of cycle) or Yin (last two weeks of cycle) Deficiency. Also seen in the postmenopausal female, is the deficient Yin menopausal pattern. Women may also present with hypertension, hyperthyroidism, and anxiety neurosis. **Treatment:** with herbs by tonify and nourish Heart and Kidney Yin; with acupuncture: HT-6, HT-7, PC-6, SP-6, KI-6, Ren-4, Ren-15 with tonification.

4. **Heart Yang Deficiency** — Caused by the preceding Deficiency patterns especially Heart Qi Deficiency as well as being derived from Kidney Yang Deficiency.

  Symptoms are those of Heart Qi Deficiency with the addition of Coldness due to Yang Deficiency. Chest pain and tightness may be more prevalent in this picture as the deficient Heart Yang cannot move the Heart Qi through the chest and it becomes blocked in the chest area. This picture is a more depleted and colder clinical picture than Heart Yin Deficiency and lacks the False Heat seen in that more active picture. The patient may present with cardiac insufficiency, angina pectoris, or shock if the Yang totally collapses. **Treatment:** with herbs by tonifying and warming Heart and Kidney Yang; with acupuncture: HT-5, PC-6, BL-15, Ren-17, Ren-6, Du-6 with moxa.

5. **Heart Fire Blazing** — This represents a more chronic and severe bodily reaction to excess stress, anxiety, depression, and anger with full excess Heat derived from Liver Fire and extending into the Heart. It is a more penetrating and pervasive presentation of Heart Yin Deficiency.

  Symptoms are more pronounced in the mental sphere and interfere with daily life. They include mental restlessness, agitation, insomnia, impulsiveness, hyperactive, palpitations, thirst, feeling hot, red face, dark urine, a bitter taste in the mouth, and mouth and tongue ulcers.

  These symptoms are seen classically in drug detoxification patients with moderate withdrawal symptoms. They may also be seen in the manic phase of bipolar disorders (Heart Phlegm and Heart Fire, see next pattern), alternating with the depressive phase, also an Excess condition (Heart Phlegm and Heart Qi Stagnation). It may be seen in combination with other Yin organs such as with Liver Fire in hypertension and hyperthyroidism, with Small Intestine Heat in some hematurias, with deficient Kidney and Heart Yin in insomnia, and with Phlegm Fire of Heart in some manias. **Treatment:** with herbs by clearing Heat and pacifying the Shen; with acupuncture: HT-7, HT-8, HT-9, Ren-15 in dispersion. SP-6 and KI-6.

6. **Phlegm–Fire in the Heart** — This is an end stage mental condition of chronic depression and emotional dysfunction produced from Spleen Qi Deficiency in combination with Internal Heat causing the Fluids to be transformed into Phlegm. In TCM, the obstruction of the orifices of the Heart by Phlegm with the disturbance of Shen is the origin of all mental disturbances. Here we have both Fire and Phlegm coming together to cause a somewhat psychotic picture.

  Symptoms include a biphasic picture of mania (uncontrolled laughter, restlessness, crying, violent behavior, incoherent speech, and dream-disturbed sleep); and depression (mental dullness and muttering, coma, and aphasia). This pattern is seen in morbid depression and in psychotic individuals. **Treatment:** with herbs to clear Heart-Fire, purge Phlegm, and pacify the mind; with acupuncture: PC-5, PC-7, HT-7, HT-8, HT-9, Ren-12, BL-15, BL-20, ST-40, SP-6, LR-3, LR-2, GB-13, Du-20, and Du-24 (all in dispersion except Ren-12 and BL-20).

7. **Phlegm Misting the Mind** — This pattern is seen as an inherited problem in children with mental retardation or speech difficulties and in adults associated with Wind stroke or Internal Wind from the Liver, resulting in stroke, aphasia, or paralysis. The pattern is

similar to Phlegm–Fire in the Heart, but is not associated with any Heat. This condition can result from long-term emotional problems and chronic anxiety. It has a Phlegm pattern and a Cold pattern.

The Phlegm pattern symptoms include rattling in the throat with mucus congestion in the lung, vomiting, aphasia, mental confusion, and unconsciousness. The Cold pattern includes slow pulse and pale and cold extremities. This pattern may be seen in stroke, head injuries, low brain perfusion, epilepsy, and mental retardation in children. **Treatment:** with herbs by warming and opening the Heart and resolving Phlegm; with acupuncture: HT-9, PC-5, BL-15, ST-40, Du-26, Ren-12, BL-20 (disperse all except Ren-12 and BL-20).

8. **Heart Blood Stagnation** — This is an end product of prolonged chronic anxiety, grief, resentment, or oppressed anger that has already manifested as Heart Yang, Blood Deficiency, or Heart Fire. Symptoms include the classical symptoms of severe angina pectoris or of actual myocardial infarction. The patient experiences excruciating chest pain with pressure, both radiating to the left arm down the Heart Meridian. There is associated Coldness of the extremities with blue lips and nail beds. **Treatment:** with herbs by invigorating congealed Blood and pacifying Shen; with acupuncture: PC-6, PC-4, HT-7, BL-14, BL-17, Ren-17. Disperse in an acute attack.

As can be seen by the above-mentioned patterns, the Heart, although at the center of the organism, is strongly influenced by its interrelationships with the pathology of the Lungs, Liver, Spleen, and Kidneys. It is rarely itself impinged upon by external stressors or evils, but derives its pathology from the pathology of the Yin organs, Qi (the Lung), Blood (the Liver), and Vital Fluids (the Spleen). Shen (its interrelationship with the Kidney essence) and Blood can be seen as its most important aspects. Kidney and Heart have a direct relationship with each other in the Five Element Theory as the Heart Fire descends and warms the Kidney Water, and the Kidney Water ascends and controls the Heart Fire. Heart Fire causes insanity, and Phlegm causes mental confusion and unconsciousness.

## Small Intestine (SI)

The Small Intestine receives the transformation products of food and drink from the Stomach and separates the pure from the impure. The pure portion is sent to the Spleen and the impure or turbid part is sent to the Large Intestine. The Small Intestine is also involved in the movement of Fluids in the body in conjunction with the kidney.

### Small Intestine Patterns

The Small Intestine, like the Stomach and Spleen, is affected by the heat or coldness of ingested foods and drink. Deficient Cold in the Small Intestine is almost identical to Spleen Qi Deficiency, and Stagnant Small Intestine Qi is equivalent to Stagnant Liver Qi.

1. **Full Heat in the Small Intestines** — Caused by excessive anxiety and being spread too thin in one's activities. It usually derives from transmitted Heart Fire that invades the Small Intestine and causes a disturbance in the function of separating Fluids in the Lower Burner (pelvic area) resulting in scant, dark urine. It may even cause hematuria. Deafness may result from Fire in the Small Intestine channel. Symptoms include mental restlessness, tongue ulcers, thirst, scant and painful urination, and lower abdominal pain. **Treatment:** with herbs by clearing Heat and Small Intestine Fire; with acupuncture: SI-2, SI-5, HT-5, HT-8, ST-39.

2. **Small Intestine Qi Pain** — Caused mainly by Liver Qi Stagnation invading the Spleen. This is aggravated by ingestion of cold and raw foods. If acute, it is an excess condition

(Liver Qi Stagnation); if chronic, it is a deficiency condition (deficient Spleen Qi). Symptoms include cramping lower abdominal pain, flatulence, and bloating. This pattern is seen in irritable bowel syndrome. **Treatment:** with herbs by moving Qi in the Lower Burner and harmonizing the Liver; with acupuncture: LR-3, LR-13, GB-34, Ren-6, ST-27, ST-29, SP-6.

## Kidney (KI)

The Kidney represents the most important energetic organ in the body with regard to the root of energy and the will to live, develop, and reproduce, represented as the Jing or Essence. The Kidneys are the foundation of Yin (left Kidney) and Yang (right Kidney) in the body. The Jing and the fluids are associated with the Kidney Yin as well as being the foundation of the Heart and Liver Yin. The Kidney Yang is the source of the Spleen and Lung Yang. The Kidneys never show an excess pattern as the Jing is depleted and difficult to replenish. In urinary tract infections (Damp-Heat) there is an associated excess in the Bladder. Men get Kidney Yang Deficient (physical work) while women get Kidney Yin Deficient (in menopause).

The Kidneys store Essence and govern birth, maturation, and reproduction. The Kidneys are the source of the pre-heaven Qi because they store the Essence or Jing. A deficiency in Jing will diminish fertility and sexual performance and retard growth and maturation in children.

The Kidneys produce "marrow" for the brain, spinal cord, and bones. The "Sea of Marrow" (brain and spinal cord) nourishes the brain and supports memory, critical thinking, and concentration. Weak Kidney Essence will cause brittle bones and loose teeth as well as poor bone development in children.

The Kidney houses the "Will," the Zhi. Weak Kidneys cause a wavering and weak will power.

The Kidneys grasp and root the Qi. The Kidneys grasp the descending Lung Qi and root it. If the Kidneys are unable to grasp and root the descending Lung Qi, then the Qi will rebel and ascend causing Kidney Deficient asthma.

The Kidneys together with the Spleen and intestines govern the water. The Kidneys act as a gate in the Lower Burner, opening and closing to control urination. When Kidney Yang is deficient, the gate stays open too long causing profuse clear urination. In a Yin deficient gate, the urine becomes dark and scanty.

The Kidneys control the lower orifices. The urethra, spermatic duct, and anus are related to the Kidney Qi (same mesodermal derivation). If the Kidney Qi is weak there will be leaking orifices — urinary incontinence, spermatorrhea, or diarrhea.

The Kidneys also control the ears. Repetitive ear infections, deafness, or tinnitus are a reflection of weak Kidney Essence.

The Kidneys manifest in the head hair. The Jing and Yin of the Kidneys nourish the head hair. The hair will become brittle, gray, and fall out with Kidney weakness.

The *Ming Men* or "Gate of Vitality" is situated between the Kidneys. It is the source of all motivational original Qi and Yang in the body. It warms and is the source of Fire for all the internal organs. It keeps the Lower Burner warm and dry, warms the Stomach and Spleen to aid in digestion, harmonizes sexual function and warms the Jing and uterus, and assists the Kidney Yang in grasping the Lung Qi from the chest.

### Kidney Patterns

Your Kidney constitutional strength is governed by the amount of Kidney Jing given to you by your parents. Fear, anxiety, shock, and prolonged stress are the major emotional issues that deplete Kidney energy. In children this makes the Qi descend with the appearance of enuresis. In adults the Qi ascends causing the symptoms of deficiency Kidney Fire with dizziness, feeling hot, tinnitus, palpitations, night sweats, and insomnia.

Kidney Jing is depleted by excessive sexual activity involving ejaculation. In females it relates more to multiple childbirth. Chronic illness always eventually drains the Kidney Yin and Yang. In old age the Kidney Jing starts to decrease and is manifested by decreasing libido, loss of hearing, and brittle bones. Physical excesses will deplete Kidney Yang, while mental overwork will deplete Kidney Yin.

1. **Kidney Yin Deficiency** — This and Liver Qi Stagnation and deficient Liver Blood are the most important pathological patterns seen in Western patients. As Kidney Yin is the source of Yin for all the organs, most other Yin deficient patterns are usually caused by a deficiency in, or will respond to, nourishing Kidney Yin. Kidney Yin Deficiency is caused by excessive emotional stress and overwork (a feature of our times), and also by depletion of Body Fluids, by febrile diseases, and by blood loss.

   The symptoms are those of deficient Kidney Heat or Fire — night sweats, red tongue, and feeling hot; deficient Yin causing decreased "marrow" production with associated dizziness, tinnitus, and poor memory. A deficiency of Yin not balancing the Yang allows the Yang to come out at night, leading to the inability to stay asleep. Fluids are decreased leading to dry mouth, excessive thirst, constipation, and scanty, concentrated urine. A loss of Yin-associated Jing leads to low back pain with the tongue being dry and bright red, often a magenta color.

   This pattern is commonly seen in males, and now even females, who are working two jobs, 60- to 80-hour weeks, or mothers who are working full-time and looking after the house and kids. These patients are burned out and exhausted. **Treatment:** with herbs by nourishing Kidney Yin; with acupuncture: KI-3, KI-6, KI-9, KI-10, Ren-1, Ren-4, SP-6. In tonification, no moxa (too much Heat already).

   This may take some time, even up to six months, to replenish the patient. You can see results in 10 days with a large dose of herbs, but the individual needs slow, steady tonification over a longer period of time in order not to relapse. This is very important as most of these individuals will not change their lifestyle and will quickly relapse as they resume their Yin and Jing consumptive lifestyles.

2. **Kidney Jing Deficiency** — Caused by a weak parental constitution (parents too old) in children, by excessive sexual activity in young adulthood, or by old age in adults. Symptoms are a reflection of the role of Essence in the reproduction and growth of bones, the production of marrow, which fills the brain, and the Jing, which governs fertility and head hair. Common symptoms in adults include weak legs and knees, loose teeth, low back pain, premature graying and loss of hair, poor memory, and infertility. Common symptoms seen constitutionally in children include delayed closure of fontanels, general growth retardation, weak bone development, and mental dullness and retardation.

   In adults, old age and infertility represent two states that have been vigorously attacked by Western medicine. The new medical industry of longevity with all its hype is really an issue of replacing Jing and Essence. Increasing antioxidants and squelching free radicals only goes so far in the retardation of aging, but does nothing for actual rejuvenation. Supplementation with human growth hormone may represent an aspect of Jing, but I don't really know. The most potent substance for the replenishment of Essence and Jing comes from the food provided for the creature that has to have thousands of offspring and still maintain her energy — the royal jelly for the queen bee.

   The use of Viagra to increase libido without a concomitant replenishment of Jing will cause a collapse of Yin and Yang as you artificially drive a depleted system, and it is not surprising that some of these patients die abruptly.

   The inducement of pregnancy by *in vivo* and *ex vivo* techniques in couples not exhibiting obvious anatomical impediments to conception is fraught with some bothersome unanswered questions. Is the reason for infertility a fundamental deficiency of Jing in the parents or in one parent, which is too low to maintain the offspring? This may occur in constitutionally Jing-Deficient individuals, who then pass on even less constitutional strength to their offspring. This may also occur in parents who are biologically too old to be having children. In most cultures the prime conception years are between ages 18 and 30 in females and ages 22 and 35 in males. The incidence of Jing-deficient induced pregnancies in late conceiving parents may have some biological consequences when these children are followed over time.

**Treatment:** with herbs by nourishing Kidney Jing; with acupuncture: KI-3,KI-6, Ren-4, BL-11, BL-15, BL-23, Du-4, Du-14, Du-20, GB-39. Tonify.

3. **Deficient (Empty) Kidney Fire** — Caused by the same issues mentioned with Kidney Yin Deficiency that have become prolonged and in an advanced stage with concurrent emotional distress and chronic burn out syndrome.

Symptoms are related to the excess of Yang (Heat) over Yin and are seen as malar flushing in the afternoon and feelings of heat and low-grade fever. The Empty Fire will agitate the Heart and mind and cause insomnia (waking up all through the night and early waking) and symptoms of excessive dryness including constipation, concentrated scanty dark urine (even hematuria if the Blood Heats up), and dry and sore throat. Weakening of Jing causes nocturnal emissions, lascivious dreaming, and excessive sexual desire. The tongue is red, peeled, and cracked like a dry lake bed.

This picture is seen in the extreme burn out cases discussed in Kidney Yin deficiency, but is also seen in thin females during menopause and is one of the causes for menopausal hot flashes, vaginal dryness, and memory problems. **Treatment:** with herbs by nourishing Kidney Yin, clearing Empty Heat, and calming the Shen; with acupuncture: KI-2, KI-3, KI-6, KI-9, K10, SP-6, HT-5, LU-7, Ren-4.

4. **Kidney Yang Deficiency** — Caused by the lack of Kidney Heat (the pilot light of the body) represented by Kidney Yang and characterized by Interior Cold symptoms. This absolute lack of Yang, which is usually preceded by exhaustion of Kidney Yin is seen in chronic disease, long-term physical overwork, and being exposed to excessive cold together with an overactive sexual life and old age.

Symptoms of Cold in the body include coldness and pain in the low back and knees and an aversion to cold. The body Essence is not warmed resulting in decreased sexual energy, impotence, and infertility. Fluids are not dried up resulting in excessive watery urine of low specific gravity and associated pedal edema. Deficient Spleen Yang results in loose stool and weak legs.

There is a logical clinical progression of Qi depletion from Kidney Yin Deficiency to deficient Kidney Fire to Kidney Yang Deficiency. The deficient Kidney Fire individual may seem to have a lot of energy due to the excessive out-of-balance Yang Heat, but this represents a hollow energy pattern that will collapse at any time. This same picture is seen in the false energy seen in "uppers" and the use of caffeine and other more potent stimulants. **Treatment:** with herbs by tonifying Kidney Yang; with acupuncture: BL-23, BL-52, KI-3, KI-7, Du-4, Ren-4, Ren-6. Use moxa for tonification.

5. **Deficient Kidney Qi** — Caused by excessive sexual activity, old age, or, in women, by having had too many children too close together. It is a Cold pattern caused by Kidney Yang Deficiency but the effects are concentrated in the Lower Burner (pelvis) because the Kidneys cannot deliver enough Qi to the bladder, with all the consequent Bladder symptomatology.

Symptoms include sore weak back, frequency with clear pale urine, weak stream, enuresis, incontinence, nocturia, prolapse of the uterus, and chronic vaginal discharge. Many of these symptoms are seen in benign prostatic hypertrophy in older men and in organ-related atrophic and prolapsing menopausal changes. **Treatment:** with herbs by reinforcing and stabilizing Kidney Qi; with acupuncture: BL-23, BL-52, Du-4, KI-3, Ren-4. Tonify with moxa.

6. **Kidney Unable to Hold and Receive Qi** — This is a constitutional weakness of the Lung and Kidneys exacerbated by strenuous physical exercise, lifting, and standing. Its basis is an inability of the Yang Kidney to receive Qi descending from the Lungs, which accumulates in the Lungs resulting in an excess pattern causing shortness of breath (Kidneys control inhalation) and asthma (Lungs control exhalation). Facial edema occurs in advanced cases due to excessive fluid accumulation (no Yang to dry it out). The Lung always manifests in the face.

   Symptoms include shortness of breath on exertion, rapid and weak breathing, difficult inhaling, sweating, cold limbs, facial edema, mental listlessness, and clear urine during an asthma attack. This pattern is seen classically in the excess syndrome of exercise-induced asthma, and in asthma brought on by stress or emotion. **Treatment:** with herbs by warming Kidneys, stimulating Qi reception of Qi, stimulating descending function of Lung; with acupuncture: KI-3, KI-7, KI-25, Ren-6, Ren-17, Du-4, Du-12, ST-36, LU-7, BL-23.

7. **Kidney Yang Deficient, Water Overflowing** — Caused by extreme Kidney Yang Deficiency without transformation of any Fluids leading to generalized edema. Both the Heart and Lung are affected by this process leading to chronic retention of Dampness with the excess fluid symptoms outlined below.

   Symptoms include edema of legs and ankles (Kidney), Cold feeling in legs and back (Kidney), clear scanty urine (Kidney), abdominal distention (Kidney), palpitations (Heart), cold hands (Heart), watery, frothy sputum (Lung), and cough and asthma (Lung). The pattern is seen in congestive heart failure, nephrosis, and protein malnutrition. **Treatment:** with herbs by tonifying Kidney Yang, draining fluids, warming the Spleen, and augmenting Heart Yang; with acupuncture: BL-20, BL-22, BL-23, Du-4, Ren-9, ST-28, SP-9, KI-7. Use moxa for tonification.

The Kidney has many combination patterns with other organs as it is the source of Yin and Yang in the whole body. The most important ones include:

1. **Kidney and Liver Yin Deficiency** — seen in the perimenopausal patient with dry eyes and throat, night sweats, irregular or scanty menstruation, headaches, and insomnia.

2. **Disharmony of Kidney and Heart** — a Kidney Yin and Heart Yin Deficiency presentation with emotional overlay, and seen as palpitations, insomnia, night sweating, anxiety, and low back pain.

3. **Kidney and Lung Yin Deficiency** — seen in chronic, unresolved viral lung invasion and pulmonary tuberculosis with dry cough, evening heat, night sweats, and shortness of breath.

4. **Kidney and Spleen Yang Deficiency** — seen in chronic parasitic infestation such as giardia or candida overgrowth, with symptoms of chronic diarrhea, poor appetite, coldness, and low back pain.

## Bladder (BL)

The bladder transforms and excretes fluids from the body. It uses the Qi from the Kidney for this purpose. Bladder deficiencies are usually a result of Kidney deficiencies, mostly Kidney Yang Deficiency. Because the Kidneys have no excess patterns, all the excess patterns in the urinary tract system are manifested in the Bladder (the Fu or Yang organ). It is quite common for the Yin organs not to manifest clinically, but to leave it to its corresponding Yang organ to manifest with symptoms, e.g., the Gall Bladder manifests for the Liver, the Stomach for the Spleen. An accumulation of Dampness is the most common pathological pattern in the Bladder.

*Bladder Patterns*

The Bladder is extremely sensitive to climatic changes. Excessive exposure to damp or cold weather will cause induced patterns of Cold–Damp or Damp–Heat in the Bladder. The Bladder, like the Kidney, is affected by fear. In anxious and insecure children, this is exhibited by the sinking of Qi resulting in bedwetting. Excessive sexual activity affects and exhausts the Kidney Yang with associated bladder incontinence and nocturia.

1. **Damp–Heat in the Bladder** — Caused by exposure to Cold or Dampness that can turn into a full blown Interior-Heat. The Heat in the Bladder and fluid-obstructing action of Dampness lead to the common symptoms.

   Symptoms include burning on micturition, frequency, dark and turbid-smelling urine, hematuria, and dysuria. This pattern is seen classically in all UTIs. Damp–Heat in the Lower Burner (pelvis) includes pelvic inflammatory disease, specific and nonspecific vaginitis, leukorrhea, genital herpes, prostatitis, and cervical dysplasia. **Treatment:** with herbs by resolving Damp–Heat in the Lower Burner; with acupuncture: SP-6, SP-9, BL-22, BL-28, BL-63, BL-66, Ren-3.

2. **Cold–Damp in the Bladder** — Caused by exposure to Damp, Cold weather causing obstruction of the water passages with dysuria and feeling of heaviness. Symptoms include frequency and urgent urination, dysuria, feeling of heaviness in the lower pelvis or over the bladder, and pale turbid urine. This pattern partially explains chronic interstitial cystitis, which, however, may have a more complex mixed Cold and Hot pattern. **Treatment:** with herbs by resolving Dampness and Cold in the lower burner; with acupuncture: SP-9, SP-6, BL-22, BL-28, ST-28, Ren-9.

3. **Deficient Bladder and Cold** — Caused by Kidney Yang and Qi deficiency in old age and associated with atrophy of the organ. Symptoms include frequent pale urination, incontinence, enuresis, low back pain. This pattern is seen in old and chronically ill individuals. **Treatment:** with herbs by astringing the Kidney and Bladder to stop leakage; with acupuncture: KI-2, KI-6, BL-15, BL-23, Ren-4, Ren-14, Ren-17.

## Liver (LR)

The Liver is the central organ of the body and is known as the "general." It is primarily responsible for the storage of Blood and the smooth distribution of Qi throughout the body. When the Liver is healthy, a person is courageous and resolute.

The Liver has a marked influence on many other organs in the body. It aids the Spleen Qi to ascend and the Stomach Qi to descend and stimulates the excretion of bile from the Gall Bladder. The Liver has a strong influence on the flow of Qi to the Large Intestines and influences a normal bowel action. It is also responsible for Qi flow to the uterus and thus has a strong influence of the menstrual flow and dysmenorrhea.

The Liver is not involved in the production of Qi, only in the distribution of Qi, and therefore it is never Qi Deficient. However, Liver Blood and Liver Yin can become deficient or stagnant and disturb the distribution of Qi.

The Liver ensures the smooth flow and distribution of Qi upwards and outwards in the body. The flow of Qi from the Liver can influence emotions, digestion, secretion of bile, and the menstrual flow.

Obstructed Liver Qi causes frustration, depression, and repressed anger. Physically this is seen as abdominal distention, alternating diarrhea and constipation, a feeling of a "lump" in the throat (plum pit Qi), hypochondriac pain, and chest tightness. This problem manifests in females as PMS, breast distention, irritability, and irregular menses. The obstructed Liver Qi will invade the Stomach and cause the Stomach Qi to ascend. The ascending Stomach Qi will cause nausea, belching, vomiting, and GERD. Invasion of the Spleen causes diarrhea. In the Gall Bladder the flow of bile is obstructed giving rise to a bitter taste, belching, jaundice, and pasty stools.

The Liver stores the Blood and regulates the blood volume of the body. This storage capacity regulates flow to the muscles during exercise and to the uterus during menses. When active, the Blood flows to the muscles, and when at rest, the Blood returns to the Liver for replenishment and restoration of energy. If this cycle is disturbed, the muscles become weak and painful and the patient is very fatigued after exercise. This pattern is commonly seen in fibromyalgia. The external muscular flow of Blood is also important in the maintenance of the Wei Qi, the external surface immune barrier to external invasion. If this is not good, the patient becomes very susceptible to invasion by the Six Evils. The Liver Blood has a marked influence on the menses. If the Liver Blood is deficient, there will be minimal bleeding or amenorrhea. If the Blood is in excess or heated up, there may be menorrhagia. Liver Qi stagnation leads to stagnation of Blood in the uterus with associated dysmenorrhea and clotted dark blood.

The Liver Blood moistens and nourishes the tendons and sinews enabling them to contract and to relax. If Liver Blood is deficient, the muscles and tendons become tight, contracted, and inflexible causing numbness of the limbs, muscle cramps, tremors, tetany, or limb weakness.

The Liver Blood manifests in the quality of the nails. If deficient, the nails are ridged, brittle, and break easily. The Liver opens to the eyes and is responsible for moistening and nourishing them. When Liver Blood is deficient, the eyes will manifest with blurred vision, color blindness, myopia, and dryness. If there is Liver Heat or Fire, then the eyes will become painful, burning, and bloodshot or red. If Liver Wind is involved you will see involuntary eye movements. Kidney Jing also has some affect on aging eyes.

The Liver houses the Ethereal Soul or Hun. The Hun represents the spiritual aspect of the Liver, is Yang in nature, and survives the death of the host to flow back into the ethereal nonmaterial energies that were the template for the body. The Hun influences the capacity of planning and finding a direction in life. When Liver Blood is full, the Hun is firmly rooted in the body and we can plan our lives with wisdom and vision; if not, we have no sense of direction in our lives. The Hun may become detached from the body at night and is characterized by a sensation of floating apart from our bodies especially in those moments just before falling asleep. If this occurs, the Yin is too weak to hold onto the Yang Hun and the patient will have a disturbed, dream-filled sleep. The Hun is rooted in the Blood and the Yin.

*Liver Patterns*

Exterior Wind can interfere with the smooth flow of Qi and stir up the Blood stored in the Liver to exacerbate Internal Liver Wind and cause skin rashes of sudden onset that move around the body, often seen in viral exanthema, drug rashes, and hives. This is seen as Liver Heat.

The emotion associated with the Liver is anger. This includes feelings of frustration, resentment, repressed anger, and irritability. Anything that causes Liver Qi Stagnation will cause anger, and anger induced by situational issues will cause Liver Qi Stagnation with all its problems and a vicious cycle is set up. A chronic state of Liver Qi Stagnation will lead to a state of depression, repressed anger, and constant resentment. These emotions are physically manifest in a tight chest, frequent sighing, a lump in the throat, and tension in the rib cage and Stomach. If Liver Qi rebels upwards and causes Liver Yang to rise, symptoms such as headache and violent outbursts of anger will result. Long-term Liver Qi Stagnation leads to the formation of Liver Fire.

The most important external physical influence on the Liver is diet. Greasy, hot, spicy foods lead to Liver Fire. Lamb, beef, curries, deep fried foods, alcohol, caffeine, and sugar are all considered hot foods. Vegetarians, lacking warming foods such as meat, can end up with Liver Blood Deficiency.

1. **Liver Qi Stagnation** — Caused by repressed anger and emotions. This is, together with Kidney Yin Deficiency, the most common imbalance seen in Western patients and reflects our angry, dysfunctional society.

   A recent study in *Lancet*[37] entitled "Functional Somatic Syndromes: One or Many?" examines the commonalties between irritable bowel syndrome, nonulcer dyspepsia, PMS, chronic pelvic pain, fibromyalgia, atypical or noncardiac chest pain, hyperventilation syndrome, CFIDS, tension headache, TMJ dysfunction, globus hystericus, and multiple chemical sensitivity syndrome. In fact, there is substantial overlap between all these syndromes and the similarities outweigh the differences. The interesting issue is that they all have Liver Qi Stagnation as the prime cause of their manifestation.

   The main manifestation of Liver Qi Stagnation is in the hypochondrium with associated left upper quadrant (LUQ) pain and bloating. In the chest there is tightness. Sighing is a mechanism for releasing stagnant Qi. Hiccup is due to stagnant Qi in the diaphragm. Liver Qi invading the Stomach causes nausea, vomiting, belching, and pain. Stagnant Qi in the throat causes "Plum Pit Qi" a sensation of a lump in the throat, often seen in emotional states such as globus hystericus. Liver Qi Stagnation causes an irregular menstrual flow with dysmenorrhea, PMS, and breast swelling and tenderness. **Treatment:** with herbs by dispersing Liver Qi and by regulating Qi; with acupuncture: GB-34, LR-3, LR-13, L1-4, TH-6, PC-6.

2. **Liver Blood Stagnation** — Caused by issues surrounding anger. Always due to stagnant Qi, as Qi controls the Blood. The focus on the Blood rather than the Qi manifests in the uterus with large clots and dark menstrual Blood. Stagnant Blood also always causes pain that is fixed in position and stabbing in quality. If it is prolonged, it will form a mass such as fibroids in the uterus.

   Symptoms include irregular, heavy, painful menses with large dark clots. Abdominal pain with abdominal masses may be seen over time. If the Liver starts to heat up, epistaxis and hematemesis may occur. **Treatment:** with herbs by dispersing the Liver and regulating the Blood; with acupuncture: GB-34, LR-3, BL-17, BL-18, SP-10, Ren-6 (disperse, no moxa).

3. **Liver Fire Rising** — Caused by a chronic emotional state of anger, repressed anger, and resentment. The addition of hot foods such as alcohol, sugar, greasy, and spicy foods will exaggerate the situation.

   Symptoms are seen in the upper part of the body, as Liver Fire tends to flare upward causing red face and eyes, headache, dizziness, disturbed sleep, and irritability. Liver Fire ascending causes tinnitus and deafness of a particular type — sudden deafness with a high-pitched whistle. The oral cavity experiences a day-long bitter taste. Heart Fire produces a bitter taste only in the morning after a bad night's sleep. Liver Fire may also cause bleeding such as epistaxis and GI bleeding. The tongue is red and dry with a yellow coating.

   This picture is seen in the type-A individual who gets red in the face with anger and is explosive and unpredictable, with the associated physical findings. Explosive migraines may be seen. The patient may be hypertensive and suffer a stroke if there is associated Phlegm. This is seen in hepatitis, usually acute. **Treatment:** with herbs by sedating the Liver and quelling the Fire; with acupuncture: LR-2, LR-3, GB-13, GB-20, EX-2 (Tai Yang). All in dispersion.

4. **Liver Damp–Heat** — Caused by a combination of Liver Heat and Spleen Dampness. Dampness is heavy and tends to move downward and settle in the Lower Burner where the Damp–Heat produces its classic symptoms.

The Qi in the Liver is restricted and this causes hypochondrial pain and distention. The Dampness retards bile formation and flow leading to jaundice and sticky, floating stools. Because the Spleen is weak, the Liver invades it causing nausea, vomiting, loss of appetite, and abdominal distention. The Heat causes a low-grade continual fever, which can be distinguished from a Yin-Deficient fever, which occurs in the afternoon or at night. Damp-Heat in the Lower Burner causes vaginal discharge and itching, pain and swelling of the testicles, and genital herpes.

This picture is common and seen in patients with recurrent or chronic disease such as nonspecific vaginitis, bowel yeast overgrowth syndromes, chronic prostatitis, nonspecific urethritis, gonorrhea, trichomoniasis, chlamydial infections, pelvic inflammatory disease, chronic UTIs, and mucocutaneous candidiasis (the axillas, groin, and under the breasts are areas of Heat and Dampness). This is seen in chronic hepatitis, cholelithiasis, and cholecystitis. It is most important to treat the Spleen Dampness and its causes before treating the Liver Heat. **Treatment:** with herbs by resolving Dampness, dispersing Liver and Gall Bladder, and dispersing Heat; with acupuncture: LR-2, LR-14, GB-24, GB-34, BL-18, BL-19, Du-9, Ren-12, SP-3, SP-6, SP-9, LI-11. Disperse all except Ren-12, do not use moxa.

5. **Cold Stagnation in the Liver Channel** — Caused by the invasion of External Cold into the Liver channel. Cold tends to descend in the body and the Liver channel goes through the external genitalia, such that the symptoms are concentrated in that anatomical area. External Cold invasion occurs with being improperly dressed for the weather, sitting on cold surfaces, or having bare legs when the cold wind blows.

   Symptoms include fullness and distention in the hypogastrium, pain referred to scrotum and testes, contraction of the scrotum and retraction of the testes, and pain that feels better when warmth is applied. This picture is uncommon but can be seen with any dysfunction in the Lower Burner that is made worse with Cold invasion including hernias, dysmenorrhea, and anorectal spasm. **Treatment:** with herbs by warming the Liver and alleviating Cold; with acupuncture: Ren-13, LR-1, LR-5. Disperse with moxa.

6. **Liver Blood Deficiency** — Liver Blood Deficiency is a multifactoral pattern. The Spleen does not make enough Blood if you are a vegan or vegetarian (important in menstruating females). There is not enough Blood to be stored by the Liver. Deficiency of Kidney Jing and Qi can also decrease the amount of available Blood. Severe hemorrhage or prolonged bleeding can also cause Liver Blood Deficiency.

   Symptoms are associated with the lessening of the Liver's physiological functions: blurred vision, dizziness, weak and numb limbs, scanty menses or amenorrhea, pale complexion and tongue, muscle cramps and spasms, brittle nails, and postmenstrual headache. Liver Blood Deficiency is the root cause or at least part cause of a number of other patterns including Liver Qi Stagnation, Liver Blood Stagnation, Liver Yang rising, Empty Heat, Heart Blood Deficiency, chronic Wind–Damp pain, unrooted Hun, Kidney Yin Deficiency, Kidney Yang Deficiency, Wind–Heat in the skin, Cold in the uterus, and Qi deficiency. These symptoms are very common and relate to the associated patterns already discussed. **Treatment:** with herbs by tonifying Liver and Kidney and Blood; with acupuncture: BL-17, BL-18, BL-20, BL-23, LR-8, SP-6, ST-36, Ren-4. Tonify with moxa.

7. **Liver Yang Rising** — This is similar to Liver Fire blazing but comes from an underlying deficient pattern of deficient Liver Yin and Kidney Yin. This deficiency causes the Liver to heat up and causes the out of control Liver Yang to rise.

   Symptoms include all the symptoms of Liver Fire blazing (headaches, dizziness, tinnitus, dry mouth, insomnia, irritability, shouting, and anger) except the true Heat symptoms of constipation, dark urine, and bitter taste in the mouth. Liver Yang headaches occur on the left side of the head (TCM holds that excess symptoms occur on the right side of the body, while deficient conditions occur on the left).

This pattern is the classical migraine or cluster headache patient. Hemiplegia and facial paralysis may occur if the Liver Yang invades the channels of the head and face. **Treatment:** with herbs by tonifying Yin and subduing Liver Yang; with acupuncture: LR-3, LR-8, TH-5, SP-6, KI-3, GB-6, GB-8, GB-9, GB-20, GB-38, GB-43, BL-12. Disperse all points except Kidney - no moxa.

## Liver Wind (Internal Wind)

*Liver wind* is generated by three different mechanisms: extreme Heat, deficient Liver Yin with Yang rising, and deficient Liver Blood.

1. **Heat-Generated Wind** — Caused by the invasion of Exterior Wind–Heat or by Heat penetrating to the Blood level and generating Wind. This pattern is usually due to viral or bacterial invasion with febrile response.

   Symptoms of this very excess type of Wind (severe) include tremors and convulsions and opisthotonus and nuchal rigidity caused by drying of the neck sinews by a dry Liver with no moistening ability and may lead to a disturbed effect with somnolence and coma.

   This pattern is seen in febrile convulsions, in the encephalitic complications of measles, and in encephalitis and meningitis. **Treatment:** with herbs by clearing Heat, dispersing the Liver, and subduing Wind; with acupuncture: LR-2, LR-3, SI-3, Du-16, Du-20, GB-20.

2. **Liver Yang Rising Causing Wind** — Caused by Liver Yin and Kidney Yin Deficiency creating an excessive Liver Yang that is bad enough to generate Wind. Liver Blood Deficiency may make things worse especially in women with menorrhagia. The emotional components of anger, resentment, and frustration are also needed for the development of this severe pattern.

   Symptoms are acute and excessive and include sudden unconsciousness, convulsions, deviation of mouth and eyes, hemiplegia, aphasia, difficult speech, and dizziness. This pattern can best be described as an "apoplexy" and may be seen in intracranial disasters or as hysterical conversion reactions. **Treatment:** with herbs by nourishing Yin, subduing Liver Yang and Wind; with acupuncture: LR-3, LR-8, SP-6, KI-3, Du-16, GB-20, BL-18. Tonify LR-8, SP-6, KI-3, disperse LR-3, Du-16 and GB-20.

3. **Deficient Liver Blood Causing Wind** — Caused by chronic Liver Blood Deficiency not being able to fill the blood vessels and nourish the muscles and sinews.

   Symptoms include chronic low-grade headaches (Wind filling the half empty blood vessels), numbness in the muscles, and some mild tics or tremors. This pattern is seen in women with headaches and menorrhagia, some cases of MS, Parkinson's disease, and benign familial tremor. **Treatment:** with herbs by nourishing Liver Blood and subduing Wind; with acupuncture: LR-3, LR-8, KI-3, Du-16, BL-17, Bl-18, Bl-20, Bl-23. LI-4. Disperse LR-3, LI-4, GB-20, Du-16, tonify others.

# Gall Bladder (GB)

The main function of the Gall Bladder is to store and secrete bile. It is very dependent on the state of the Liver, and the smooth flow of Liver Qi is important to its function. The Gall Bladder is very susceptible to Dampness originating in the Spleen (diet).

## Gall Bladder Patterns

Diet affecting the Spleen is very important in the Gall Bladder. The excessive ingestion of greasy or fatty foods leads to Dampness that becomes lodged in the Gall Bladder. The emotions of anger, repressed resentment, and frustration cause Heat and, over a period of time, Liver and Gall Bladder Fire, and when mixed with Dampness, give Damp–Heat. Climactic changes of Heat and Dampness from the exterior will induce elements of Damp–Heat in the Gall Bladder.

1. **Gall Bladder Damp–Heat** — Caused by feelings of anger over time coupled with poor dietary choices of fats, hot foods, and sugar.

   Symptoms occur due to the Spleen Dampness extending into the Gall Bladder causing Liver Qi Stagnation and associated hypochondrial pain. The Liver invading the Spleen causes nausea, while the belching and vomiting is caused by the Stomach Qi rebelling and ascending. The bitter taste in the mouth, dark urine, and fever are all signs of Heat. The combination of Dampness and Heat in the Gall Bladder over time turns into Phlegm (gallstones).

   This is a typical pattern seen in the fat, fatigued, fertile, forty-year-old female — all signs of Spleen Dampness and Liver Yin deficiency — who has acute or chronic cholecystitis with or without stones. Cholecystectomy only removes the stones and the physical site of Damp-Heat, but does not change the pain (Liver Qi Stagnation) or the underlying problem: anger with Damp-Heat, which then invades the Liver channel and focuses on the breast where Phlegm will again form (tumor), or it will descend into the Lower Burner with the Phlegm forming in the uterus (fibroids) or the ovaries (tumor). Many patients who have had their gallbladders out still have LUQ pain. **Treatment:** with herbs by resolving Dampness, clearing Heat, and stimulating the smooth flow of Qi; with acupuncture: GB-24, GB-34, LR-14, Ren-12, Du-9, BL-18, BL-19, BL-20, LI-11, TH-6.

2. **Deficient Gall Bladder** — Constitutional or environmental mental state characterized by extreme timidity, lack of courage, and difficulty in making decisions. It may be treated as a Liver Blood Deficiency. All these symptoms relate to the Ethereal Soul's not being housed with Liver Blood. Best described by the English term "lily livered." The Zulu in South Africa eat the lion's Liver to attain courage. **Treatment:** with herbs by tonifying Blood and warming the Gall Bladder; with acupuncture: GB-40 with moxa.

## OTHER PATTERNS OF DIAGNOSIS IN TCM

The two patterns of diagnosis that were not dealt with in this section on TCM and acupuncture were the Six Stages and the Four Levels.

### Patterns According to the Six Stages

This diagnosis was formulated by Zhang Zhong Jing in the second century A.D. in his Discussion on Cold-Induced Diseases.[40] This diagnosis relates to the penetration of the External Evils — mostly Cold, Heat, and Wind — into the body from the superficial layers to the deeper layers, from external Yang to internal Yin. In order of penetration from outside to inside they are: Tai Yang → Shao Yang → Yang Ming, then deeper — Tai Yin → Shao Yin → Jue Yin. Each of these stages has associated clinical signs and symptoms that characterize the penetration of, for instance, a viral illness that starts with fever and myalgia (Tai Yang → Shao Yang) to high fever, thirst, sweating, and constipation (Yang Ming), to abdominal discomfort, vomiting, no appetitie, diarrhea (Tai Yin), to coldness and chills, diarrhea, no thirst, abundant pale urine (Shao Yin), to heat and fever, insomnia, dry mouth, scanty urine, feeling of energy rising into chest (Jue Yin).

### Patterns According to the Four Levels

This diagnosis was described by Ye Tian Shi (1667–1746) in his book *Discussion of Warm Diseases*.[51] This pattern describes the pathogenesis of the the Evil Wind–Heat and describes the state of progress of a febrile infectious disease, in much the same way as described in the Six Stages, but using the TCM terms of defensive Qi–Wei Qi (superficial — mild symptoms), Qi (deeper — high fever), nutritive Qi–Rong Qi (deeper still — insomnia and mental symptoms), and Blood level–Yuan Qi (the deepest — vomiting and loss of Blood and convulsions).

## Clinical Use of Six Stages and Four Levels

These diagnoses are somewhat important as they indicate at what level and intensity the patient needs to be treated. If the disease is still superficial, a little tonifying input into Wei Qi is sufficient, but if deeper, you do not want to tonify Wei Qi for fear of energizing the disease, and deeper tonification of the organs is necessary. Use your clinical judgment as to how deep the disease has penetrated by looking at what meridians and organ systems seem to be showing symptoms — Yang are superficial and Yin are deep.

This ends the discussion of organ patterns in TCM, probably the most important but difficult concepts to master for the uninitiated. These patterns will start to fall into place as they are utilized with the diagnostic tools in Chapter 13 on real patients. Because we have been advocating the use of Chinese herbs in the organ patterns, before we launch into acupuncture, it would be useful to understand how Chinese herbs are combined to form a clinical formula.

# 6 Chinese Herbal Prescribing

## INTRODUCTION

Practically speaking, no one reading this book is going to go to the trouble, time, and expense of learning how to put together a Chinese herbal formula from scratch for each individual patient. There are many companies selling well-constructed, thought out, prepared formulas in tablets, capsules, powders, and liquids. Each line has its own formulators who have their own thoughts on how to "Westernize" the classical Chinese formulas. The company or preparation of herb you use for a particular patient or condition is a matter of taste and experience. Classically, Chinese herbs were and are still given to patients to prepare as a boiling tea or decoction, but many volatile oils and volatile components are lost with this method. Modern techniques use a water–alcohol extraction system in a closed container to preserve any volatiles. In a subsequent volume, I will discuss my preferences in this regard.

The Chinese patent formulas from China are cheap and work well, but you never quite know their level of quality, or if any adulterants have been added, although some manufacturers have bowed to pressure and allowed the FDA to inspect and sanction their factories and processing plants. I still prefer to use herbs that are formulated in the U.S., because there are strict purity and quality checks on the raw herbs. Powders from Taiwan are equally pure and quality controlled. I have never had a single instance of contamination or an irregular batch in ten years of herbal prescribing.

I think that it is useful to have some idea how the Chinese think when they are putting together a formula. The TCM diagnosis is made first and, according to the pattern, an herbal combination is constructed to oppose the excesses or deficiencies seen in the patient. If the patient is hot, then cooling herbs are used; if Blood is deficient, then Blood nourishing herbs are used, etc. Each patient may have a mixture of patterns such that the herbal combination will have to take into consideration each pattern encountered to harmonize the whole.

**Dosages** — Herbs may be used for short time periods in increased doses for acute disease (3 to 10 days) or in lower doses for long periods in chronic disease (3 to 6 months or longer). The Chinese say that it takes one month for every year that you have had your disease, to rectify and stabilize the imbalance. Each manufacturer has guidelines for dosage because each tablet or liquid has different herbal concentrations according to the mode of manufacture. Some tablets are just ground up herbs that are compacted and tableted. You will need more of these for an equivalent dose of, say, a freeze-dried, powder-compacted tablet from a liquid concentrate. In general an adult dose is 2 to 3 tablets 3x/day of a 750 mg tablet, but will increase for an acute syndrome to 4 to 6x/day and decrease for slow tonification to once a day. Children and the elderly usually take proportionally less herb according to body weight or age. When a patient is on constitutional tonification and experiences an acute disease syndrome, such as a virus, the patient should stop the constitutional therapy, otherwise the acute Evil will be tonified. The patient can restart the constitutional therapy after the acute problem has subsided. The timing of taking the herb may be significant, although any compliance is better than none. For example, herbs for morning sickness need to be taken in the morning, herbs for afternoon fatigue taken in the afternoon, and herbs for insomnia just before bedtime. Herbs to strengthen an organ should be taken during the two-hour peak of activity, and those that are calming or decongesting an organ, may be taken just before maximum activity or at the two-hour nadir. Spleen tonics should be taken with food.

Many patients cannot tolerate herbs and will experience nausea and bloating, even abdominal pain. Most of these patients have weak spleens, and you may either have to address that pattern first with liquid or chewed herbs or by administering the Spleen herb together with a reduced dosage of the therapeutic herb.

Herbs should be taken 2 to 3 hours away from regular drugs to prevent any interactions between them. Herbs should be taken on an empty stomach to enhance absorption, but may be taken with food if there is associated gastro-intestinal (GI) intolerance. Herbs will keep for 1 to 2 years, after which they will lose some of their efficacy, but are still useable.

The dose for each person should be tested, and even then some patients will aggravate on the first day. Most aggravations and intolerances will disappear within 24 to 48 hours of stopping or reducing the herbal dose. Chinese herbs are pretty forgiving and you rarely can cause much harm with them. This not the case with Western herbs, which are used singly as a drug substitute.

## CLASSIFICATION OF CHINESE HERBS

Chinese herbs may be classified according to four principles: (1) energy and effects; (2) element, taste, and color; (3) action; and (4) therapeutic categories.

### ENERGY AND EFFECTS

| Energy | Effects |
|---|---|
| Cold | Quells fire (anti-inflammatory/spasmodic, sedative) |
| Cool | Subdues Heat (reduces fever, detoxifies, lowers BP) |
| Neutral | Gentle effects (does not alter Hot or Cold conditions) |
| Warm | Enhances circulation (alleviates chills, improves organ function) |
| Hot | Dispels Cold (breaks Qi blockages, warms the center) |

Note: Cool and Cold herbs do overlap, as do Hot and Warm herbs.

### ELEMENT, TASTE, AND COLOR

| Element | Taste | Color | Effect |
|---|---|---|---|
| Earth | Sweet | Yellow | Nourishing, tonifying |
| Metal | Acrid | White | Dispersing, decongesting, stimulating |
| Water | Salty | Black | Diuretic, purgative, softening |
| Wood | Sour | Green | Astringent, absorbing, circulation |
| Fire | Bitter | Red | Sedating, anti-inflammatory/Fire, soothing |

### ACTIONS

1. **Ascending** — upward circulation of Qi.
2. **Descending** — downward circulation of Qi.
3. **Opening Channels** — opens the meridian circulation of Qi
4. **Invigorating Blood Flow** — improves Blood circulation.
5. **Sedative** — calms Shen and reduces Yang.
6. **Drying** — eliminates accumulations of moisture.
7. **Moisturizing** — treats dryness of skin and mucous membranes.
8. **Breaks Up Blockages** — disperses blockages of Qi.
9. **Normalize Qi Flow** — treats nausea, vomiting, bloating, and flatulence.

10. **Yang Tonic** — nourishes Yang.
11. **Yin Tonic** — nourishes the Yin.
12. **Moves Dampness** — normalizes the distribution of water.
13. **Astringent** — reduces excess sweating and leakage of fluids.

## THERAPEUTIC CATEGORIES

This section will deal with the individual actions of classes of herbs. These include: release exterior conditions, clear heat, downward draining, drain dampness, expel wind dampness, aromatic herbs that transform dampness, relieve food stagnation, regulate the qi, regulate blood, warm the interior and expel cold, transform phlegm and stop coughing, tonifying, astringents, calm the spirit, aromatics that open the orifices, extinguish wind and stop tremors, expel parasites, external application. The next section on the *Eight Methods of Herbal Therapy* will deal with their clinical application.

1.  **Release Exterior Conditions:** diaphoretics for the treatment of exterior symptom complexes, subdivided into warming and cooling herbs.
    A.  *Wind Heat:* Fever, headache, and sore throats with mild chills. Viral infection of hot virus. **Herb:** Chrysanthemum — Jua Hua (spicy, cool).
    B.  *Wind Cold:* Chills, neck pain, and sneezing with runny nose with clear discharge. Caused by Cold Wind, in and out of air conditioning. Wearing a scarf around the neck will prevent the entry of Wind-Cold into the Gall Bladder channel at the back of the neck. **Herb:** Angelica — Bai Zhi (spicy, warm).
2.  **Clear Heat:** antipyretics, herbs for clearing Internal Heat subdivided into five categories.
    A  *Quell Fire:* Chronic hypertension, high fevers. **Herb:** Anemarrhena — Zhi Mu (bitter, cold).
    B.  *Cool Blood:* Skin rashes, chronic epistaxis (due to Blood Heat), dry nose (Yin Deficiency of Lungs), excess menstrual bleeding, and hematuria or malena. **Herb:** Rehmannia, raw — Sheng Di Huang (sweet, bitter, cold).
    C.  *Clear Heat and Dry Dampness:* Oozing skin lesions, herpes, poison oak and poison ivy, and acute urinary tract infections. **Herb:** Gentiana — Long Dan Cao (bitter, cold).
    D.  *Clear Heat Poisons:* Bacterial infections with cellulitis and carbuncles, any toxic swelling such as spider bite. **Herb:** Honeysuckle (Lonicera) — Jin Yin Hua (sweet, cold).
    E.  *Clear and Relieve Summer Heat:* Fever, sweating and diarrhea — the summer Stomach flu or dysentery. **Herb:** Dolichos — Bai Bian Dou (sweet, neutral).
3.  **Downward Draining:** Purgatives, lubricating herbs, and strong diuretics.
    A.  *Purgatives:* Act fast like salt water. **Herb:** Rhubarb (Rheum) — Da Huang (bitter, cold).
    B.  *Moist Laxative:* Moistens the intestines in deficient individuals. **Herb:** Cannabis Seeds — Huo Ma Ren (sweet, neutral).
    C.  *Harsh Expellents:* Used to drain ascites and acute pleuritic edema. **Herb:** Morning Glory Seeds — Qian Niu Zi (bitter, acrid, cold, poisonous).
4.  **Drain Dampness:** Diuretics, cooling and warming herbs. Most useful for edema below the waist and for increasing urinary output. **Herbs:** Poria Cocos — Fu Ling (sweet, bland, neutral); Alisma — Ze Xie (sweet, bland, cold).
5.  **Expel Wind Dampness:** Antirheumatics for the Bi syndrome. These herbs have analgesic, anti-inflammatory, antipyretic, and circulation promoting actions. Usually due to invading wind. Different types of pain are appreciated according to the herbal pattern:
    A.  *Wind* — pain that migrates from joint to joint.
    B.  *Damp* — lingering, swelling with numbness (also Blood Stagnation).
    C.  *Cold* — fixed severe pain, better for heat and associated with decreased mobility.

D. *Hot* — joint pain with swelling and heat; responds favorably to cold; fever, thirst, and yellow, coated tongue.

E. *Congealed Blood* — fixed and sharp pain.

The *choice of herbs* in Bi syndromes depends on the presentation, age, and site of the arthritic pain. Some herbs, such as Angelica — Du Huo, are tonifying and warming and should be used in older patients, while others, such as Mulberry twigs (ramulus Mori Albae) — Sang Zhi, are mild and useful in children. Some herbs, such as radix Notopterygii — Qiang Huo, are used for the neck and shoulders, while others, such as Angelica — Du Huo, are used in the lower back and hips.

6. **Aromatic Herbs that Transform Dampness:** Herbs with fragrant odor for resolving Dampness. These herbs work primarily on the Spleen–Stomach Dampness with abdominal fullness, nausea, vomiting, and diarrhea. These usually occur with food poisoning or acute gastroenteritis. These herbs are acrid, warm, aromatic, and dry. They can exhaust the Qi and dry out the Yin. **Typical herbs:** Cardamon — Bai Dou Kou, Magnolia — Hou Po, and Atractylodes — Cang Zhu.

7. **Relieve Food Stagnation:** These are digestives, increase gastrointestinal secretions, have enzymatic functions, and optimize peristalsis for better digestion. Symptoms include indigestion, fullness in the stomach, bloating, and abdominal pain. These manifestations are really a subtype of stagnant Qi and these herbs are usually given together with Qi-regulating herbs. Food stagnation is seen clinically most often in children who have a poorly developed Spleen function causing food Stagnation with otitis media and sinusitis. If food stagnation is chronic, then Blood Stagnation in the stomach ensues. **Typical Herbs:** Hawthorn (Crataegus) — Shan Zha, and Sprouted Barley Malt — Mai Ya.

8. **Regulate the Qi:** The two primary disorders of Qi are deficient Qi and stagnant Qi. Deficient Qi will be dealt with under tonification of Qi. Stagnant Qi results in pain, usually in the head and extremities. This section deals with the pain and organ dysfunction seen in the chest and abdomen. There three major types of stagnant Qi, depending on the major organ involved:

A. *Stagnant Spleen and Stomach Qi:* The primary symptoms are epigastric and abdominal pain, belching, gas, acid regurgitation, nausea, vomiting, and diarrhea or constipation. Most of these herbs aid in digestion and function of the GI tract. **Herb:** Aged Tangerine Peel — Chen Pi (acrid, bitter, warm, aromatic).

B. *Constrained Liver Qi:* Due to repressed anger and causes a constricted feeling in the chest, flank pain, loss of appetite, depression, and irritability. In women this can manifest as irregular menses or swollen, tender breasts. **Herb:** Green Citrus Peel — Qing Pi (bitter, acrid, slightly warm).

C. *Stagnant Lung Qi:* Primary symptoms are wheezing and coughing with shortness of breath and a sense of tightness in the chest. **Herb:** Lignum Aquilariae — Chen Xiang (acrid, bitter, warm, aromatic).

9. **Regulate Blood:** Homeostatics and herbs that activate (invigorate) Blood circulation.

A. *Herbs that Stop Bleeding:* Used for hematemesis, epistaxis, hemoptysis, malena, hematuria, menorrhagia, or bleeding from trauma. These herbs are not usually used alone, but in combination with herbs to cool Blood, tonify Yin, tonify Spleen, etc. **Herb:** Pseudoginseng — San Qi (sweet, slightly warm).

B. *Herbs that invigorate the Blood:* Used for problems of congealed Blood. They include:
   • Pain from congealed Blood — Pain is fixed in a precise location, is deep, colicky, and of long duration. This pain is seen in the lower abdomen, chest, trauma, and internal bleeding.
   • Abscess and ulcers — Stagnation of Qi and Blood are involved in the pathogenesis of ulcers, abscesses and necrotic inflammations, suppurative and slow-healing

inflammation of soft tissues, and intestinal abscesses (a diagnosis that overlaps with appendicitis).

- Abdominal masses — There are two types of abdominal masses appreciated: the hard, immobile abdominal masses (zheng) seen as hepato- and splenomegally, abdominal or pelvic tumors or cysts; and the visible, mobile abdominal masses seen as distention and bloating.

**Herb:** There are many herbs for moving Blood including Turmeric — Yu Jin (acrid, bitter, cool); Corydalis — Yan Hu Suo (acrid, bitter, warm) the most important herb for any pain; and Safflower (Carthamus) — Hong Hua (acrid, warm). In general, Western medicine regards these herbs for use in hemorrhage, congestion, ecchymoses, thrombosis, and local ischemia and tissue masses. Invigorating herbs can also be used for therapeutic abortion.

10. **Warm the Interior and Expel Cold:** Herbs for dispelling Internal Cold. Patterns of Interior Cold arise, if mild, from Internal Cold and are seen as cold extremities, aversion to cold, pale complexion, lack of thirst with craving for warm or hot fluids, and loose stools. More serious Cold is usually caused by invasion of Cold from the exterior and is seen as a collapsed Yang and Qi with ice-cold extremities, fear of cold, sweating, watery stool, and weak pulse. This is seen in shock. The organs usually invaded by Cold are the Stomach, Spleen, and uterus. In the gastrointestinal system, Cold invasion is seen as Cold in the Middle Burner, with nausea, belching, and diarrhea — acute gastroenteritis and gastritis in Western medicine. These herbs have a Yang-tonifying action that can be interpreted as being cardiotonics that reflexively stimulate the vasoactive centers of the CNS, thereby stimulating blood flow. **Herb:** Ginger — Gan Jiang (acrid, hot) for the Spleen and Stomach; Cinnamon — Rou Gui (acrid, sweet, hot) for the Kidney Yang; and Evodia — Wu Zhu Yu (acrid, bitter, warm, poisonous) for Cold dysmenorrhea and Cold testicles.

11. **Transform Phlegm and Stop Coughing:** Herbs for resolving Hot and Cold Phlegm and resolving cough. Phlegm is formed in the Spleen from excessive Dampness and is stored in the Lungs, the "receptacle of Phlegm." Phlegm is seen in the Lungs, Stomach, channels, and misting the orifices of the Heart.

    A. *Phlegm in the Lungs:* When Phlegm accumulates in the Lungs it leads to cough, wheezing, and a feeling of constriction or tightness in the chest. Cold Phlegm is clear or white with a loose rattle. Hot Phlegm is yellow, brown or green, thick, coagulated, and tenacious. The breasts are in close proximity to the lung, and Phlegm in the breasts (tumors, cysts, and cancer) is treated with the same Lung herbs. **Herb:** Hot Phlegm and breast tumors (Fritillaria) — Chuan Bai Mu (bitter, sweet, cool); Cold Phlegm (Inulae) — Xuan Fu Hua (bitter, acrid, slightly warm).

    B. *Phlegm in Stomach:* Accompanied by nausea, vomiting, loss of appetite, bloating, sometimes with cough. Mucus can be seen in the stool. **Herb:** Pinellia — Ban Xia (acrid, warm, poisonous).

    C. *Phlegm in the Channels:* Causes numb, stiff, and swollen joints and tumors such as goiter and cysts. **Herb:** Arisaematis — Tian Nan Xing (bitter, acrid, warm, poisonous).

    D. *Turbid Phlegm Misting the Orifices:* Causes stroke, coma, epilepsy, and Shen disturbances. **Herb:** Acorus — Chang Pu (acrid, slightly warm, aromatic).

12. **Tonifying:** Tonifying herbs are used to strengthen deficiencies in weak and fatigued patients. In strengthening the body's defense against disease they are used together with herbs to expel external pathogenic influences. If you tonify a patient with an pathogenic influence without combining the tonification with pathogenic expelling herbs, you run the risk of strengthening the external pathogen. The Rule of Tonification is: clear first, then tonify.

The deficiency problems addressed in tonification include Deficient Qi, Blood, Yang, and Yin. In patients with weak digestions or who are Yin Deficient, tonifying herbs may be too rich, especially Yang tonics, which may lead to Empty Heat syndromes.

A. *Tonify Qi:* The Spleen and the Lungs are the two organs most affected by Qi deficiency because of their function in producing Qi. Patients are generally fatigued, weak, pale, and cold; have a feeble, weak voice and weakness in the muscles and limbs. *Spleen Qi Deficiency* is seen as lethargy, weakness in the extremities, lack of appetite, abdominal distention or pain, and loose stool or diarrhea. *Lung Qi Deficiency* is seen as shortness of breath, shallow breathing, dyspnea on exertion, weak voice, pallid complexion, and spontaneous sweating. Qi is responsible for the generation and circulation of Blood, and so there is always a component of Blood Deficiency with Qi Deficiency. These herbs are very rich and need to be combined with herbs that move and regulate the Qi, otherwise they will lead to congestive chest symptoms and Heat.

   **Herbs:** Ginseng — Ren Shen (sweet, slightly bitter, slightly warm). Astragalus — Huang Qi (sweet, slightly warm); Codonopsis — Dang Shen (sweet, neutral).

   Note: In most cases of Qi Deficiency, Codonopsis should be used. Ginseng is only preferred in cases of Qi and Yang collapse. Astragalus is more important in generation of Wei Qi, the protective, superficial Qi. Codonopsis and Ginseng tonify the organ and source Qi and work well together. Chinese, Korean, and Red Ginseng are all warm or hot in nature, while American Ginseng is cool and moistening and may be used for extended periods of time, especially for dry Lungs with dry cough. In fatigue you need to tonify Blood, Lung and Spleen Qi, Yin Deficiency and Yang Deficiency, and move stagnant Liver Qi and Blood.

B. *Tonify Blood:* These herbs nourish the Blood. The clinical signs of Blood Deficiency are pallid face and lips; dizziness and vertigo (not enough Blood to fill the head); diminished vision; lethargy; palpitations; dry skin, hair and nails; menstrual irregularities; and pale tongue. The two organs most impacted are the Heart (directs the Blood) and the Liver (stores the Blood).

   Deficient Blood is seen not only in anemia but also in psychosomatic disturbances, CHF, and chronic hepatitis, to name a few. Most of the herbs do not have a direct marrow and hemopoietic effect, but improve nutrition and bodily strength, thereby increasing the marrow activity. Blood tonifying herbs are not used alone, but usually in combination with Qi and Yin tonifying herbs. Blood tonifiers tend to cause digestive upset and should be used with Spleen and Stomach herbs.

   **Herbs:** Angelica — Dang Gui (sweet, acrid, bitter, warm); Polygonum — He Shou Wu (bitter, sweet, astringent, slightly warm); Rehmannia — Shu Di Huang (sweet, slightly warm).

C. *Tonify Yang:* These herbs tonify primarily Kidney Yang, the source of Yang in the body. Others organs that need Yang tonification include the Spleen and Heart. The principal symptoms include systemic exhaustion, withdrawal from society, aversion to cold, cold extremities, sore and weak lower back, pale tongue, habitual miscarriages, impotence, enuresis, polyuria, wheezing, and cockcrow diarrhea.

   From a Western biochemical standpoint these herbs regulate the function of the adrenal cortex, energy metabolism, and sexual functions and promote growth and strengthen resistance.

   **Herb:** Eucommia — Du Zhong (sweet, slightly acrid, warm).

D. *Tonify Yin:* Herbs are used to tonify, nourish, and nurture the Yin of the Lung, Stomach, Liver, and Kidneys. In combination with other herbs they can be used for moistening Dryness and transforming Phlegm, moistening the Large Intestines in constipation, producing fluids to alleviate thirst, calming the Shen, tonifing the Blood, stopping bleeding, and increasing strength.

*Lung Yin Deficiency* — seen as dry cough, loss of voice, thirst, dry throat, dry skin, and sometimes yellow, thick sputum. If the Yin Deficiency worsens, then it is called *Consumptive Lung* with chronic cough, low-grade afternoon fevers, night sweats, and hemoptysis.

*Stomach Yin Deficiency* — is a lack of Fluids in the Stomach. This often occurs in severe febrile diseases with lowered appetite, irritability, thirst, dry mouth, and constipation. Lung Yin tonifying herbs are used. These herbs have antipyretic, diuretic, laxative, and expectorant properties.

*Liver Yin Deficiency* — similar to Liver Blood Deficiency with the addition of low-grade sensation of Heat. If Ascendant Liver Yang is associated with the Liver Yin deficiency, then additional symptoms include vertigo, tinnitus, dry mouth and throat, insomnia, and red tongue.

*Kidney Yin Deficiency* — is seen in many chronic diseases, especially in chronic stress. Clinical symptoms include fatigue, anxiety, insomnia (cannot stay asleep), dizziness, tinnitus, weak and painful lower back and knees, halitosis, warm palms and soles, afternoon low-grade fevers, reduced sexual function, scant and dark urine, and a red and dry tongue. These herbs regulate fluid metabolism, and some lower blood pressure and serum cholesterol.

**Herbs:** Ophiopogonum — Mai Men Dong (sweet, slightly bitter, slightly cold); Lily Bulb — Bai He (sweet, slightly bitter, slightly cold).

13. **Astringents:** These herbs are used for treating disorders of fluid loss or organ slippage. These disorders include diarrhea, excessive urination, excessive sweating, hemorrhage, and prolapse of rectum, bladder, or uterus. These disorders are due to autonomic nervous dysfunction or weakening of the elasticity of smooth muscle slings. **Herb:** Schisandra — Wu Wei Zhi (sour, warm) is a very important adaptogen, that is, it regulates many body functions and increases the organism's ability to deal with stress.

14. **Calm the Spirit:** These are used either to settle and calm the spirit or to nourish the Heart and calm the spirit. Symptoms are mainly irritability and insomnia.

   A. *Substances that Settle and Calm the Spirit:* These herbs are all made of heavy, dense substances (minerals, shells, or resins) that will "ground" the Shen. They weigh upon the Heart and calm the Shen (palpitations, anxiety, sweating, vivid dreams, and insomnia), the floating Liver Yang (headaches, dizziness, bad temper, flushed face), the Lung to contain the leakage of Lung Qi (coughing and wheezing), and the Stomach to redirect Rebellious Qi downwards (vomiting, hiccups, or belching). These herbs have sedative and tranquilizing effects. Most herbal mixtures will contain herbs for tonifying the Spleen, which these substances can easily injure. **Herb:** Dragon Bone — Long Gu (sweet. astringent, neutral); Oyster Shell — Mu Li (salty, astringent, cool).

   B. *Herbs that Nourish the Heart and Calm the Spirit:* Used for palpitations with anxiety and for insomnia with deficient Heart Blood and deficient Liver Yin. **Herb:** Polygala — Yuan Zhi (bitter, acrid, warm).

15. **Aromatics that Open the Orifices**: Used mostly for strokes and coma, which may be either Hot or Cold syndromes.

   A. *Hot Closed Syndrome* — delirium, irritability, convulsions, red face, and heavy breathing. Seen in deep Heat invasion such as meningitis, encephalitis, severe pneumonia, and systemic sepsis. Can also occur in heat stroke, end-stage liver disease, uremia, and cardiovascular accidents (CVAs). **Herbs:** Water Buffalo Gall Bladder — Niu Huang (very bitter, sweet, cool); Borneal — Bing Pian (acrid, bitter, cool).

   B. *Cold Closed Syndrome* — ashen face, cold and limp body, sudden collapse, foaming at mouth, coma, CVAs, and poisoning. **Herbs:** Musk — She Xiang (acrid, warm, aromatic); Acorus — Chang Pu (acrid, slightly warm, aromatic).

These herbs stimulate the CNS and lead to revival from coma. They also tranquilize and stop spasms and irritability.

16. **Extinguish Wind and Stop Tremors:** Wind, one of the evils, has both external (virus, bacteria) and internal manifestations. The Internal Wind is generated from pathogenic organ changes, usually in the Liver or Kidneys. Internal movement of Liver Wind is caused by deficient Liver and Kidney Yin with ascending Liver Yang, deficient Blood, or high fevers.

   A. *Internal Movement of Liver Wind* — seen as headache, dizziness, blurred vision, tinnitus, and in more severe cases irritability, vomiting, palpitations with anxiety, and muscle twitches or tics. Clinically seen as hypertension, restless legs, eye twitches, and tics. These herbs exhibit antihypertensive, mild sedative, and antispasmodic activity.

   B. *Windstroke* — the pattern may progress to tremors (Parkinson's disease), tonic-clonic spasms (grand mal seizures), sudden loss of consciousness, facial paralysis (Bell's palsy), hemiplegia, and aphasia. The herbs improve Blood circulation and rehabilitate nerves.

   C. *Internal Wind–Heat* — opisthotonus from high fevers such as childhood febrile convulsions (need to use Heat clearing herbs — Anemarrhenia or Silk Worms).

   D. *Deficient Blood Internal Wind* — seen as dizziness, blurred vision, ataxia, tinnitus, and numb extremities (an MS pattern).
   **Herb:** Gastrodia — Tian Ma (sweet, slightly warm).

17. **Expel Parasites:** These herbs are not as fast acting or strong as Western drugs, but their effects are longer lasting, more prolonged, and less toxic. They also have some Spleen tonic action and may be used in the weaker patient. Most patients susceptible to parasite infestation are Spleen deficient and Damp — especially in children with their underdeveloped Spleens. **Herbs:** Garlic — Da Suan (acrid, warm); Betel Nut (Areca Seeds) — Bing Lang (acrid, bitter, warm); Artemesia — Qing Hao (bitter, acrid, warm); Aquilaria — Chen Xiang (acrid, bitter, warm, aromatic).

18. **External Application:** All are toxic and are used for inflammation, swelling, pain, rashes, and oozing fluids. **Herbs:** Toad Skin Neurotoxin — Chan Su (sweet, acrid, warm, poisonous); Hornet Nest — Ban Mao (acrid, cold, poisonous).

## THE EIGHT METHODS OF HERBAL THERAPY

These are the clinical actions that are required of the herbs in balancing dysfunctions (disease) and returning the patient to homeodynamic equilibrium (health). These actions include resolving, tonification, heat dispelling, chill dispelling, harmonization, diaphoresis, purgation, and emesis.

1. **Resolving:** used to break up accumulations of Dampness, Phlegm, Qi, or Blood in the body. Resolving therapies are contraindicated when there is severe weakness or hemorrhage

   A. *Qi-Correcting:* When the flow of Qi is either entangled or disrupted.
      • An energetic lump (can be felt, but negative on ultrasound) in the throat or the abdomen. Seen in Globus Hystericus, esophageal spasm, breast swelling, bloating, PMS, etc.
      • A gastrointestinal disturbance that is functional, such as irritable bowel syndrome (IBS), bloating and gas, vomiting, and hiccup (all Rebellious Stomach Qi).
      • Wandering pains in body or joints or muscles.

   B. *Blood-Correcting:* When Blood stagnates.
      • Skin ailments such as venous stasis ulcers, varicose veins, ecchymoses, blue-purple acne, Kaposi's, etc.
      • Pain, especially in abdomen and pelvis.

- Gyne problems such as prolonged cycles, dysmenorrhea, fibrocystic breast disease, and scanty dark flow with clots.
- Mental illness such as schizophrenia or psychosis.

   C. *Interior-Resolving:* When moisture and Phlegm accumulate in the digestive system.
- Weak digestion due to deficient Spleen and Stomach Qi.
- Nausea due to Stomach and Spleen Qi Deficiency and Dampness.
- Gallstones due the Damp Heat leading to Phlegm formation (stones).
- Diarrhea due to Spleen Qi Deficiency and Spleen Yang Deficiency leading to Dampness.

   D. *Expectorants:* When Fluid and moisture accumulate in the Lungs. This is seen clinically as Lung congestion with white or clear mucus that is thick and difficult to expectorate.

   E. *Moisture-Moving:* Generalized edema or localized accumulations of moisture.

2. **Tonification:** A long, gentle therapy to strengthen the body by supplementing the Yang, Yin, Qi, and Blood.

   A. *Yang Tonification:* Used when there is a lack of vital Heat with Internal Cold and Dampness. Tonification should be done during the season before winter.
- Coldness with pale features and lack of circulation.
- Weak colon function with no desire to defecate or only passes small incomplete amounts.
- Impotence.
- Edema both dependent and generalized with anasarca.
- Frequent urination with abundant clear, watery urine.
- Diarrhea due to Spleen Dampness, seen in the early morning, cock's crow diarrhea.

   B. *Yin Tonification:* Used when there is Internal Dryness and Deficient (False) Heat. They are cool and moist herbs, but too much use leads to Spleen Dampness and gastrointestinal problems.
- Night sweats.
- Dry skin, no available moisture.
- Dizziness.
- Afternoon tidal fevers of a mild nature.
- Constipation due to dryness of the stool.

   C. *Qi Tonicification:* Used for general body Qi tonification.
- Fatigue — use Spleen tonics.
- Lethargy.
- Prolapse of organs, a Spleen Qi Deficiency.
- Poor circulation, Qi's dependence on Blood.
- Shallow breathing, a Lung Qi Deficiency.

   D. *Blood Tonification:* Used when there is Blood Deficiency.
- Anemia.
- Menstrual disorders, usually irregular menses, amenorrhea, or scant menses.
- Skin ailments, the skin being nourished by the Blood.
- Dizziness, not enough Blood to fill the cranium.
- Infertility.

3. **Heat Dispelling:** Used for dispelling Internal Heat. Use only for short periods of time (2 to 3 weeks) as they are very bitter and cold and will damage the Spleen and cause digestive problems by putting out the "digestive Fire" and cause bloating and diarrhea.
- Acute fever.
- Infection.
- Skin diseases seen as eczema — Blood Heat.

- Sunstroke.
- Hemorrhage, as most all bleeding is Fire related.
- Thirst.
- Inflammation.

4. **Chill Dispelling:** Warms the body and augments the Yang. It is used when organ functions are deficient.
    - Chills and fevers.
    - Coldness below the waist and hot above the waist. Yang Deficiency and empty Tchong Mo.
    - Cold and pain, always responds to heat (hot water bottle).
    - Yang deficient.

5. **Harmonization:** Used for three types of disharmonies.
    A. *When Condition is Exterior and Interior:*
    - Fever/chill.
    - Sinus/Lung congestion.
    - Cold/flu with diarrhea and vomiting.
    B. *Liver Disturbance with Internal Wind:*
    - Nervousness.
    - Convulsions.
    - Anger.
    - Migrating skin rash, as in hives and urticaria.
    - Headache.
    - Menstrual disorders.
    C. *Wood (Liver) Invading Earth (Spleen):*
    - Nausea.
    - Vomiting.
    - Flatulence.
    - Bloating.

6. **Diaphoresis:** Increases the peripheral circulation at the surface of the body, opening the pores to increase sweating and thereby expelling the invading External Wind and relieving exterior symptoms. Only used for 1 to 5 days in acute disease. However, may be used years later to evict virus from of a joint, for example.
    - Colds and flus in the initial stages.
    - Acute skin eruptions.
    - Arthritis, in the early stages.
    - Headache associated with invading External Wind.
    - Fever associated with External Wind.

7. **Purgation:** Stimulates the elimination through the colon. Purgatives are divided into categories of warming/cooling, slow-acting/fast-acting, and lubricating/drying.
    A. *Warming:*
    - Poor colon function
    - Deficient bile production.
    - Chill in digestive tract.
    - Stagnating Blood in lower abdomen.
    B. *Cooling:*
    - Heat in colon.
    - Gallstones.
    - Hypertension.
    - Blood toxicity.

C. *Slow-Acting:* Have a mild effect and can take up to several days to be effective. They are used when constipation is chronic and elimination is incomplete.

D. *Fast-Acting:* Produce an effect within about 24 hours of administration and are used short term for 1 to 2 weeks only.

E. *Lubricating:* Bring moisture to the colon and the stool, and are employed when there is intestinal dryness.

F. *Drying:* Used to treat severe edema by eliminating water through the colon.

8. **Emesis:** Induces vomiting.
   • Food poisoning.
   • Food allergy.

## HERBAL ACTION

Each herb has several therapeutic actions and may be used for one or for many of its individual actions in combination with other herbs used for their action or actions. The following is an explanation of all the descriptive herbal actions.

*Ascending:* Causes energy or Qi to move to the top of the body. Used in prolapses and hemorrhoids, equivalent to using the acupuncture point GV-20.

*Descending*: Causes activity to move downwards in the body, such as diuretics, purgatives, and Lung herbs. Also good for rising Rebellious Qi.

*Channel Opening*: Moves energy through the channels to expel substance lodged in the channels, such as Phlegm and Wind–Damp.

*Invigorates Blood:* Helps the circulation and nourishment of Blood in symptoms such as menstrual problems and fixed pain.

*Sedates:* Good for sleep and anxiety with disturbance of the Shen. These are all cold, heavy minerals or resins.

*Drying:* Is able to dry and resolve moisture and Dampness.

*Moisturizes:* Adds to the moisture of the body such as in Yin and Blood tonics.

*Breaks up Blocks:* Used in Qi stagnation, blockage in pain, etc.

*Normalizes Flow:* Moves Qi in the correct direction. Seen in vomiting, nausea, flatulence, and all Rebellious Qi.

*Yang Tonics:* Tonifies the Yang and vital Heat of the body.

*Yin Tonics:* Moisturize and cool the body.

*Moving and Draining Dampness:* All the diuretics.

*Astringing:* Consolidates Qi and fluids of the body and stops excessive perspiration, bleeding, and incontinence.

### QUALITIES OF HERBS

Each herb has certain physical qualities or properties that are discernible by smell or taste by the selecting herbalist, or by clinical experience. These qualities and actions are:

**Temperature Properties:** There 5 temperatures that tell you how the herb is going to behave in the body in terms of heating it up or cooling it down.

1. *Hot* (Yang tonics) — dispels Cold (breaks Qi blockages, warms the center).
2. *Cold* (heavy metals) — quells Fire (anti-inflammatory, antispasmodic, sedative).
3. *Warm* (Qi tonics) — enhances circulation (alleviates chills, improves organ function).
4. *Cool* ( Yin tonics) — subdues Heat (reduces fever, detoxifies, lowers blood pressure).
5. *Neutral* (medicinal mushrooms) — gentle effects (will not alter hot/cold aspect of patient, can be taken for long periods of time).

It is very important to match the temperature of the total herbal combination with the clinical picture.

**By Taste:** Herbs are classified by their taste, which indicates their therapeutic properties. The tastes are:

1. *Sweet* (yellow) — tonifies, harmonizes, and may moisten.
2. *Bitter* (red) — sedating, purges Fire, anti-inflammatory, drain moisture, and dry.
3. *Acrid* (white) — disperse, decongest, stimulate, and move.
4. *Sour* (green) — are astringent and absorbing, and alter blood circulation.
5. *Salty* (black) — diuretic, purge, and soften.
6. *Bland* — calming and soothing, leach out Dampness, and promote urination.

**By Channel Entered:** Many herbs, on the basis of the Organ they influence, are said to enter the channel or meridian of that organ group. This provides a kind of herbalized acupuncture, where the herb is acting as needles would, if placed in the acupuncture points of that meridian. This means that inclusion of that particular herb will focus the action of the herbal mixture in a particular channel or meridian. For example, Bleupurum is said to enter Jue Yin, the Liver meridian or channel.

## PARTS OF THE HERB

The parts of the herb used for therapy are separated into those parts above the ground, and those below the ground.

Parts above the Ground:

Herba = tops (leaves and stems)
Flos = flowers
Cortex = bark
Caulis = stem
Semen = kernel of seed
Calyx = part attaching fruit to stem
Lignum = wood
Ramulus = branch
Fructus = fruit
Pericarpium = peel
Folium = leaves

Parts below the Ground:

Bulbus = bulb
Radix = root
Radicis cortex = root bark
Rhizoma = rhizome

## THEORY OF HERBAL COMBINING

We have learned the uses of the herbs from three different aspects. Now we need to have a small understanding of how herbal formulas are constructed. There are four components to the average herbal combination. They are named in order of importance:

1. *The Emperor:* One or two herbs that give the herbal combination its basic characteristic actions. They may not be the greatest percentage of the formula, just the most important clinical herbal directive; they act as leader of the script.

2. *The Minister:* Up to 5 herbs in number. Their job is to help the Emperor herbs in their activities. They enhance, augment, or broaden the effect of the Emperor.
3. *Assistant:* Between 7 and 10 herbs to counteract any side effects of the first two combinations and to further customize the blend to the patient's picture. They will modify the energy of the formula closer to neutral and can also address secondary symptoms.
4. *Servant:* Enables the mixture to increase circulation and to be harmonious, well absorbed, and tolerated by the patient. The servant may be used as a dispensing agent or to give flavor or texture. It is usually Liquorice — Gan Cao.

## HERBS — CLINICAL DISCUSSION

Chinese herbal therapy has thousands of years of clinical- and patient-based data to back up its theory and usefulness. In other words, it is solid evidence-based therapy. The constituent herbs, numbering in the thousands, have all stood the test of time in terms of usage, efficacy, and toxicity. The herbal combinations were built up from very basic recipes, dealing with common disease patterns, encountered every day in the practitioner's office. Over time, the recipes have become more sophisticated and subtle as man's existence has changed, such that any patient or disease manifestation can be treated. This is a very comprehensive and forgiving medical philosophy and herbal system.

The same cannot be said for Western herbs. These herbs are, for the most part, poorly characterized as to constituents, efficacy, usage, and toxicity. Even the German Commission E Monographs[42] are somewhat speculative and offer very little clinical information. Very little has been done in terms of herbal combining, and usually individual herbs are used as a substitute for a Western-oriented drug or disease process. An example of this is St. John's Wort (Hypericum perforatum), which is used as a substitute for the serotonin uptake inhibitors in depression; or Kava Kava or Valerian Root, used as replacements for bedtime soporifics. There is no medical philosophy that goes with the use of Western herbs, so they have to be used in an allopathic sense. There are Western, Ayuverdic, and Tibetan herbs that have definite utility, but they do not compare to the all-encompassing understanding of man and his disease within his greater environment that TCM affords us. These herbs will be discussed as their use comes up in the disease monographs.

As a practicing clinician, you must take the time to master the elements of TCM diagnosis and herbal prescribing, and you will have a clinical tool that will solve any and every problem you encounter, irrespective of the Western label or nonlabel put on that disease or patient. No need to know what the serum rhubarb is, just treat what you see in front of you, and the body with its nonlinear dynamics will do the rest.

# 7  Acupuncture

"Acupuncture works because it works.
I don't think it needs more validation."

Candice Pert, Ph.D.

## INTRODUCTION

Acupuncture is the alter ego of herbal prescribing. At one time in China, due to political infighting, acupuncture was only allowed as an adjunct to herbal therapy, and the selection of acupuncture points had to mimic herbal patterns of prescribing. This is still true to a certain extent in Chinese acupuncture and this adherence to herbal pattern points makes Chinese acupuncture somewhat less useful than French energetic acupuncture or Japanese acupuncture, which are both energetic systems in their own right. Certainly, you may practice either herbal medicine or acupuncture alone, but you must use both to get a truly comprehensive response over time at both a superficial and deeper level.

I will not discuss the scientific basis for acupuncture. The details of this large body of scientific work can be found in numerous books, to which I refer the reader.[41,42] What is more important is not how it works, but that it does work, and very well. There are many ways to practice acupuncture, put forward by various schools and societies, each of which has its strengths, weaknesses, and clinical utility. The different acupunctural approaches can be subdivided according to the philosophical bent of the different proponents. They are:

1. **Traditional Chinese Acupuncture** — as part of TCM, taught and practiced in Asia and by Chinese practitioners around the world, including non-M.D. practitioners of acupuncture in the U.S.
2. **Energetic Acupuncture** — as practiced by the French, Vietnamese, Japanese, and American medical doctors taught by Joseph Helms, M.D. through U.C.L.A. (French Energetics); Mark Seem, Ph.D. at the Tri-State Institute (Acupuncture Osteopathy and Imaging); and Yoshio Manaka, M.D. (Ion Pumping), Kiiko Matsumoto, Stephen Birch, and Miki Shima (Japanese Meridian Acupuncture) in private practice.
3. **Psycho-Spiritual-Emotional Acupuncture** — the "Five Element School of Acupuncture," as taught by the English acupuncturist, J. R. Worsley and by the Institute for Traditional Acupuncture in Maryland; Terrains and Diathetic issues in acupuncture by Yves Requena, M.D.
4. **Neuroanatomical Acupuncture** — as practiced and taught by George A. Ulett, M.D., Ph.D., and for pain relief by William F. Craig, M.D., (P.E.N.S.); Joseph Wong, M.D. (Neuropathic Pain); P. E. Baldry, M.B., B.S., F.R.C.P. (Trigger Point Treatment); Yoshio Nakatani, M.D. (Ryodoraku); and Ronald M. Lawrence, M.D. (Osteopuncture).
5. **Reflexive Micro-Mapping Somatotrophic Acupuncture** — as taught in the Auriculo-Therapy of P. M. F. Nogier; Korean Hand Acupuncture of Tae-Woo Yoo, O.M.D., Ph.D.; and Yamamoto New Scalp Acupuncture by Toshikatsu Yamamoto, M.D.

In TCM herbal prescribing the issues of Qi, Blood, Fluids, and Spirit in regards to the Zang/Fu organs were paramount, but in acupuncture only the Qi and the balance between Yin and Yang in the channels and meridians are of importance. Acupuncture may be regarded as an external means of maintaining and restoring the normal balance of Yin and Yang and the circulation of Qi through the meridian system by resolving blocked or constrained Qi. Acupuncture is especially good at regulation, equilibration, and biological point setting and pain control. I will concentrate on the meridian energy imbalances as they relate to the Organs and their associated symptomatic manifestations, but not on the Organs themselves (dealt with under TCM herbology).

No single or combination of physiological mechanisms totally explains acupuncture's activity. Although much of our therapeutic point selections in acupuncture will be linear thinking, when dealing with these somewhat linear acupuncture constructs (meridians and Five Element Theory), the actual outcomes will be conjectural at best, and may often be quite surprising. A good example is the correlation of MRI of severe disc disease to acupuncture efficacy in low back pain. Injured backs that appear hopeless on MRI may improve in one treatment, whereas backs with a normal MRI may be refractory to acupuncture. The model of acupuncture energetics offers a unique linear insight into the nature and working of nonlinear dynamics and chaos theory within the body. The system of primary, curious, and secondary acupuncture meridians/channels, or energy lines, offers one of the only examples of a truly linearly appearing biological system that can be utilized in a purely linear fashion, but still produces a nonlinear result. By virtue of their organizational coherence, the acupuncture meridians manifest a logical system of biological intent. I am always amazed at the clinical changes that occur with a simple ten-minute acupuncture treatment.

I have already discussed the critical importance of initial conditions, such that very small inputs (such as the acupuncture needle) will cause major shifts in the apparent superficial chaos with its underlying implicate order. Also, a multiplicity of small inputs may lead to a surprisingly larger response. The key in acupuncture is to identify the major competing chaotic patterns (acupuncture diagnoses) and to design an input to favor the stabilization of the chaotic pattern you wish to predominate.

Now let us look at the models upon which acupuncture is based and see how we can diagnose the chaotic imbalance (disease pattern) and work out an input to stabilize our preferred "chaos."

The acupunctural concepts will be presented as they are thought to occur in the developing embryo, from the inside the body to the outside, and in reverse order of the penetrance of disease. Each system will be explained fully as to its functions, anatomical trajectories, associations, acupunctural points, and clinical use.

Note: This deliberate movement from the inside of the body to the outside, as we discuss the various acupunctural systems, will give you a feeling of the multiple-layer concept of acupunctural Qi energy and at what energetic level the patient is presenting. It is very important to treat at the presenting level and not deeper, lest you allow a superficial disease to gain access to a deeper layer in the body.

## EMBRYOLOGICAL AND ENERGETIC ANATOMY

The *Meridian Energetic System* is thought to develop from the moment of conception, and, indeed, there is evidence that this energetic system may be the biological organizer that directs the formation of the three elementary embryological layers and the cellular differentiation that results in the somatic form of the fetus. The *curious meridians* are used as a multifactoral input into the global energy matrix of the body, are able to balance and regulate multiple meridians, and are useful for specific functional and pain syndromes that are associated with their energetic trajectories. Although they are dealt with in the first section on acupuncture because they are the first to appear in the embryo, they represent a very sophisticated input and should only be used by the experienced acupuncturist. Nevertheless, they need to be understood as the basis of the more elementary meridians to follow.

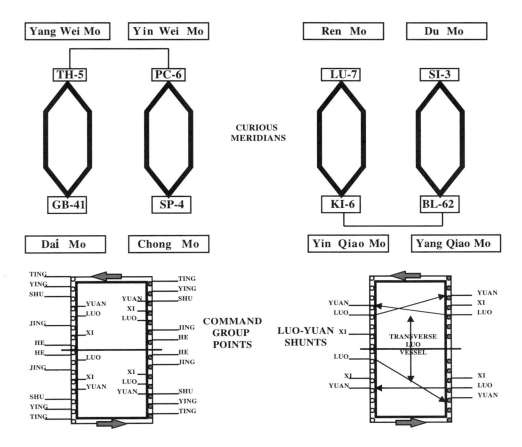

**FIGURE 7.1** Curious Meridians Command Points Luo Yuan Shunts.

## THE CURIOUS OR EXTRAORDINARY MERDIANS

The curious meridians form a network of organizing and controlling reservoirs of energy. They are able to respectively donate or accept energy in deficient and excess meridian energy states and contain the Juan Qi and the Wei Qi energy for the body. The curious meridians do not influence specific organs, but have a regional zone of influence with their associated principal meridian. Each curious meridian has a range of clinical disorders over which it has a general influence. The curious meridians represent the central homeodynamic force in the organism.

The first energy lines to appear in the embryo, probably at the level of the morula are the first three extraordinary or curious meridians, *Chong Mo, Ren Mo*, and *Du Mo*. These three serve as the body's chief energetic organizers, and each has a zone of energetic and, hence, physiological and structural influence.

Each curious meridian is activated by two acupuncture points, called the *master point* and the *coupled point*, borrowed from, and situated on, a principal meridian. One point is on a superior extremity and the other is on an inferior extremity. Each cardinal curious meridian is coupled with an energetically symmetrical complementary curious meridian, such that the master point of the one is the coupled point of the other and vice versa. In order for the body to know which of the two coupled curious meridians you are activating with the shared acupuncture points, one must use focusing points, which will indicate which of the two curious meridians is under consideration. In addition to the master and coupled point, each curious meridian has an *activation point* that is used to stimulate the meridian. This point is usually used on the complementary curious meridians and not on the cardinal curious meridians. The activation point often is the *departure point* of the coupled complementary curious meridian. The complementary curious meridians also have a designated *Xi point,* which is used for unblocking energy in that meridian. The points on the principal meridians that make up the surface trajectory of the curious meridians are called *reunion points.* These points may be used in developing a treatment if they are tender to palpation. The curious meridians are needled symmetrically on both sides of the body.

**Chong Mo (Cardinal):** Energizes the front of the body and nourishes the visceral organs and is the energetic basis of the Zang Fu organs. It is called the "Mother of the 5 Yin and 6 Yang organs" because it brings energy and Blood to the Zang Fu organs and to the meridians they create. It is also known as the "Sea of Blood" because of its influence in the abdominal and pelvic areas.. The Chong Mo represents the body's internal, vertical, and most important energetic axes. It operates as the energetic balance, regulation, and reservoir for all the meridians and obtains its energy from the Kidneys whose meridian it most closely overlies.

**Anatomical Pathway:** Energy descends from the Kidney to the perineum where it splits into 3 branches:

1. **Anterior branch** — travels close to the midline where it mingles with the principal meridian of the Kidney and the ventral, midline curious meridian, Ren Mo. It ascends into the chest, and then to the head where it surrounds the mouth and penetrates nasal passages and medial eye.
2. **Posterior branch** — ascends along the anterior aspect of the spinal column to the top of the chest.
3. **Inferior branch** — descends from the perineum along the medial thigh to the medial malleolus, the plantar surface of the foot, and the first toe.

As we can see, the energetic trajectory of Chong Mo is very similar to the Kidney principal meridian and encompasses the pelvis and genitourinary organs as well as the prevertebral autonomic ganglia, endocrine glands, and the chakras.

**Chong Mo Clinical Protocols:** Chong Mo is the most versatile of all the curious meridians. It has the capability of affecting the body's energetic, structural, and functional dimensions.

**Acupuncture Points:** (Chong Mo Signal Input)

> **Master Point** — SP-4 (Coupled point of Yin Wei Mo)
> **Coupled Point** — MH or PC-6 (Master point of Yin Wei Mo)
> **Reunion Points** — KI-3 and ST-30

**Chong Mo Endocrine Points:** SP-4 + MH-6 or PC-6 to which you add:

> **Ovaries** — CV-2 + CV-4 + ST-30 — to Yang Ming — ST-36/40/43/44.
> **Uterus** — CV-2 + CV-4 + ST-30 — to Shao Yang -GB-30/34/39.
>       — to Dai Mo — GB-26/41, TH-5, BL-63.
> **Prostate** — CV-2 + CV-4 + ST-30 — to Yang Ming — ST-36/40/43/44, LR-9 to CV-1.
>       — to Kidney-Bladder distinct meridian System.
> **Adrenal Glands** — KI-3 + BL-23 + BL-22 or CV-6 + KI-16.
> **Mammary Glands** — CV-22 + ST-13/15/25 — to Yang Ming — ST-30/36/40/43.
> **Thyroid Gland** — CV-22 + CV-23 + ST-9 — to Yang Ming — ST-11/ 12/36/40/43.
> **Anterior Pituitary** — LR-14 + GB-20 — to Shao Yang — GB-34/39.
> **Posterior Pituitary** — KI-27 + BL-10 — to Tai Yang — BL-59/60/67.

The curious meridian Chong Mo is important as the conduit of the central energy core and energy vortices making up the esoteric energy fields described by the Hindus and other Asian religions — the Chakras and Nadis.

**Chong Mo Chakra Points:** SP-4 and MH or PC-6 to which you add:

**First Chakra** — **Base Chakra** — Ren-1 — Corresponds to kidney Yin. Used for patients with deficient grounding and self-identity.

**Second Chakra** — **Polarity Chakra** — Front: Ren 2-4; Back: Du 2-4 (Ming Men) — Corresponds to Kidney Yang, Urinary Bladder, and Large Intestine and Lower Heater. Used for sexuality and relationship problems.

**Third Chakra** — **Solar Plexus Chakra** — Front: Ren-8/12; Back: Du-5/6 — Corresponds to Spleen and Liver and Middle Heater. Used for issues of personal will and emotional expression. If out of balance, it is responsible for addictions, striving for power, anger, and rage.

**Fourth Chakra** — **Heart Chakra** — Front: Ren-17; Back: Du-11 — Corresponds to the Heart and Upper Heater. Used for issues of understanding, compassion, friendliness, balancing of contrasts, striving for harmony, inner peace, and love. It represents the energetic center of the human being and is the most important integrating Chakra between the three below and the three above.

**Fifth Chakra** — **Throat Chakra** — Front: Ren-22; Back: Du-14 — Corresponds to Lung and thyroid. Used for all issues of communication and issues of speech and creativity. The suppression of this Chakra is responsible for all thyroid disease.

**Sixth Chakra** — **Third Eye** — Front: Yin Tang; Back: Du-15. Used in issues of focusing the mind, understanding, the power of discernment, intuition, and clairvoyance.

**Seventh Chakra** — **Crown Chakra** — Du-20 and Extra-6 (Sishencong) 4 points, like a star around Du-20 — Corresponds to the highest Yang in the body. Used for issues involving the understanding of the higher issues in life, providing a connection to the spirit. These points serve to harmonize the psychic functions and the whole energy balance of the body.

Note: It is customary to open the base, heart, and crown Chakras before proceeding to the other Chakras to ensure good energy flow. After needling of the appropriate acupuncture points, the patient is asked to direct his or her awareness at the relevant Chakra to facilitate the balancing of the energy. Both the practitioner and the patient focus on opening the Chakra and visualizing the flow of energy from above downward. The selection of Chakra treatment can be ascertained by patient history and muscle testing with appropriate energetic filters (see biokinesiology in Chapter 10). Chakra acupuncture can be the very first acupuncture treatment in appropriate patients, or the very last treatment to round out the entire energetic body.

Chong Mo is associated with specific clinical pictures that will lead to its use in therapy. These clinical pictures include urinary and prostate problems; uterine, tubal, and ovarian disorders; sexual dysfunction and menstrual difficulties; many gynecological problems including infertility, abortion, development of embryo and fetus, labor, and delivery. Its most important use is in the endocrine axis, for over- or underactivity. Circulatory and thermoregulatory problems can be addressed, especially cold feet. Pelvic pain, endometriosis, and pelvic inflammatory disease may addressed with Chong Mo, as well as inguinal pain and deep lumbar pain extending to the medial thigh.

Chong Mo can also be used as an entry axis to a different type of treatment circuit such as the "cerebral circulation" points, other curious meridians and all the other meridians, both principal and distinct.

**Ren Mo (Cardinal Meridian):** The Ren Mo (Ren) or Conception Vessel (CV), controls the ventral surface of the body and hence all the Yin energy of the body, especially that of the Liver and Kidney. The Ren Mo is nourished by the Yuan Qi descending from the Kidney in Chong Mo..

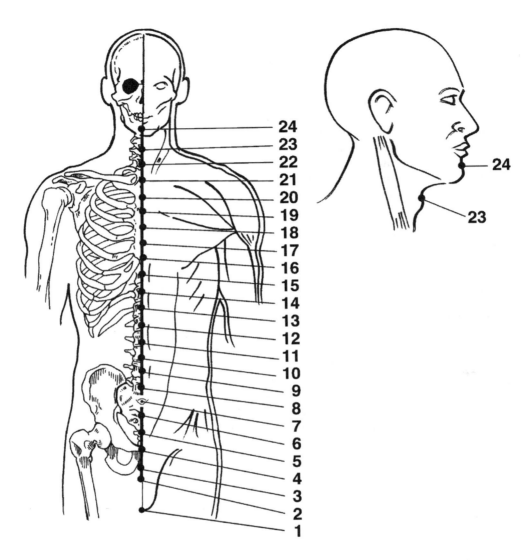

**FIGURE 7.2** Conception Vessel (CV).

Anatomical Pathway: Ren Mo originates in the perineum and ascends along the anterior midline surface, which is its energetic territory

1. **Anterior path** — it travels to the throat and jaw, and in the face it encircles the mouth before penetrating the eyes at ST-1. There are many reunion points with Chong Mo along its ascending trajectory.
2. **Deep path** — a deep pathway encircles the uterus and ascends on the anterior surface of the spine, overlapping the posterior course of Chong Mo and the Kidney.

Acupuncture Points on Ren Mo (CV) (Ren)
　　Number of Points: 24
　　Related Channel: Du Mo — Governor Vessel (GV) (Du).

Note: Ren Mo should almost never be needled in the reducing mode, especially CV-4, CV-5, and CV-6, since Ren Mo is the major source of energy in the body.

**Important Points:**

1. **CV-1 (Huiyin)**
   Location: In the center of the perinium.
   Clinical: Pelvic Problems — hemorrhoids, prostatitis, sexual dysfunction, scrotal and penile pain; genital herpes with LV-9. Emergency resuscitation of drowning victim — if urine flows, he will survive. Used with Chong Mo and Kidney–Bladder distinct meridian as a focusing point.

2. **CV-2 (Qugu)**
   Location: In the midline, just above the top of the pubic symphysis.
   Clinical: Pelvic Problems — strong point for all genitourinary and gynecological problems. Gathering point with CV-3 for the 3 Yin leg tendinomuscular meridians.

3. **CV-3 (Zhongji)**
   Location: In the midline, one inch above the pubic symphysis.
   Clinical: Mu point of the Bladder (BL). Used for increasing Yang energy, especially in Cold uterine conditions (use moxa). It is the main point for reproduction in the body. Alternate point with CV-2 as Yin leg tendinomuscular meridian gathering point. May be used in reducing method for Damp–Heat in the Lower Burner.

4. **CV- 4 (Guanyuan)**
   Location: In the midline, roughly the midpoint between the umbilicus and pubis symphysis (slightly more towards the pubis).
   Clinical: Mu point of the Small Intestine (SI). Meeting point of the Yin and Yang Qi — a very important point to input energy into the body, usually used with moxa. Part of *Dan Tien*, the storage and distribution point for energy in the energetic and physical body, with CV-5 and CV-6. Can be used for gynecological and urinary problems and for diarrhea. Used to tonify the Kidney.

5. **CV-5 (Shimen)**
   Location: In the midline, 2 inches below the umbilicus.
   Clinical: Mu point of the Triple Heater (TH). Part of Dan Tien with CV-4 and CV-6. Regulates the lower Heater and all its organs. Treat edema and ascites with CV-5, CV-9, SP-9, and BL-20.

6. **CV-6 (Qihai)**
   Location: In the midline, 1.5 inches below the umbilicus.
   Clinical: Excellent point for tonifying Qi together with CV-4. CV-6 is more for dispersing stagnant Qi, while CV-4 is used more for tonifying deficiency. Can be used with ST-36 and SP-6 for CFIDS and other fatigue issues.

7. **CV-7 (Yinjiao)**
   Location: In the midline, one inch below the umbilicus.
   Clinical: Command point for the lower Heater together with CV-5.

8. **CV-8 (Shenque)**
   Location: Center of the umbilicus.
   Clinical: It is forbidden to needle this point. The umbilicus should be filled with salt and the moxibustion done on top of the mound of salt for acute and chronic diarrhea (if Cold) such as colitis together with ST-25, CV-6, and CV-10, and other Yin disorders.

9. **CV-12 (Zhonguan)**
   Location: In the midline, halfway between the umbilicus and the xiphisternal junction.
   Clinical: Mu point for Stomach. Roe point (influential point) for all the hollow organs (Fu organs). Command point for the Middle Heater. Center of the body — a very strong

point to concentrate energy especially of the Stomach and Spleen. Is used to "ground" agitated patients together with LV-3 and HT-3. A good point for disturbances of any hollow or Fu organ, e.g., Stomach, Large Intestine, Small Intestine, Bladder, or Gall Bladder.

10. **CV-14 (Juque)**
    **Location:** In the midline, one inch below the tip of the xiphoid.
    **Clinical:** Mu point for the Heart. Used to calm the anxious patient and the Shen. Also used for local chest pain and spastic stomach, rebellious Stomach Qi, or esophageal spasm. Relates to the area described as the "solar plexus."

11. **CV-15 (Jiuwei)**
    **Location:** In the midline, at the tip of the xiphisternum.
    **Clinical:** Luo point of the Ren Mo. Source point of all Yin organs. Can be used interchangeably with CV-14.

12. **CV-17 (Shaozhong)**
    **Location:** In the midline, between the nipples, at level of 4th intercostal space.
    **Clinical:** Mu point for Pericardium (PC). Roe point (influential point) for all meridian energy in the body and command point for the Upper Heater. A very strong point for anxiety and stress, and a major point for all respiratory and Lung disorders. Use with CV-16 and CV-18, whichever is the more tender.

13. **CV-22 (Tiantu)**
    **Location:** In the midline, at the center of the suprasternal notch.
    **Clinical: Dangerous point!** You can damage anterior mediastinal structures including the aortic arch. This is the "Window of the Sky" point and is the most important point for all throat and thyroid problems. Very effective point for acute asthmatic attack, dysphagia, and hiccups.

14. **CV-23 (Lianqquan)**
    **Location:** In the midline, in the depression of the upper border of the hyoid bone.
    **Clinical:** Good for voice and speech problems. May be used after anterior cervical fusion to facilitate healing of traumatized tissue, aphonia, laryngitis, and problems of speech and swallowing.

15. **CV-24 (Chengjiang)**
    **Location:** In the midline, in the depression of the mento-labial groove.
    **Clinical:** Good for toothache and shoulder pain. Is a very effective point for calming Kidney fear and Heart anxiety.

**Ren Mo Clinical Protocols:** When the Ren Mo is disordered it creates a disturbance in the Yin meridians and organs, especially the Liver and Kidney.

**Acupuncture Points:**

**Master Point** — LU-7 (Coupled Point of Yin Qiao Mo).
**Coupled Point** — KI-6' (Command Point of Yin Qiao Mo).
**Conception Vessel Points** — CV-1 to CV-24.
**Luo Point** — CV-15.
**Upper Heater** — CV-17.
**Middle Heater** — CV-12.
**Lower Heater** — CV-5 or CV-7

Ren Mo is associated with specific clinical pictures that will lead to its use in therapy. These symptoms are anterior and midline and include pains in the genitalia and umbilicus radiating to the chest, and a tense painful abdomen. The Ren Mo is similar to Chong Mo as it can be utilized in problems of menstruation, fertility, pregnancy and labor, and menopause. Ren Mo is most often used to focus treatment on the three body Heaters.

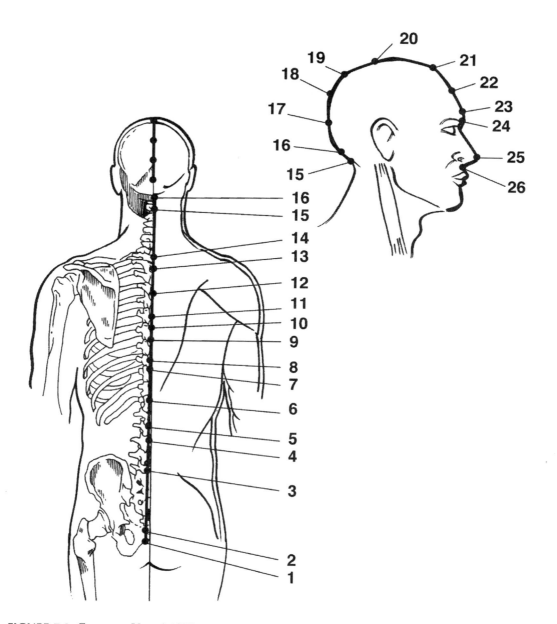

**FIGURE 7.3** Governor Vessel (GV).

**Du Mo (Cardinal meridian):** The Du Mo or governor vessel (GV) is the prime meridian in control and command of the body's Yang energy and meridians, and is called the "Sea of Yang Channels." It is also responsible for circulation of the nourishing energy, Rong Qi. All Yang meridians meet at the point GV-14, where the focus of Du Mo governs the spine, marrow, Kidney Yang, and whole dorsal aspect of the body.

**Anatomical Pathway:** Du Mo originates from the energy of Chong Mo descending to the perineum from the Kidneys. From the perineum it encircles the genitalia and then divides into two branches. The posterior branch joins the Kidney and Bladder meridians, passes through the Kidneys, and then ascends up the vertebral collumn to the base of the skull. There it enters the brain, ascends to the top of the head, and then descends in the midline to the forehead and nose. The anterior branch ascends in the midline on the surface, goes past the heart, enters the throat and chin, circles the mouth, and runs into the eyes.

## Acupuncture Point on Du Mo (GV) (Du)

Number of Points: 28
Related Channel: Ren Mo — Conception Channel (CV) (Ren)
**Important Points:**

1. **GV-1 (Changqiang)**
   **Location:** Midway between tip of coccyx and anus.
   **Clinical:** Luo point for Dai Mo. Connects with Ren Mo at CV-1. Used for hemorrhoids, rectal prolapse, and coccygeal pain.
2. **GV-3 (Yaoyuangguan)**
   **Location:** Below spinous process of L-4 vertebra.
   **Clinical:**Opposite to CV-4 and creates a shunt between upper and lower parts of body. Used for lumbar pain with sciatica.
3. **GV-4 (Mingmen)**
   **Location:** Below the spinous process of L-2 vertebra.
   **Clinical:** Is the energetic center of the body between the Yin (left) and Yang (right) Kidneys at the level of BL-23, the Shu point for the Kidneys, with which it is often used. This is the main energizing point on the body with BL-23 and is the main point for low back pain that does not radiate down the legs or to the hips.
4. **GV-6 (Jizhong)**
   **Location:** Below spinous process of T-11 vertebra.
   **Clinical:** Used for muscular relaxation in spastic states. Used with electricity with GV-2 in spastic paralysis. Also used for digestive problems with BL-20, the Shu point for Spleen.
5. **GV-8 (Jinsuo)**
   **Location:** Below the spinous proces of T-9 vertebra.
   **Clinical:** Main point for the musculature of entire spine because it is at the same level as the Shu point for Liver, BL-18, which controls the muscles and tendons.
6. **GV-14 (Dazhui)**
   **Location:** Between the spinous processes of C-7 and T-1 vertebrae.
   **Clinical:** The Sea of Yang — represents the meeting point of all the Yang meridians in the body, and is the main point for all problems in the neck, head, and arms. Good for mental disorders, local muscle problems, frozen shoulder, pain along the spine including ankylosing sponylitis, all Lung disorders, viral infections, and fever. It is an important immune-stimulating point and will immediately bring down fever in children when used with pricking of the fingertip pads.
7. **GV-15 (Yamen)**
   **Location:** Between the spinous processes of C-1 and C-2 vertebra.
   **Clinical: Dangerous point!** Sea of Marrow point. Used as a unit with GV-16.
8. **GV-16 (Fengfu)**
   **Location:** Just below the center of the external occipital protuberance, between the trapezius attatchments, the "Pithing Point."
   **Clinical: Dangerous point!** You will enter the medulla oblongata if needle goes too deep. Window of the Sky point. Used by the brave or foolish for early viral infections or local neck and brain issues.
9. **GV-20 (Baihui)**
   **Location:** In the midsaggital line on the crown, midway on a line connecting the earlobe and the ear apex.

**Clinical:** Meeting point of 100 Points. The meeting point of all the Yang lines of legs and arms and the Liver meridian. This is the best tranquilizing and sedative point in the body. Good for depression when used with electricity in a "Star" using the four Si Shen Cong points. Excellent hemorrhoid point.

10. **GV-23 (Shangxing)**
    **Location:** On median line, one inch behind the hairline.
    **Clinical:** Control point for sinus. Tonify point; if sinus improves, the sinus is Yin and chronic and continue tonification; if the sinus gets worse, then it is Yang and acute and needs dispersion.

11. **GV-24.5 EX-1 (Yin Tang)**
    **Location:** On the midline, between the supercilliary ridges.
    **Clinical:** Used for sinusitis, rhinitis, and frontal headaches. Use with BL-2.

12. **GV-26 (Shuigo)**
    **Location:** Midline of philtrum, one-third the distance down from nose to lip margin.
    **Clinical:** Emergency point to bring back patients from needle shock, loss of consciousness, and acute lumbar and cervical pain and muscle spasm. Use with Yao Tong Dian points on dorsum of hands.

**Du Mo Clinical Protocols:** Du Mo has 28 points along its posterior midline channel. Du Mo is used to control the Yang meridians at GV-14 and presents much as disturbances in the Yang meridians, Tai Yang, or Yang Qiao Mo, as all three are activated by Tai Yang command ponts. Another important point is GV-4, which represents an entry point into Ming Men.

**Acupuncture Points:**

**Master Point** — SI-3 (Coupled Point of Yang Qiao Mo).
**Coupled Point** — BL-62' (Command Point of Yang Qiao Mo).
**Activating Point** — GV-1
**Luo Point** — GV-1 ascends to GV-16 and goes top of head.

**Du Mo Clinical Pictures:** Excess in Du Mo is seen as a stiff and painful neck and low back and muscle spasms. The pain is in the midline, made worse by movement and better with rest. Deficiency in Du Mo is seen as a heavy head, urinary retention, hemorrhoids, and vertigo.

These three cardinal meridians, Chong Mo, Ren Mo, and Du Mo form the energetic organizers of the body, each having influence over its territory: Chong Mo — the ventral body and all the organs; Ren Mo — the Yin energies on the ventral surface; and Du Mo — the Yang energies on the dorsal surface. A fourth meridian, *Dai Mo*, encircles these three longitudinal meridians at the belt line, and directs the energies of the upper and lower part of the body.

**Dai Mo:** Dai or the "Belt meridian" controls the energy flow up and down the trunk, from Yin to Yang and from Yang to Yin.

**Anatomical Pathway:** Dai Mo starts at the L2 vertebra and follows the false ribs horizontaly along the iliac crest, along the anterior iliac border, and then upwards to the umbilicus.

**Dai Mo Clinical Protocols:** Dai Mo influences the entire hip, lower lumbar area, and the lower abdomen from umbilicus to pubis. The Dai Mo is closely associated with the Liver and Gall Bladder meridians.

**Acupuncture Points:**

**Master Point** — GB-41 (Coupled point for Yang Wei Mo)
**Coupled Point** — TH-5 (Master point for Yang Wei Mo)

Activation Point — GB-26
Reunion Points — GB-27, GB-28, GV-4, LV-13.

**Dai Mo Clinical Pictures:** The classic clinical picture is one of cold buttocks, or the sensation of sitting in cold water. This may be accompanied by cold legs and feet or even paralysis of the lower extremities. Radiating lumbar pain and pelvic problems are addressed with Dai Mo. These pelvic problems include vaginal inflammatory problems, cold or hot genitals, dysuria, and acute or chronic pelvic pain. Dai Mo is often coupled with Chong Mo in these clinical situations.

The other four complementary curious meridians — *Yin Qiao Mo, Yang Qiao Mo, Yin Wei Mo,* and *Yang Wei Mo* — organize the particular Yin and Yang energetics of the four quadrants, connecting upper left and lower right and vice versa.

**Yin Wei Mo:** The Yin Linking Vessel uses the same acupuncture points as Chong Mo. Yin Wei Mo is responsible for connecting and maintaining all Yin channels and their associated organs, Tai Yin, Shao Yin, and Jue Yin. These Yin organs cover the energetic areas of the chest, flanks, and abdomen and unite in Ren Mo.

**Anatomical Pathway:** Yin Wei Mo follows the medial aspect of the leg of the Yin meridians, it courses up the abdomen to the chest in two equal lateral branches and meets at CV-22, before ending under the chin at CV-23.

**Acupuncture Points:**

Master Point — MH-6
Coupled Point — SP-4
Activation Point — KI-9

**Yin Wei Mo Clinical Pictures:** Yin Wei Mo in excess is seen as chest, head, lumbar, and abdominal pain. Yin Wei Mo in deficiency is seen as Blood and Yin deficiency with insomnia, anxiety, palpatations, and restlessness. It is coupled with Yang Wei Mo to balance interior–exterior energy.

**Yang Wei Mo:** Is clinically more useful than Yin Wei Mo. As the Yang linking vessel, it connects and unites all the Yang vessels. The Yang vessels tend to produce more external physical manifestation than the more internal Yin vessels. It is paired with Dai Mo in its activation points.

**Anatomical Pathway:** It starts at BL-63 and travels along the lateral surface of the leg to the hip (GB-35 to GB-29). It continues upwards along the lateral abdomen and rib cage, behind the axilla, across the shoulder, up the lateral neck, behind the ear and to the forehead (TH-15 through GB-21 to GB-20). It then moves posteriorly to the occiput and ends at GV-16 and GV-15. You will recognize this coinciding mostly with Shao Yang channel.

**Acupuncture Points:**

Master Point — TH-5
Coupled Point — GB-41
Activation Point — BL-63
Xi Point — GB-35

**Yang Wei Mo Clinical Pictures:** The Yang channels present with muscle spasms and contractures and associated joint stiffness. Deficiency is seen as generalized aching and swelling, especially in the lumbar region. The person complains of internal chilliness and aversion to weather changes. Yang Wei Mo has a characteristic headache that starts at GB-20 in the lateral occiput, and travels anteriorly to the forehead or behind the ipsilateral eye. Neck pain, in association with sacral pain, radiating to the hip, is seen in Yang Wei Mo. This area is anatomically lower than the energetic area covered by Dai Mo. Yang Wei Mo represents the lateral surface of the body and can be used together with a Yin meridian in painful lateral conditions.

**Yin Qiao Mo:** Causes the Yin energy to move and is responsible for balance of Yin energy in the lower leg and also influences the pelvis, the eyes, and the brain. It is paired with Ren Mo.

**Anatomical Pathway:** The energy line starts from KI-6' of the Kidney meridian, along the medial surface of the leg, through the genitalia, going deep at the pubic symphysis (CV-2), up through the abdomen and chest to emerge at the mid-clavicular point, ST-12. From there it crosses the cheek from ST-9 to BL-1, where it joins Tai Yang and with Yang Qiao Mo enters the brain.

**Acupuncture points:**

**Master Point** — KI-6'
**Coupled Point** — LU-7
**Activation Point** — KI-6'
**Xi Point** — KI-8

**Yin Qiao Mo Clinical Picture:** Yin Qiao Mo is primarily used for disorders of the eyes and forehead, and secondarily for pelvic problems. Excess Yin energy will cause closing of the eyes and difficulty in staying awake. If Yang Qiao Mo is in excess, then the eyes are wide open and the patient cannot sleep. The energies of Yin and Yang Qiao Mo meet at the eyes, and so most eye disorders can be treated by balancing the Yin and Yang movement through these two meridians. Some of these disturbances include pain and inflammation starting at the medial aspect of the conjunctiva, and unilateral frontal headaches near the eye. In the genitourinary system, Yin Qiao Mo can be used to treat diffuse pelvic pain, cystitis, leukorrhea, irregular menses and sterility. In excess, Yin Qiao Mo causes spasms of the medial leg musculature.

**Yang Qiao Mo:** Causes the Yang energy to move. It is derived from Tai Yang, and hence it influences the eyes, brain, and dorsal musculature. It is used with Yin Qiao Mo to balance the Yang and Yin energy on both sides of the body. It is paired with Du Mo.

**Anatomical Pathway:** Its trajectory starts at the BL-62, ascends to BL-61 and then BL-59 to the hip along the lateral aspect of the leg. It then comingles with the Small Intestine and Large Intestine on the posterolateral aspect of the upper body at points SI-10, LI-15, and LI-16. It then goes up the neck and onto the lateral face where it joins with the Stomach points (ST-1 to ST-6), joins with Yin Qaio Mo and Tai Yang at the BL-1 point, then arches backwards over the temporalis muscle to GB-20 and enters the brain at GV-16.

**Acupuncture Points:**

**Master Point** — BL-62'
**Coupled Point** — SI-3
**Xi Point** — BL-59

**Yang Qaio Mo Clinical Picture:** The Yang Qiao Mo picture is characterized by muscular spasm on the lateral and posterolateral apsect aspect of the body, and brings Yang energy to the eyes. It is useful in the treatment of excess Yang in the head, including acute headaches, and internal wind problems such as facial paralysis and stroke. It is also useful for unilateral rigid muscular spasm in the neck or mid- or lower back. Most patients are Type-A, irritable, and excitable with red faces.

## TENDINOMUSCULAR MERIDIANS (TMM)

The second set of meridians to develop are the *tendinomuscular meridians*. These meridians are closely associated with the Liver and function as the outer protective layer of the body with the protective Wei Qi energy circulating within them. The tendinomuscular meridians have well-defined pathways that overlie the principal meridians in broad and widened energetic bands, like body armor. They represent the first line of defense against external invaders, such as the Six Evils. These *external pathogenic factors* will first penetrate:

- the *Tendinomuscular Meridians*, then enter
- the *Luo Vessels* that connect the skin to the soft tissue, then enter
- the *Principal meridians*, and finally enter into
- the *Distinct organ meridians*.

Typical relationships of external pathogenic factors to organs are:

Wind $\rightarrow$ Liver and Muscles
Heat $\rightarrow$ Heart and Spirit
Dampness $\rightarrow$ Spleen and Veins
Cold $\rightarrow$ Kidney, Joints and Bone

They are also associated with the free flow of muscular energy, the body's mesenchymal structures including the fascia and connective tissues, the diaphragm, and the serous membranes of the abdomen and thorax. The Wei Qi energy is also responsible for opening and closing the pores of the skin, and moistening, warming, and nourishing the skin, subcutaneous, and myofascial soft tissue. The Wei Qi concentrates in the external Yang channels during the day, thus protecting the body from external attack, and then concentrates in the Yin channels at night protecting the inner being from the dark side of the "Force."

The TMMs are used primarily in the treatment of acute traumatic lesions such as sprains, blunt-force trauma, abrasions, and burns. They may be used for localized rashes and eruptions, such as herpes zoster or progenitalis. The Wei Qi energy is a very potent healer of acute inflammation, bruising, and swelling.

*Timing of use is critical*, as the TMMs are most useful in the first 12 to 24 hours of an injury, but may be used up to the first 10 to 14 days with good effect. The reason for this timing is that the injury is most superficial during this time period and will be reached by the healing energy of the more superficial Wei Qi. After two weeks, if the injury is not healed, the perverse energy tends to penetrate deeper into the tissues and a different technique is required.

The location of the lesion is correlated to the broad zone of influence of the particular overlying TMM. At the most, one or two TMMs will be implicated. Using more than three TMMs does not improve treatment, as the involved TMM is usually activated unilaterely, on the side of the lesion.

The 12 TMMs (one for each associated principal meridian) are grouped according to their extremity of origin, leg or arm, and if they are on the Yin (inner or medial) or Yang (outer or lateral) surface of the extremity. There are three Yin TMMs of the leg and three Yin TMMs of the arm; three Yang TMMs of the leg and three Yang TMMs of the arm. Each TMM starts at a toe or fingertip acupuncture point (Ting point or Jing-Well point), depending on the location of the underlying principal meridian, and follows a broad band overlying the course of the principal meridian, having acupuncture points of concentration along the way (usually situated on major joints), and then ends in a gathering point situated on the trunk or face. The energetic flow of half of the TMMs may be contrary to their underlying principal meridian, because they may start at the end of the meridian and not at the begining of the meridian.

1. **Yin TMMs of Leg:**
   Spleen — SP-1
   Liver — LV-1                    Gathering Point — CV-2
   Kidney — KI-1′

2. **Yang TMMs of Leg:**
   Bladder — BL-65
   Gall Bladder — GB-44    Gathering Point — SI-18
   Stomach — ST-45
3. **Yin TMMs of the Arm:**
   Lung — LU-11
   Pericardium — PC-9    Gathering Point — GB-22
   Heart — HT-9
4. **Yang TMMs of the Arm:**
   Small Intestine — SI-1
   Triple Heater — TH-1    Gathering Point — GB-13
   Large Intestine — LI-1

The treatment protocol involves identifying the involved TMM or TMMs. Activate the flow of energy through the lesion by piquring the extremity point on the toe or finger and giving a little manual tonification (moxa or electrical stimulation may also be used). These points are in the proximal nail angle and can be quite tender, and the patient should be warned of this issue. Then, piqure the gathering point for the TMM in neutral technique. This completes the circuit. Now focus the energy on the lesion by surrounding it at 0.5 cms with as many needles as necessary, or piqure the bruised or spastic muscle at its tendermost points. One may also needle the focal energy concentrations of the TMM in the acupoints over the neighboring joints. Needles need to be left in for 20 to 40 minutes, or until any surrounding needle erythema abates.

## PRINCIPAL MERIDIANS

The *Principal Meridian (PM) System* is the main energy system that is used in acupuncture. It represents the most important access to the human energetic biology, and its acupuncture points are utilized in activating the curious meridians, the tendinomuscular meridians, the Mu-Shu system, and the distinct meridians.

The *Principal Meridians* are composed of linear energy lines that course over the surface of the body and represent the energetic signature, balance, and content at any one time of the Zang Fu organ with which each PM is associated. The Yang PM channels are situated on the dorsal surface (in reference to the anatomical acupuncture position, arms outstretched upward to heaven, palms facing forwards) and course downward toward the earth, while the Yin PM channels are on the ventral surface and course upward toward heaven. Thus the Yang and Yin PM channels create a closed loop around the body that changes from Yang to Yin and Yin to Yang at the fingertips and toes, respectively. The coupling of Yin and Yang channels at the extremities creates a set of bilaterally symmetrical pairs of energy subcircuits that divide the body into three parasagittal planes. Each subcircuit represents a territory of influence over the skin, muscles and structural tissues through which it flows, and the Organs and organ functions with which it is associated.

Each of the three symmetrically paired subcircuits is composed of a couplet, consisting of a Yin and Yang channel connected at the extremities. The upgoing Yang channel is composed of two parts, a Yang channel of the leg associated with one Organ and a Yang channel of the arm associated with another Organ. The same is true for the connected Yin energy channel. So, we have a continuous energy loop of two continuous Yin channels (leg and arm) connected with two continuous Yang channels (leg and arm). This loop constitutes one of the three symmetrical energtic subcircuits, for example, Kidney (Yin of leg)–Heart (Yin of arm)–Small Intestine (Yang of arm)–Bladder (Yang of leg) form one of the three subcircuits. These subcircuits are called the *Six Axes* and can be used to delineate the predominant characteristic "pole" of a patient and his or her disease. There is a "coupled" relationship between the Yin and Yang energy lines of a subcircuit in the leg and in the arm, such that, for example, Kidney and Bladder are coupled meridians (a Yin–Yang pair) and Heart

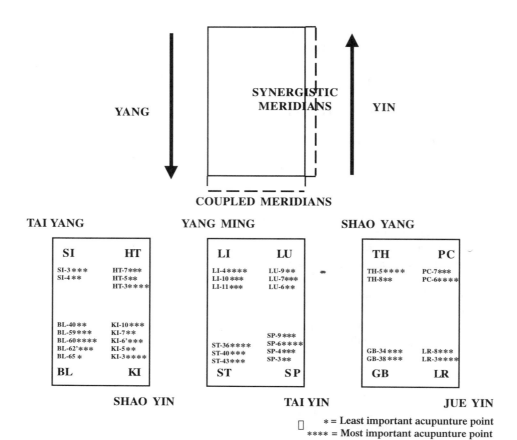

**FIGURE 7.4** Principal Meridians and Points.

and Small Intestine are coupled meridians. This is important, as an imbalance in one will cause an equal, usually opposite imbalance in the other. The two Yin organs are said to be synergistic, an imbalance in one causing a similar added imbalance in the other, and the same is true for the two Yang organs (Fig. 7.4).

The synergistic Yin pairs and Yang pairs are given Chinese names according to the relative amount of Yin or Yang that they contain, remembering that in every Yin element there is a little Yang and vice versa.

Tai — the most or greater
Shao — intermediate or lesser
Jue — the least

## Principal Meridian Subcircuits — The Six Axes

1.  Small Intestine (SI)          ←          Heart (HT)
    ↓ Tai Yang                                ↑ Shao Yin
    Bladder (BL)                              → Kidney (KI)

2.  Triple Heater (TH)           ←          Pericardium (PC)
    ↓ Shao Yang                               ↑ Jue Yin
    Gall Bladder (GB)            →          Liver (LV)

3.  Large Intestine (LI)        ←        Lung (LU)
    ↓ Yang Ming                          ↑ Tai Yin
        Stomach (ST)            →        Spleen (SP)

So, as you can see in the diagrams above, the following are the couplets of Yin and Yang:

| Energy | Axis Energy | Meridians | Anatomy |
|---|---|---|---|
| 1. Tai Yin | Greatest Yin | SP+LU | Most ventral Yin |
| 2. Shao Yin | Lesser Yin | KI+HT | Medial Yin |
| 3. Jue Yin | Least Yin | LV+PC | Most lateral Yin |
| 4. Tai Yang | Greatest Yang | SI+BL | Most dorsal Yang |
| 5. Shao Yang | Lesser Yang | TH+GB | Lateral Yang |
| 6. Yang Ming | Least Yang | LI+ST | Most ventral Yang |

Note: Yang Ming should have been called Jue Yang, but has been given the name "Bright Yang" or Yang Ming. Pericardium (PC) is sometimes refered to as "Master of the Heart."

## The Concept of Triple Heater (TH)

The *Triple Heater* (San Jiao) or *Triple Warmer* or *Triple Energizer* has no correlation in Western anatomy or physiology. *San Jiao* has been said to be a name without a bodily shape and a function without a structure. The *Three Heaters* refer to the three body cavities and their associated organs and linked bodily functions:

1.  Upper Heater — Thoracic cavity (HT, LU, and PC)
    • Access point: CV-17
    • Energy association: Yang of Jue Yin, Tai Yin and Shao Yin
2.  Middle Heater — Abdominal cavity (SP, ST, GB, and LR)
    • Access point: CV-12
    • Energy association: Yang Ming and Tai Yin
3.  Lower Heater — Pelvic cavity (KI, BL, SI, and LI)
    • Access point: CV-5 and CV-7
    • Energy association: Jue Yin and Shao Yin

The Triple Heater in TCM terms has to do with fluid, water, and energy metabolism in each of the three Heaters. The workings of the San Jiao are essential for the smooth flow of Qi, Blood, and Body Fluids in the body. Without a coordinated three Heater physiology, the body's nourishment, production, and distribution of energy would be deficient. The Triple Heaters balance the Yin energies of nourishing, moistening, and cooling with the Yang energies of transformation, movement, and warming. A fluid metaphor is used to describe each cavity: the Upper Heater has a mist, the Middle Heater has a pool, and the Lower Heater has a swamp.

Each of the Heater command points energizes that cavity and the functions of its constituent organs. These command points can be used frequently in the clinic with other acupuncture treatment inputs. The Middle Heater has three CV points that connect the Middle Heater to the Upper Heater (CV-13) to the Lower Heater (CV-10) which reinforces itself (CV-12). The point CV-5 is the Mu point for the Triple Heater acupuncture principal meridian and is important for body energy in general. It warms the Kidney and reinforces the Lower Heater influences of CV-7.

In describing the principal meridians and their acupuncture points, each point on the extremity below the knee and elbow will be given different elemental qualities such as Earth, Metal, Water, Wood, and Fire, and also have command point (Ting-Ying–Shu-Jing-He) and special point (Tsri, Xi-Cleft, Hui, Roe, Horary, Luo, Yuan, Mu, Shu) names. The meaning of these points and their individual uses will follow the description of the principal meridians.

## Tai Yang Subcircuit

This subcircuit consists of the two Yang meridians, Small Intestine in the arm and Bladder in the dorsal aspect of the body and leg. This subcircuit is used for the movement of Yang energy through the surface regions of their structural influence. The listed acupuncture points will move energy through the Tai Yang side of the Tai Yang–Shao Yin major circuit and are used mainly for pain problems represented by energy blockage. The medial Bladder line, running the length of the back, is the access point for the back *Shu points* located between T-3 and S-1vertebrae and allows direct access to the energetic, metabolic, and transport functions of their associated Zang Fu organs. These Shu points are used with the ventral Mu points. This *Shu–Mu system* of direct organ access will be discussed later.

*Small Intestine (SI)*

The Small Intestine meridian is useful for pathology and symptomatology of the underlying skin, muscles, soft tissue, and bony structures that mark its course over the arm, shoulder, and side of the face. It is rarely used for dysfunction of the digestion or its assimilatory function. The Tai Yang Fire biopsychotype is a very imposing and assured personality.

**Anatomical Course:** It originates from the nail angle of the fifth finger at SI-1, courses down the ulnar edge of the little finger and hand (SI-2 to SI-5), across the wrist (SI-6), up the Yang surface of the ulnar (SI-7), crosses the elbow (SI-8), up the arm along the edge of triceps, across the deltoid, to involve the scapula (SI-9 to SI-13). It then passes across the trapezius (SI-14 to SI-16), sternocleidomastoid (SI-17), to the mid-ramus of the mandible (SI-17), forward to the zygomatic arch (SI-18), and finally ends just anterior to the tragus (SI-19).

**Acupuncture Points of the Small Intestine (SI)**

Number of Points: 19
Coupled organ: Heart (HT)
Element: Fire
Sense organ: Tongue
Active Time: 1 to 3 P.M.
Alarm — Mu Point: Ren-4
Shu Point: BL-27 (first sacral foramen)

1. **SI-1 (Shazoe)**
   **Location:** Ulnar nail angle of 5th finger.
   **Clinical:** Ting point. Metal point on Fire meridian. Start of TMM point to gathering point GB-13. Used for acute febrile disorders to break fever. Causes breast to lactate.
2. **SI-2 (Qiangu)**
   **Location:** In a depression anterior to the 5th metacarpal, ulnar side.
   **Clinical:** Ying point. Water point on Fire meridian.
3. SI-3 (Houxi)
   **Location:** At the medial end of the main transverse crease of the palm on clenching the fist.
   **Clinical:** Shu point — Wood point on Fire meridian
      Mother point — tonification point.
      Master point of Du Mo. Coupled point of Yang Qiao Mo. Used clinically for pain along the entire Tai Yang axis, including neck, mid-back, and lower back. Used with N → N+1 circuits involving Tai Yang and Shao Yin.
4. **SI-4 (Wangu)**
   **Location:** Ulnar side of palm in depression formed by base of 5th etacarpal and triquetral bone.

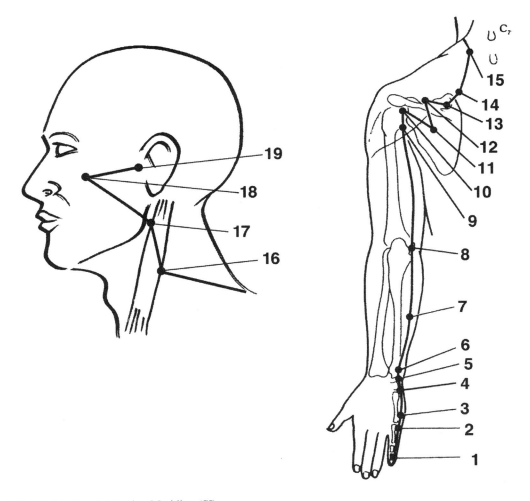

**FIGURE 7.5** Small Intestine Meridian (SI).

   **Clinical:** Yuan point. Source point that receives Luo vessel from Heart meridian from
   HT-5. A good second choice to SI-3 to move energy through the SI meridian and to take
   excess energy from the Heart meridian.
5. **SI-5 (Yangu)**
   **Location:** Ulnar side of wrist, in depression between styloid process of ulnar and pisiform
   bone.
   **Clinical:** Jing point. Fire point on Fire meridian. Horary point.
6. **SI-6 (Yanglao)**
   **Location:** Dorsal aspect on head of ulnar, in cleft on radial side of styloid process.
   **Clinical:** Tsri point. Barrier point. Useful for acute painful disorders along the meridian.
7. **SI-7 (Zhizheng)**
   **Location:** Just less than halfway (5/12) between line joining SI-5 and SI-8 on the ulnar
   border.
   **Clinical:** Luo point — sends branch to Iunn point HT-7.
8. **SI-8 (Xiaohai)**
   **Location:** Between the olecranon of the ulnar and tip of medial epicondyle when elbow
   is flexed.

Clinical: He point. Earth point on Fire meridian.
Sedation point — son point.

9. **SI-9 (Jianzhen)**
Location: One inch above the dorsal end of the axillary fold with arm hanging by side.
Clinical: Excellent point for all arm and shoulder pain, frozen shoulder, any inflammation stopping abduction of the arm. Used with LI-15 and TH-14.

10. **SI-10 (Naoshu)**
Location: With the arm abducted, directly above SI-9 in depression inferior and lateral to scapular spine.
Clinical: Accessory Iu for shoulder and upper arm. Excellent for shoulder, neck, scapular, and arm pain.

11. **SI-11 (Tianzong)**
Location: Center of infrascapular fossa, forming an equlateral triangle with SI-9 and SI-10.
Clinical: Barrier point commanding entire scapular area. Important trigger point for this region.

12. **SI-12 (Bing Fen)**
Location: Center of suprascapular fossa directly above SI-11 in a depression that forms when one abducts the arm.
Clinical: Barrier point. Good point for upper arm and shoulder pain.

13. **SI-15 (Jian Zhonshu)**
Location: Two inches lateral to C-7 vertebra spinous process (GV-14).
Clinical: Good for shoulder pain when tight. Also used for asthma and Lung problems.

14. **SI-16 (Tran Chuang)**
Location: Posterior border of sternocleidomastoid, 1/2 inch posterior to LI-18, at level of upper border of thyroid cartilage.
Clinical: Window of the Sky point. In Meridian Stress Assessment (MSA) is the point for the anterior pituitary point. Used for cervical pain and stiffness. Useful in torticollis.

15. **SI-17 (Tianrong)**
Location: Posterior to the angle of the mandible in the depression on the anterior border of the sternocleidomastoid.
Clinical: Window of the Sky point. Used for local pain and tinnitus.

16. **SI-18 (Quanliao)**
Location: Directly below the lateral canthus of the eye, in depression under the zygomatic arch.
Clinical: Connecting point to BL-1. Gathering point for Yang TMMs of the leg. Used for local pain and eye disorders.

17. **SI-19 (Ting Gong)**
Location: Directly anterior to the tragus, in depression that forms when mouth is open.
Clinical: Cerebral circulation of Kidney — receives a branch. Needle with mouth open. Used for TMJ, all ear problems, Meniere's, and trigeminal neuralgia.

*Bladder (BL)*

The Bladder meridian is a very usefull meridian because it encompases the whole dorsal aspect of the body, from the forehead to the toes. It is the longest and most complex meridian in the body. Its points are used to directly access and direct input into all the Zang Fu organs via the back Shu points. It is used for eye and sinus problems on the face, muscular and fascial pain problems of the neck, back, buttocks, and posterior leg. The organ function of the Bladder is governed by the energy of the paired Kidney meridian. The biopsychotype of the Bladder meridian is one of indecisiveness and excessive analytical thinking without action.

**Anatomical Course:** The cephalic division starts at the inner canthus of the eye (BL-1), travels to the forehead on a level with Yin Tang (BL-2), upward over the head to the vertex at GV-20 (in between BL-7 and BL-8), back and downward to posterior occiptal protuberance (BL-9), into the nape of the neck (BL-10) where it splits into a medial line situated 1.5 inches from the spinal midline and a lateral line 3 inches from the midline. The inner line is used for physical and physiological problems (via the Shu and local points), the outer line for more emotional and mental problems related to the organ at that somatic level. The two lines traverse the upper (BL-12/41 and BL-13/42), mid (BL-18/47 and BL-20/49), and lower back (BL-23/52 — on level with GV-4 and BL-25), cross the medial buttocks (BL-30/54) (lateral buttocks belongs to the Gall Bladder meridian) and reunite in the popliteal fossa (BL-40). The conjoined line then courses between the heads of gastrocnemius (BL-55), and the mid-body of gastrocnemius (BL-56) to the lateral lowest aspect of gastrocnemius in a line above BL-60 (BL-58), to the lateral superior insertion of the achilles tendon (BL-59), down to the achilles tendon fossa on a level with the lateral malleolus (BL-60), around the back of the lateral malleolus (BL-61) along the lateral border of the foot, passing the underside of the lateral malleolus (BL-62′) to the lateral nail angle of the fifth toe (BL-67).

### Acupuncture Points of the Bladder (BL)

Number of Points : 67
Related organ: Kidney (KI)
Element: Water
Sense organ: Ear
Active Time: 3 to 5 P.M.
Alarm — Mu Point: Ren-3
Shu Point: BL-28 (second sacral foramen)

1. **BL-1 (Jingmung)**
   **Location:** Just medial and superior to the inner canthus of the eye.
   **Clinical:** Dangerous point — you need to push the globe of the eye laterally before inserting needle. Connection point from SI-18. Reunion point for curious meridians Tou Mo, Yin Qiao Mo, and Yang Qiao Mo. Distinct meridian superior point for Spleen–Stomach and Heart–Small Intestine distinct meridians. Used for all local eye problems.
2. **BL-2 (Zanzhu)**
   **Location:** One-third length of the eyebrow from the medial end, in the supraorbital notch.
   **Clinical:** Should be used instead of BL-1. A main point for frontal sinusitis and headaches. Angle needle toward Yin Tang (EX-1). Good point for sneezing and tearing.
3. **BL-10 (Tianzhu)**
   **Location:** About one inch lateral to GV-15 in the deepest point in the midneck.
   **Clinical:** Window of the Sky point. Superior access point for the Kidney–Bladder distinct meridian. Very good point for all cervical problems including stiff neck, neck pain, and cervical headaches.
4. **BL-11 (Dazhu)**
   **Location:** Inner Bladder line at level of the T-1 spinous process.
   **Clinical:** Roe, Hui, or influentual point for bone. Intersection point of the upper Yang meridians SI, BL, TH, GB, and Du Mo. Good point for dispersing excess Yang in the head. Use Ding Chuan point, 1/2 inch lateral to GV-14 to calm asthma.
5. **BL-12 (Fengmen)**
   **Location:** Inner Bladder line, at the level of T-2 spinous process.
   **Clinical:** Most important point to expel External Wind. Use with GB-20 to treat early viral invasion. Good for tonifying Lung and for urticaria (Lung controls skin).
6. **BL-13 (Faishu)**
   **Location:** Inner Bladder line, at level of T-3 spinous process (OBL BL-42).

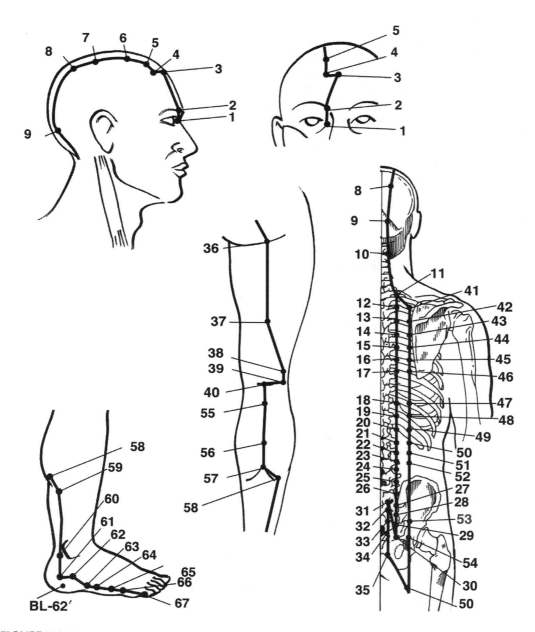

**FIGURE 7.6** Bladder Meridian (BL)

**Clinical:** Shu point for Lung (Mu point — LU-1). Used for all Lung energy and Lung organ disturbances. Use with ST-40 to purge Phlegm.

7. **BL-14 (Jue Yinshu)**

   **Location:** Inner Bladder line, at level of T-4 spinous process (OBL BL-43).

   **Clinical:** Shu point for Pericardium or Master of the Heart (Mu point — CV-17). Is used for all Heart problems relating to its pumping activity, including angina, palpitations, CCF, and any excess Yang symptom in the chest.

8. **BL-15 (Xinshu)**
   **Location:** Inner Bladder line, at level of T-5 spinous process (OBL BL-44).
   **Clinical:** Shu point of the Heart (Mu point — CV-14). Used for disturbances of the Heart Shen, with HT-3 or HT-5 or HT-7 for stagefright or depression, insomnia (cannot get to sleep). Also useful for angina and other heart physiological problems. Is a potent point to disperse all Fire activity.

9. **BL-17 (Geshu)**
   **Location:** Inner Bladder line, at the level of the T-7 spinous process (OBL BL-46).
   **Clinical:** Roe, Hui, or influential point for Blood. Accessory Shu point for diaphragm and esophagus. Major reflex point for the epigastric area. Strongly influences the movement of the diaphragm, and a good point for hiccups with BL-16. Good for spasmodic cough and globus hystericus.

10. **BL-17.5**
    **Location:** Inner Bladder line, on level with T-8 spinous process
    **Clinical:** Accessory Shu point for pancreas. Use this point for neural therapy or homeopuncture in pancreatitis and chronic pancreatic pain.

11. **BL-18 (Ganshu)**
    **Location:** Inner Bladder line, at level of T-9 spinous process (OBL BL-47).
    **Clinical:** Shu point for the Liver (Mu point — LR-14). Used for all Liver energy and organ problems. Also useful for excess Liver Yang or Fire causing eye problems, muscular spasms, and tendon problems. Good for lateral rib pain and external genitalia problems.

12. **BL-19 (Danshu)**
    **Location:** Inner Bladder line, at the level of the T-10 spinous process (OBL BL-48).
    **Clinical:** Shu point of Gall Bladder (Mu point — GB-24). Good for all energetic and organ problems of the Gall Bladder. Also good for bitter taste in the mouth, cholecistitis, and cholelithiasis. Disperses Liver and Gall Bladder Heat and Fire.

13. **BL-20 (Pishu)**
    **Location:** Inner Bladder Line, at level of T-11 spinous process (OBL BL-49).
    **Clinical:** Shu point for Spleen (Mu point — LR-13). Addresses all Spleen energy and organ problems. Use in dispersion to disperse excess Yang; in tonification for Spleen Qi Deficiency and Dampness. Also for internal bleeding, prolapses, and most Stomach problems.

14. **BL-21 (Weishu)**
    **Location:** Inner Bladder line, at the level of the T-12 spinous process (OBL BL-50).
    **Clinical:** Shu point for Stomach (Mu point — CV-12). Used for all gastric disorders.

15. **BL-22 (San Jiaoshin)**
    **Location:** Inner Bladder line, at the level of L-1 spinous process (OBL BL-51).
    **Clinical:** Shu point of Triple Heater — San Jiao (Mu point — CV-5 or CV-7). Can be used as a Shu point for the adrenal gland. Always used with BL-23, the Kidney Shu point for all digestive and energy problems in all the Zang Fu abdominal organs.

16. **BL-23 (Shenshu)**
    **Location:** Half an inch lateral to GV-4 at the inferior border of L-2 spinous process (OBL BL-52).
    **Clinical:** Shu point for Kidney (Mu point — GB-25) and is the major point on the back for all Shu point stimulation. Used for all Kidney energy and organ problems. Used for all sexual and infertility problems. Used for all energy and fluid disturbances in the body (KI — pedal edema; SP — central edema and ascites; LU — facial and upper extremity edema). Used for all ear and bone problems; all menstrual irregularities and problems with Bladder. Used for all low back problems. Used with BL-52 of the outer Bladder line.

17. **BL-25 (Dachangshu)**
    **Location:** Inner Bladder line, on level with L-4 spinous process (on a line level with the iliac crest).

**Clinical:** Shu point for Large Intestine (Mu point- ST-25). Used for all intestinal disturbances, pain, distention, constipation, or diarrhea. Local low back pain.

18. **BL-26 (Guanyuanshu)**
   **Location:** Inner Bladder line, at level of L-5 spinous process.
   **Clinical:** Accessory Shu point for energy and Blood. Controls the Lower Heater with CV-4, 5, 7.

19. **BL-27 (Xiaochangshu)**
   **Location:** Inner Bladder line, at level of first sacral foramen, overlying sacroiliac groove.
   **Clinical:** Shu point for Small Intestine (Mu point — CV-4). Used for local sacroiliac and radiating lumbar pain.

20. **BL-28 (Pangguanshu)**
   **Location:** Inner Bladder line, at level of second sacral foramen, in the depression between the medial aspect of the posterior superior iliac spine and the sacrum (OBL BL-53).
   **Clinical:** Shu point of Bladder (Mu point — CV-3). Excellent point for all urine excretory problems including stones, UTIs, incontinence, prostatitis, and impotence.

21. **BL-30 (Baihuanshu)**
   **Location:** Inner Bladder line, at the level of the fourth sacral foramen, on level with GV-2.
   **Clinical:** Accessory Shu point of the "White Circle." Used for disorders of the uterus and prostate.

22. **BL-35 (Huiyang)**
   **Location:** On either side of the tip of the coccyx, 1/2 inch lateral to GV-1.
   **Clinical:** For problems involving coccyx, anus, and rectum.

23. **BL-36 (Chengfu)**
   **Location:** At base of buttock in middle of gluteal fold.
   **Clinical:** Sciatica with local tenderness.

24. **BL-37 (Yinmmen)**
   **Location:** Tender point in middle of biceps of upper leg in a line joining Bl-36 and BL-40.
   **Clinical:** Sciatica and local pain and tenderness; spasm of biceps femoris.

25. **BL-39 (Weiyang)**
   **Location:** On popliteal crease, lateral to BL-40 on medial border of biceps femoris tendon.
   **Clinical:** Lower Ho point of Triple Heater. When lower Heater empty, piqure for incontinence; when Lower Heater is excessive, piqure for anuria.

26. **BL-40 (Weizhong)**
   **Location:** At midpoint of crease in popliteal fossa.
   **Clinical:** He point of Bladder meridian. Earth point on Water meridian. Lower Ho point for Bladder. Lower access point for Kidney–Bladder distinct meridian. Controls the whole lower lumbar and renal area (just as LU-7 controls the neck, LI-4 controls the face and mouth, and ST-36 controls the abdomen). All Kidney, Bladder, and local knee problems may be addressed with BL-40.

27. **BL-58 (Feiyang)**
   **Location:** On posterior border of fibula, 7 inches above BL-60, on the lateral inferior border of gastrocnemius.
   **Clinical:** Luo point of Bladder meridian and sends branch to Yuan point of the Kidney, KI-3. Dispels Tai Yang channel pathogens, transfers energy from Bladder to Kidney channel.

28. **L-59 (Fuyang)**
   **Location:** Three inches directly above BL-60.
   **Clinical:** Tsri or Xi point of Yang Qaio Mo. Dispels Tai Yang channel pathogens. Strong polarizing point to bring Tai Yang or Yang Qaio Mo energy.

29. **BL-60 (Kunlun)**
    **Location:** In the depression between the highest point of the lateral malleolus and the Achilles tendon.
    **Clinical:** Ying point. Fire point on Water meridian. Is the major inferior polarizing and extraction point for Tai Yang energy. "The Garbage Dump" of the body for energy extraction.

30. **BL-62 and 62′ (Shenmai)**
    **Location:** In depression below lateral malleolus (BL-62) or directly below the tip of the lateral malleolus at the red–white border at the entrance to the tarsal sinus (BL-62′).
    **Clinical:** Master point of Yang Qiao Mo and coupled point of Du Mo. Used for sensations of energy rising to top of head, sedation and tranquilization, and for all dorsal muscular and pain problems and Kidney problems. Bl-62′ is used in preference to the classically decribed Bl-62.

31. **BL-63 (Jinmen)**
    **Location:** At the calcaneo–cuboid articulation, in a depression immediately proximal to the tuberosity of the base of of the fifth metatarsal at the red–white border.
    **Clinical:** Tsri or Xi point of the Bladder meridian. Used with GB-41 for Yang Wei Mo issues including frontal headaches starting at the back of the head, neck and sacral pain, hip pain.

32. **BL-64 (Jinggu)**
    **Location:** On the distal side of the fifth metacarpal tuberosity.
    **Clinical:** Yuan point — receives Luo branch from KI-4. Used for medial eye pain.

33. **BL-65 (Shugu)**
    **Location:** On the lateral side of the dorsum of the foot, proximal to the head of the 5th metatarsal bone, on the red–white border.
    **Clinical:** Shu point. Wood point on Water meridian. Son point and dispersion point. Fear and aversion to Wind and Cold.

34. **Bl-66 (Tonggu)**
    **Location:** In the depression distal and slightly inferior to the fifth metatarsophalangeal joint, in the skin crease.
    **Clinical:** Jing point. Water point on Water meridian. Horary point.

35. **BL-67 (Zhiyin)**
    **Location:** Lateral nail angle of the fifth toe.
    **Clinical:** Jing-Well point (Ting point). Metal point on Water meridian. Mother point and tonification point. TMM start point that gathers at SI-18 (Yang TMMs of the Leg). Strong point that can be used for acute Bladder problems; in tonification with moxa for repositioning the breech presentation and with ST-36 for inducing labor. Good point for pain anywhere in the body.

## Shao Yin Subcircuit

The *Shao Yin* subcircuit is composed of the Yin, Water Kidney meridian, and the polar opposite Yin, the Fire Heart meridian. These patients will show mixed elements of both polar opposites, with one or the other pole predominating.

### Kidney (KI)

The *Kidney meridian biopsychotype* is dominated by fear, anxiety, and chilliness with a desire for salt. Clinical uses include genitourinary disorders, low back pain, excess Lung disorders (Water — KI is the Son of Metal — LU), edema and excessive sweating (disorders of the element Water), convulsions and acute emergencies (using K-1), bone, cartilage, nail, hair, and ear disorders. Channel-structured symptoms relate to the lumbosacral area with pain improved by movement and heat (Rhus tox. of homeopathy). If deficient, these patients will exhibit chest pain, low back pain, knee problems, tinnitus and deafness, throat inflammations, and difficulty staying asleep. The Yang aspect of the Kidney is seen as disorders of the adrenal with adrenal exhaustion and the endocrine side of the Kidney (the renin-angiotensin system) with associated fluid and electrolyte abnormalities and hypertension. The Kidney meridian is closely associated with curious meridian, Chong Mo. See Kidney under TCM patterns.

**Anatomical Course:** The principal meridian of the Kidney starts on the plantar surface of the foot (KI-1), travels to the medial surface of the ankle under the pantar arch (KI-2), does an overhand loop around the medial malleolus, going past the depression between the Achilles tendon and the medial malleolus (KI-3), the insertion of the Achilles tendon into calcaneus (KI-4), up toward the malleolus (KI-5), under the midpoint of the medial malleolus (KI-6 and KI-6′), and around to the anterior medial ridge of the Achilles tendon (KI-7), anterior to the medial tibial border (KI-8), to the lower medial belly of gastrocnemius (KI-9), over the gastrocnemius to the medial edge of the politeal fossa (KI-10), along the posterior aspect of the medial thigh to the pubic tubercle at a level with CV-2 (KI-11). From there it ascends vertically up the anterior abdominal wall, lateral by one-half inch, and parallel to the conception vessel (KI-11 through KI-21) until it reaches the level of CV-14 where it moves laterally along the costosternal border to its final point at the sternoclavicular junction (KI-27). It joins HT-1 in the axilla. The cerebral Kidney division ascends internally through the trachea and tonsils to the optic chiasm and the inner and middle ear.

## Acupuncture Points of the Kidney (KI)

Number of Points: 27
Related organ: Bladder (BL)
Element: Water
Sense organ: Ear
Active Time: 5 to 7 P.M.
Alarm — Mu Point: GB-25
Shu Point: Bl-23 (L-2)

1. **KI-1 (Yong Quan)**
   **Location:** In the depression on the sole of the foot when it is in plantar flexion. The medial nail angle of the fifth toe is usually used as an alternate KI-1.
   **Clinical:** Jing-Well point (Ting point). Wood point on Water meridian. Son point, dispersion point. TMM departure point gathering at CV-2 (TMM Yin of the Leg). Extremely useful point for reviving patients from coma, shock, fainting, hysteria, seizures, vomiting, etc. Also used in plantar fascitis, plantar warts, and excessive foot sweat.
2. **KI-2 (Rangu)**
   **Location:** Anterior and inferior to the medial malleolus, on the inferior ridge of the navicular–cuneiform joint, in a depression on the red–white border.
   **Clinical:** Jing point. Fire point on Water meridian. Good for traumatic genital pain, sore throat. Is a secondary dispersion point for the Kidney.
3. **KI-3 (Taixi)**
   **Location:** Halfway between the most prominent point of the medial malleolus and the Achilles tendon, in a depression overlying the posterior tibial artery.
   **Clinical:** Shu point. Earth point on Water meridian. Yuan point receiving Luo vessel from BL-58. The strongest and most versatile point on the Kidney meridian. Can be used for Kidney energy movement, reinforcement, or dispersion. Good for all Kidney disease aspects — urinary frequency, menstrual disorders, sexual dysfunction, lumbar pain, pedal edema, arthritic and degenerative diseases, fever without sweating, agitated states, and insomnia. Good for excessive asthma together with KI-7.

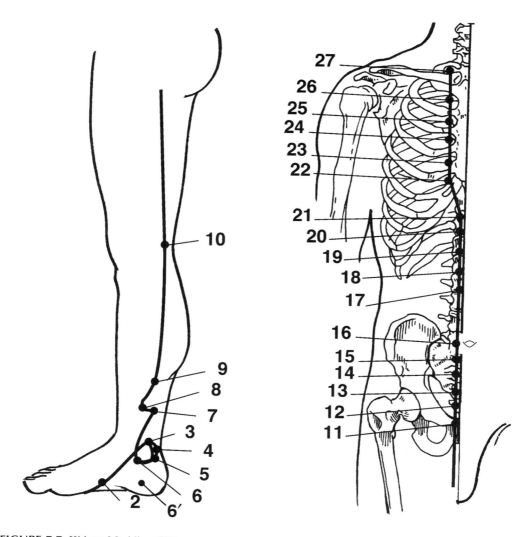

**FIGURE 7.7** Kidney Meridian (KI)

4. **KI-4 (Dazhong)**
   **Location:** In the depression formed by the insertion of the Achilles tendon into the calcaneum.
   **Clinical:** Luo point — sends vessel to Yuan point BL-64. Good for local heel pain.
5. **KI-5 (Shuiquan)**
   **Location:** In the depression midway between the tip of the medial malleolus and KI-4.
   **Clinical:** Tsri or Xi-Cleft point. A very strong point for influencing Kidney organ dysfunction such as nephritis, renal colic, nephrolithiasis, Kidney failure, and dysuria. Also useful for dysmenorrhea, irregular menses, and uterine prolapse.
6. **KI-6 (Zhaohai) and KI-6' (Six Rein Bis)**
   **Location:** KI-6 is one inch below the medial malleolus. KI-6' is directly below the tip of the medial malleolus, in a depression overlying the medial tarsal sinus on the red–white border.

**Clinical:** Master point of Yin Qiao Mo and coupled point of Ren Mo. A very strong point to bring Kidney energy into play with the curious meridians.

7. **KI-7 (Fuliu)**

   **Location:** In a hole, two inches proximal to KI-3, along the anterior ridge of the Achilles tendon.

   **Clinical:** Jing point. Metal point on Water meridian. Mother point, tonification point. Very good tonification point especially if electrified with KI-3. Tonifies Yuan Qi, Wei Qi, and Yin. Used for excessive sweating together with LI-4 and HT-6. For sweaty palms add LU-10, PC-8 and HT-8; sweaty axilla add HT-1; for sweaty soles add KI-1.

8. **KI-10 (Yingu)**

   **Location:** On the medial side of the popliteal fossa level with BL-40, between the tendons of semimembranosis and semitendonosis tendons with the knee flexed.

   **Clinical:** He point. Water point on Water meridian. Horary point. Distinct meridian access point for the Kidney–Bladder distinct meridian. Direct access to Bladder and Kidney organs and their local and regional functions — nephritis, renal colic, cystitis, prostatitis, urinary difficulties, deep lumbar stiffness and pain, lower abdominal pains, colitis, and hemorrhoids.

   KI-11 at level of CV-2
   KI-16 at level of umbilicus and CV-8
   KI-19 at level of CV-12
   KI-21 at level of CV-14
   KI-23 at level of CV-17

   All the above Kidney points are used to reinforce the associated CV point functions as well as the activity of Chong Mo, with which they all communicate.

9. **KI-27 (Shufu)**

   **Location:** In the depression on the lower border of the clavicle, two inches lateral to CV-22.

   **Clinical:** Access to the cerebral circulation of the Kidney meridian.

## Heart (HT)

The *Heart principal meridian* has a biopsychotype that is expansive, talkative, and happy to be alive. These patients are very creative thinkers and idealists and tend toward melodrama and mania.

Heart channel structural symptoms are uncommon. They may occur as the typical cardiac-referred pain down the ventral aspect of the arm. Central sternal pain at CV-16, CV-17, or CV-18 may represent Heart channel symptoms, but are more representative of Kidney Yin deficiency with False Heat propagated up the Heart channel. More energetic problems relate to insomnia due to nervousness with difficulty falling asleep. Frequent anger of an explosive character can be seen. Disturbance of the curious meridian Yin Wei Mo may often accompany Heart disturbances.

**Anatomical Course:** The principal meridian of the Heart starts in the middle of the axilla (HT-1) and travels down the anterior surface of the arm between the biceps and brachialis muscles (HT-2), to the medial limit of the antecubital crease (HT-3), along the antero-lateral aspect of the ulnar to the area of the wrist (HT-4, HT-5, HT-6, HT-7) and crosses over the palmar surface of the hand, across the "Heart Line" (HT-8) to the radial nail angle of the little finger (HT-9).

**Acupuncture Points of the Heart (HT)**

Number of Points: 9
Related organ: Small Intestine (SI)

Element: Fire
Sense organ: Tongue
Active Time: 11 A.M. to 1 P.M.
Alarm — Mu Point: Ren-14
Shu Point: BL-15 (T-5)

1. **HT-1 (Jiquan)**
   **Location:** Center of axilla, medial to axillary artery.
   **Clinical:** Use with discretion. Used for access to distinct meridian of Heart–Small Intestine.
2. **HT-2 DO NOT USE.** You risk direct cardiac influence.
3. **HT-3 (Shaohai)**
   **Location:** When the elbow is flexed at the medial end of the transverse cubital crease in the depression anterior to the medial epicondyle of the humerus. HT-3′ is one-half inch closer to the bone on the transverse crease.
   **Clinical:** He point. Water point on Fire meridian. The most important Heart point. Has a positive influence on the psyche and emotions. Good for all depressive and agitated symptoms. Used with LR-3 to create an excellent sedating couplet. Used with PC-6 and HT-7 for paroxysmal atrial tachycardia (PAT). HT-3 may be double piqured at HT-3′, which is one-half inch nearer to the bone on the transverse crease, to increase the sedative and Fire dispersing quality of the treatment. Piqure with LI-10 for numbness in the arms. Good for tremors of the forearm.
4. **HT-4 (Lingao)**
   **Location:** 1.5 inches above HT-7 (wrist crease) on the radial side of the tendon of flexor carpi ulnaris.
   **Clinical:** Jing point. Metal point on Fire meridian. Local tendonitis and sudden stiffness of tongue.
5. **HT-5 (Tongli)**
   **Location:** One inch proximal to HT-7 on the radial side of the tendon of flexor carpi ulnaris.
   **Clinical:** Luo point that sends branch to Yuan point at SI-4. Strong psychological action when combined with HT-7. Use for stage fright, exam phobia, and all complaints of psychological origin. Add ST-41 for depression.
6. **HT-6 (Yinpi)**
   **Location:** One-half inch above HT-7 on the radial side of the tendon of flexor carpi ulnaris.
   **Clinical:** Tsri or Xi-Cleft point. Used for energy obstruction of the Heart organ or the meridian. Clears Heart Fire.
7. **HT-7 (Shenmen)**
   **Location:** On the transverse crease of the wrist, in the articular region between the pisiform bone and the ulnar, in a depression on the ulnar side of the tendon of flexor carpi ulnaris.
   **Clinical:** Shu point. Earth point on Fire meridian. Son point, sedation point. Receives Luo vessel from SI-7. Strong point for dispersing Heart Fire. Used for hysteria, insomnia, agitation, palpitations, and Heat in the palms. Use with PC-7 and and HT-3 to calm a very agitated person.
8. **HT-8 (Shaofu)**
   **Location:** Between the fourth and fifth metacarpals at the "Heart Line," or where the flexed little finger contacts the palm.
   **Clinical:** Jing point. Fire point on Fire meridian. Horary point. Excellent point for dispersing excess Heat or Fire symptoms. Used for sweating, Heat in the palms, burning sensation in the hands (peripheral neuropathy).

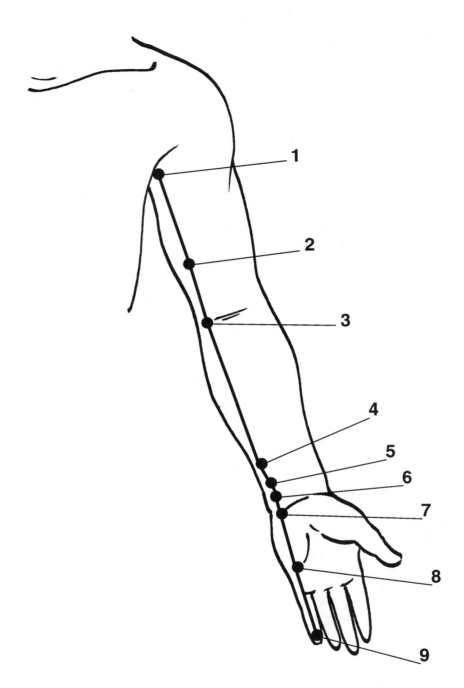

**FIGURE 7.8** Heart Meridian (HT).

9. **HT-9 (Shaochong)**
   **Location:** Radial nail angle of the little finger.
   **Clinical:** Jing-Well point (Ting point). Wood point on Fire meridian. Mother point, tonification point. Departure point for TMM Yin of hand gathering at GB-22. Used for tonification of the Heart (Yin pump or Yang spirit). Used for acute myocardial infarction.

## The Shao Yang Energy Subcircuit

The *Shao Yang energy subcircuit* consists of the Gall Bladder meridian in the lateral and lower part of the body and the Triple Heater meridian of the arm and face. Shao Yang is the Middle Yang, and as such is the hinge between Yin and Yang and governs all lateral presentations on the side of the body between the ventral Yin and the dorsal Yang. The most common presentation is that of myofascial spasm, trigger points, and superficial pain syndromes involving the side of the head (migraine, headaches, ear pain); neck and shoulder pain; lateral rib cage and hip pain; lateral epiconylitis, dorsal wrist, and lateral knee and ankle pain. The Triple Heater meridian is not used to activate the three burners of the body, which are accessed by the CV points. The physiological and organ disturbances are reflected in the coupled meridians of the Jue Yin energy subcircuit, the Liver and Pericardium (Master of the Heart). Energetic theory places the Triple Heater meridian as the energetic equivalent to the parasympathetic system and the Pericardium or Master of the Heart as the equivalent of the sympathetic nervous system.

### Gall Bladder (GB)

The *Gall Bladder biopsychotype* is one of erratic behavior (much like the course of the meridian) with explosive anger, evasiveness, indecision, and enduring resentment. These patients prefer the spring, early morning, and sour flavors. The Gall Bladder meridian is, with the Bladder meridian, the most often used for muscle spasm and pain syndromes. All of the manifestations occur on the lateral aspect of the body. The Gall Bladder meridian is almost never tonified, most of its manifestations being due to excess. If pain in the meridian has become chronic, it is acceptable to use electricity on the meridian, not to tonify, but to blast through the blockage.

**Anatomical Course:** The Gall Bladder meridian is the second longest of the Yang prinicipal meridians after the bladder, and it follows a very tortuous route from the head to the foot, on the lateral aspect of the body. It starts at the outer canthus of the eye (GB-1), runs posterior to the tragus and TMJ (GB-2), then follows a backward and forward course from the forehead (GB-14) to the lateral occiput (GB-20) covering most of temporalis (GB-3 to GB-12) and the parieto-ocipital area of the scalp (GB-15 to GB-19). From the occiput it runs down the lateral trapezius to the shoulder (GB-21), around the anterior aspect of the shoulder to a point in the mid-axillary line just under the axilla (GB-22). It then courses downward and forward to the lateral anterior abdomen and to the gallbladder itself (GB-24), then reverses direction to a point at the tip of the 12th rib in the mid-axillary line (GB-25), and then makes a forward loop across the lateral iliac crest from the mid-axillary line (GB-26) to the anterior superior iliac spine (GB-27 and GB-28) and then backward to the sciatic notch (GB-30). From the buttock it courses down the lateral side of the leg passing the fascia lata (GB-31 and GB-32), the lateral knee (GB-33), the head of the fibula (GB-34), and the lateral calf (GB-35 to GB-39), in front and below the lateral malleolus (GB-40) and the foot ray between the 4th and 5th metatarsals and phlanges (GB-41 to GB-43), and ends in the lateral nail angle of the fourth toe.

## Acupuncture Points of the Gall Bladder (GB)

Number of Points: 44
Related organ: Liver (LR)
Element: Wood
Sense organ: Eye
Active Time: 11 P.M. to 1 A.M.
Alarm — Mu point: GB-24
Shu Point: BL-19 (T-10)

1. **GB-1 (Tongziliao)**
   **Location:** In a depression, one-half inch lateral to the outer canthus of the eye.

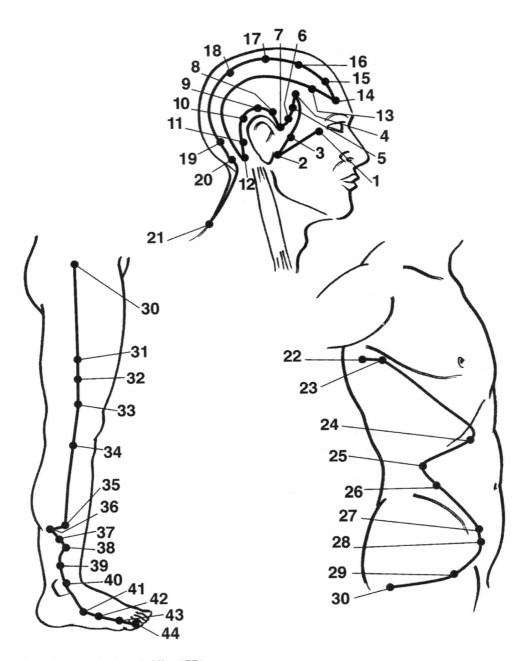

**FIGURE 7.9** Gall Bladder Meridian (GB).

**Clinical:** Access point for Liver–Gall Bladder distinct meridian. Used for all eye problems, headache, facial numbness, and tics.

2. **GB-2 (Tinghui)**
   **Location:** Anterior to the intertragic notch, directly below SI-19, at the posterior border of the condyloid process of the mandible.

**Clinical:** The point is taken with the mouth open until the needle is felt. It is used for TMJ problems, toothache, trismus, facial numbness, and Bell's palsy. Ear problems are dealt with by adding TH-17, TH-19, and TH-20 together with GB-8.

3. **GB-8 (Shuaigu)**
   **Location:** One and one-half inches above the apex of the auricle, in line with GV-20.
   **Clinical:** Used for paritotemporal headaches and vertigo. Is an important point in anti-smoking protocol.

4. **GB-13 (Benshen)**
   **Location:** On a line ascending from the lateral corner of the eye, 1/2 inch behind frontal hairline.
   **Clinical:** Gathering point for Yang TMMs of the arm.

5. **GB-14 (Yangbai)**
   **Location:** On the forehead, one inch above the midpoint of the eyebrow, at approximately one-third the distance from the eyebrow to the anterior hairline, in a depression.
   **Clinical:** Excellent point for frontal headaches, frontal sinusitis, and all frontal problems.

6. **GB-18 (Chengling)**
   **Location:** Three inches lateral to GV-20 on an imaginary line from GV-20 to apex of ear.
   **Clinical:** Used in antismoking protocol.

7. **GB-20 (Fengchi)**
   **Location:** At base of occipital bone in a depression between the sternocleidomastoid and trapezius.
   **Clinical:** Excellent point for early Wind invasion (myalgias of viral infection). Major point for treatment of headaches, migraines, cervical muscle spasm and pain, and stiffness in the shoulders. Used for occipital pain radiating to the eye, high Blood pressure, and stroke.

8. **GB-21 (Jianjing)**
   **Location:** Midway between C-7 (GV-14) and the bony prominence above LI-16 at the highest point on the shoulder.
   **Clinical:** Major regional point for trapezius and cervical tension, pain and rigidity, including cervical and occipital headaches, torticollis, and any blockage of Qi in the head. Used for all upper extremity pain.
   Note: Can cause *needle shock* if piqured in sitting position; use ST-36 if this happens.
   **Do not needle during pregnancy** — very potent labor induction point.

9. **GB-22 (Yuanye)**
   **Location:** On the mid-axillary line at the level of the nipples in the 4th intercostal space, three inches below the axillary crease.
   **Clinical:** Gathering point for the Yin TMM of the arms. Entry point into the thorax for the distinct meridians of the Lung, Heart, and Pericardium. Used for excess Yang or fullness or weakness in the chest.

10. **GB-24 (Riyue)**
    **Location:** In the 7th intercostal space in the mid-clavicular line, one rib space below and slightly lateral to LR-14.
    **Clinical:** Mu point of the Gall Bladder. Useful in all hepatobiliary problems. Good for rebellious Qi.

11. **GB-25 (Jingmen)**
    **Location:** At the tip of the 12th rib on the lateral side of the abdomen in the mid-axillary line.
    **Clinical:** Mu point of Kidney. Good for Kidney input, especially renal angle and flank pain.

12. **GB-26 (Daimai)**

    **Location:** In the mid-axillary line, below the 11th rib, just above the iliac crest, level with the umbilicus.

    **Clinical:** Dai Mo point. Puts Dai Mo into action for pain radiating in a belt-like fashion from the lumbar region to the front. All gynecological and menstrual disorders, pelvic problems, and lower lumbar pain. Used for distended abdomen with heaviness in the pelvis and cold buttocks.

13. **GB-30 (Huantiao)**

    **Location:** In a depression one-third the distance between the most prominent aspect of the greater trochanter to the sacrococcygeal ligament.

    **Clinical:** Access point for Liver–Gall Bladder distinct meridian. Main point for low lumbar, sacral and hip pain, and for sciatica that radiates down the side of the leg (BL line for back of leg). All lateral thigh and leg pain. Use with local needles over the hip joint.

14. **GB-34 (Yanglingquan)**

    **Location:** In the depression anterior and inferior to the head of the fibula.

    **Clinical:** He point. Earth point on Wood meridian. Lower uniting He point of the Gall Bladder. Roe, Hui, or influential point for tendons and muscles. A very strong point to be used for local knee, lumbar, lateral leg, and foot problems. Can be added as treatment for all myalgias, contusions, strains, leg weakness, posttraumatic muscular atrophy. Facilitates labor — **do not use in pregnant females**. Strong point for pulling down Gall Bladder energy from the head or upper body.

15. **GB-37 (Guangming)**

    **Location:** Five inches above the prominence of the lateral malleolus, on the anterior border of the fibula.

    **Clinical:** Luo point of the Gall Bladder — sends vessel to Yuan point LR-3. Good for eye disorders and shunting excess energy in the Gall Bladder meridian into the Liver meridian.

16. **GB-38 (Yangfu) or GB-39 (Xuanzhong)**

    **Location:** There is some dispute regarding which of these two points is the main GB point of the body. Pick the larger hole about 3 to 4 inches above the prominence of the lateral malleolus on the anterior border of the fibula on the lateral side of extensor digitorum longus.

    **Clinical:** Jing point. Fire point on Wood meridian. Son point, sedation point. Roe, Hui, or influential point for marrow and brain. Intersection point for the three Yang channels of the leg (just as SP-6 is the intersection point for the three Yin channels of the leg). GB-38/9 can be used with SP-6, just as TH-5 and PC-6 are used as inside–outside balancing points in cases of Yin–Yang disturbances. The most important concentration of Gall Bladder energy and strongest inferior polarizing point on the Shao Yang channel. Used clinically for dispersion of muscular and vascular spasm, general leg aches and pains, sciatica, swollen feet and ankles.

17. **GB-40 (Qiuxu)**

    **Location:** Anterior and inferior to the lateral malleolus, in the depression on the lateral side of the tendon of the extensor digitorum longus.

    **Clinical:** Yuan point — receives Luo vessel from LR-5. Good for local ankle sprains and pain.

18. **GB-41 (Zu Linqi)**

    **Location:** In the depression distal to the junction of the 4th and 5th metatarsal bones, on the lateral side of the tendon of the extensor digitorum brevis.

    **Clinical:** Shu point. Wood point on Wood meridian. Horary point. Master point of Dai Mo. Coupled point of Yang Wei Mo. Used for curious meridian movement and local foot pain. Any disorder in the cephalic course of the Gall Bladder meridian.

19. **GB-43 (Jiaxi)**
    **Location:** Between the 4th and 5th phalanges, 1/2 inch proximal to the web margin.
    **Clinical:** Ying point. Water point on Wood meridian. Mother point, tonification point. Rarely used as a tonification point, as Gall Bladder is rarely deficient. Tonify the Yin organ first — Liver.
20. **GB-44 (Zu Qiaoyin)**
    **Location:** Lateral nail angle of the 4th toe.
    **Clinical:** Jing-Well point (Ting point). Metal point on Wood meridian. Departure point for Yang TMM of the leg gathering at SI-18.

*Triple Heater (TH)*

The *Triple Heater biopsychotype* is one of excess energy and irritable nervousness on one side, or boredom, shyness, insomnia, and depression on the other. The meridian is used mainly to move obstructions in the Shao Yang meridian and has little to do with its energy and metabolic activity in the three Heaters (which are accessed by CV points).

**Anatomical Course:** The Triple Heater starts at the ulnar nail angle of the fourth finger (TH-1), and travels across the dorsum of the hand and knuckles (TH-2 and TH-3) to the middle of the dorsal aspect of the wrist (TH-4), up the middle of the arm between the LI and SI meridians in the groove between the radius and ulnar (TH-5 to TH-9), to the dorsal aspect of the elbow (TH-10), up the back of the arm between the long and lateral heads of the triceps muscle (TH-11 to TH-13), to the acromion (TH-14), across the trapezius (TH-15) to the neck and mastoid process (TH-16), and to the angle between the maxilla and root of the ear (TH-17). It then encircles the ear from behind (TH-18 to TH-20) to the tragus (TH-21), courses anterior and upward onto the lateral face and forehead (TH-22), and ends just lateral to the superciliary ridge (TH-23).

**Acupuncture Points of the Triple Heater (TH)**

Number of Points: 23
Related organ: Pericardium (PC) — Master of the Heart
Element: Fire
Sense organ: Tongue
Active Time: 9 to 11 P.M.
Alarm — Mu Point: Ren-5, (CV-5)
Shu Point: BL-22 (L-1)

1. **TH-1 (Guanchong)**
    **Location:** Ulnar nail angle of the 4th finger.
    **Clinical:** Jing-Well point. Metal point on Fire meridian. Departure point for Yang TMM of arm, which gathers at GB-13. Reduces Heat in the three body Heaters. Used to defervesce fever by bleeding, together with LU-11, LI-1, and PC-9.
2. **TH-2 (Yemen)**
    **Location:** Between base of 4th and 5th finger, proximal to the margin of the web.
    **Clinical:** Ying point. Water point on Fire meridian. Clears Fire and Heat in the Triple Heater meridian. Used with TH-3.
3. **TH-3 (Zhongzhu)**
    **Location:** On the dorsum of the hand between the 4th and 5th metacarpals, in the depression proximal to the metacarpophalangeal joint.
    **Clinical:** Shu point. Wood point on Fire meridian. Mother point, tonification point. Used to tonify and move energy down the whole Shao Yang line. Used as a distal point for ear and eye disorders. Also useful in arm pain and paralysis.

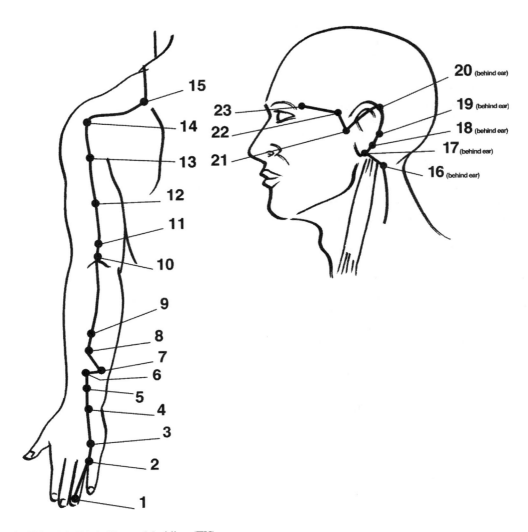

**FIGURE 7.10** Triple-Heater Meridian (TH)

4. **TH-4 (Yangchi)**
   **Location:** At the junction of the ulnar and wrist in the depression lateral to the tendon of the extensor digitorum communis.
   **Clinical:** Yuan point — receives Luo vessel from PC-6. Used for local wrist pain.
5. **TH-5 (Waiguan)**
   **Location:** In a large hole, at the dorsal midpoint between the ulnar and radius about two inches above the wrist crease.
   **Clinical:** Luo point — sends vessel to Yuan point PC-7. Master point of Yang Wei Mo and coupled point of Dai Mo. An important balancing point between Yin and Yang and internal and external imbalances. Used with PC-6 and similar to the balancing action in the lower extremity of SP-6 and GB-38. Distal point for head problems. Indicated in occipital headaches that radiate to the forehead or behind the eye. Used for ENT problems, torticollis, and pain and stiffness in the forearm and wrist.

6. **TH-6 (Zhigou)**

   **Location:** In a depression midway between the ulnar and radius about three inches proximal to the dorsal wrist crease.

   **Clinical:** Jing point. Fire point on Fire meridian. Horary point. A good point to disperse for Heat related problems such as constipation, IBS, pneumonia, dermatitis, and fever without sweating. Also used in acupuncture analgesia for thoracic surgery.

7. **TH-8 (Sanyangluo)**

   **Location:** Four inches proximal to the dorsal wrist crease in between the ulnar and radius.

   **Clinical:** Intersection point of the three Yang vessels of the arm. Used for pain problems of the hand, wrist, arm, and shoulder. Also used for all pain syndromes of the chest wall, such as intercostal neuralgia, herpes zoster, and Coxsackie myalgia. Used with TH-6 in thoracic acupuncture analgesia.

8. **TH-10 (Tianjung)**

   **Location:** In a depression about one inch superior to the tip of the olecranon, with the elbow flexed.

   **Clinical:** He point. Earth point on Fire meridian. Son point, sedation point. Used for local elbow problems and dermatitis, pharyngitis, and lymphadenitis.

9. **TH-14 (Jianliao) and TH-15 (Tianliao)**

   **Location:** TH-14 — Between the acromium and the greater tuberosity of the humerus in the more posterior position with the arm abducted to the horizontal position. TH-15 — Midway between GB-21 and SI-13 on the superior angle of the scapula.

   **Clinical:** For shoulder problems involving the TH channel. May be used with surrounding channels if also involved.

10. **TH-16 (Tianyou)**

    **Location:** Posterior and inferior to the mastoid process, on the posterior border of the sternocleidomastoid, level with SI-17 and BL-10.

    **Clinical:** Window of the sky point. upper meeting point for Triple Heater–Pericardium distinct meridian. Used to dispel Heat problems in head and face.

11. **TH-17 (Yifeng)**

    **Location:** Posterior to the lobule of the ear, in the depression between the mandible and mastoid process.

    **Clinical:** This is the most used and effective point for all ear problems. It is used for ear problems with GB-8, SI-19, TH-18, TH-19, TH-20, and TH-21. It can also be used for parotitis and facial paralysis. It is a great point for eustachian tube blockage and ear pain that radiates to the throat.

12. **TH-21 (Ermen)**

    **Location:** In a depression anterior to the supratragic notch, above SI-19.

    **Clinical:** For all ear problems and TMJ problems. Can be used together with SI-19 and GB-2.

13. **TH-23 (Sizhukong)**

    **Location:** In a depression at the lateral end of the eyebrow.

    **Clinical:** For lateral eye problems and temporal and lateral migraines.

## The Jue Yin Energy Subcircuit

The *Jue Yin energy subcircuit* is composed of two very similar meridians, Liver (LR) and Pericardium (PC) or Master of the Heart (MH). Liver, a Yin meridian, tends towards Yang problems and Pericardium is a Yin, Fire meridian. So, the differences between them are not great, and their fundamental biopsychotypes are similar. Liver has to do with hepatobiliary problems, while Pericardium is looked upon as being the sympathetic nervous system and used to indirectly affect the physical Heart. Most of the functions of Jue Yin have to to to do with the general adrenergic activity of the body.

## Pericardium (PC)

The Chinese concept of this meridian is one of a Protector of the Heart. The Pericardium regulates the functions of Heart Shen, Heart organ, and Heart energy. As protector of the Heart, it is concerned with activities of the vagus nerve on the Heart, and is used with all arrythmias. The Heart and Pericardium are also associated with the brain and its functions. Most TCM disorders relate to Heat and febrile problems. The structural channel influences of Pericardium relate to the forearm and wrist, seen as tendonitis, muscle spasm, or contractions such as wrist pain, carpal tunnel, and Dupuytrens contracture. The *biopsychotype of the Pericardium* is partial to dark chocolate and coffee and is somewhat agitated, tense, and enclosed within a tight emotional and physical framework.

**Anatomical Course:** The Pericardium meridian starts in the 4th intercostal space, one inch lateral to the nipple (PC-1). It ascends to the anterior axillary fold and does a U-turn, proceeds distally, between the LU and HT meridians, down the arm between the heads of biceps (PC-2) to the midpoint of the antecubital crease (PC-3), down the volar aspect of the forearm over the median nerve, between the tendons and muscles of palmaris longus and flexor carpi radialis (PC-4 to PC-6), crosses the midpoint of the wrist (PC-7) to the center of the palm (PC-8), and ends in the radial nail angle of the middle finger (PC-9).

**Acupuncture Points of the Pericardium (PC)**

> Number of Points: 9
> Related organ: Triple Heater (TH)
> Element: Fire
> Sense organ: Tongue
> Active Time: 7 to 9 P.M.
> Alarm — Shu Point: CV-17
> Shu Point: BL-14 (T-4)

1. **PC-1 (Tianchi)**
   **Location:** One inch lateral to the nipple in the 4th intercostal space, but pratically the tender point above the anterior axillary crease.
   **Clinical:** Window of the Sky point. Pericardium–Triple Heater distinct meridian access point. Opens up the chest. Used for intercostal neuralgia and angina. Used for axillary swelling with Bl-39.

2. **PC-3 (Quze)**
   **Location:** In the antecubital crease, on the medial (ulnar) side of the biceps tendon.
   **Clinical:** He point. Water point on Fire meridian. Used to disperse Fire symptoms with CV-17, such as palpitations, anxiety, and energy rising to the head. Good for elbow pain and to access the brachial artery and median nerve.

3. **PC-4 (Ximen)**
   **Location:** Five inches above the wrist crease, in the cleft between the tendons of palmaris longus and flexor carpi radialis.
   **Clinical:** Tsri or Xi-Cleft point. It is used to treat acute cardiac and circulation disorders, such as angina, cardiac arrythmias, tachycardia, pericarditis, and chest pain. Also used as a point for cardiac anesthesia. Effective for hemoptysis when used with LI-11 and TH-8.

4. **PC-5 (Jianshi)**
   **Location:** Three inches above the wrist crease, between the tendons of palmaris longus and flexor carpi radialis.

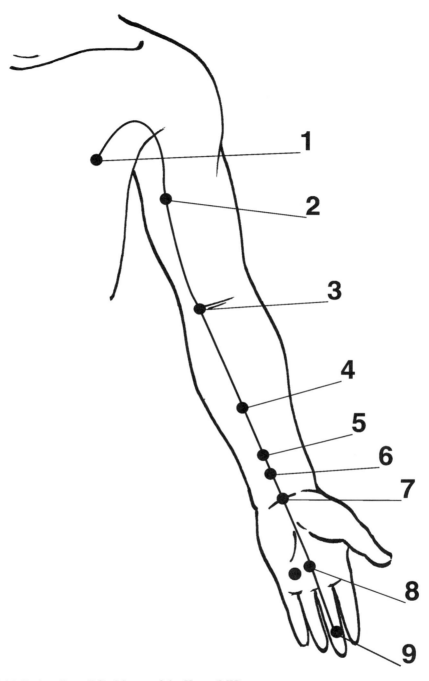

**FIGURE 7.11** Pericardium (PC); Master of the Heart (MH).

**Clinical:** Jing point. Metal point on Fire meridian. Used for Phlegm in the Heart — psychiatric disorders.

5. **PC-6 (Neiguan)**
**Location:** Two inches above the wrist crease between the tendons of palmaris longus and flexor carpi radialis.

**Clinical:** Luo point — sends vessel to Yuan point, TH-4. Master point of Yin Wei Mo and coupled point of Chong Mo. One of the major points of the body for inside–outside equilibration with TH-5 and the couplet SP-6/GB-38. Allows general excesses and deficiencies to adjust. Is the most important distal point for disorders of the epigastrium and anterior chest wall. Important for the mental–emotional disturbances of excess Fire, as well as the physical symptoms of excess Fire, such as cardiac irregularities, respiratory dysfunction, gastritis and gastric and duodenal ulcers, hiccups, and motion sickness and vomiting. As it commands the Upper Heater, it should be used in all cardiac and respiratory problems. Big point for postoperative or postchemotherapy nausea with ST-36. Used for morning sickness and hyperemesis gravidarum and for carpal tunnel syndrome. Acupuncture analgesia for chest and upper abdominal surgery.

6. **PC-7 (Daling)**
    **Location:** In the depression in the middle of the tranverse wrist crease, between the tendons of palmaris longus and flexor carpi radialis over the median nerve and flexor retinaculum.
    **Clinical:** Yuan point — receives Luo vessel from TH-5. Earth point on Fire meridian. Son point, sedation point. Shu point. Used as an important sedation point for excess Fire and excess Yang symptoms such as anxiety, manias, chest pain, and hysteria (can be coupled with HT-3 and HT-7). Used for Heat-type skin rashes. Used for local wrist pain together with LU-9 and HT-7. Important point for carpal tunnel syndrome and any medial nerve compression syndrome.

7. **PC-8 (Laogong)**
    **Location:** With the fingers bent, where the tip of the 3rd finger meets the palm, on the radial side of the 3rd metacarpal.
    **Clinical:** Ying point. Fire point on Fire meridian. Horary point. Major Fire dispersion point, but very painful to needle. Used for excess Fire in the head symptoms such as madness, epilepsy, epistaxis, insomnia, anger, headaches, and fear. Good point for peripheral neuropathy and Dupuytren's contracture.

8. **PC-9 (Zhongchong)**
    **Location:** Radial nail angle of the middle finger.
    **Clinical:** Jing-Well (Ting) point. Wood point on Fire meridian. Mother point, tonification point. Departure point for Yin TMM of arm gathering at GB-22. Used in acute emergencies for collapse, fainting, and stroke with syncope together with GV-26.

*Liver (LR)*

The *Liver meridian* is responsible for smooth flow of Qi and for the storage of Blood, especially in menstruation. The Liver rules the muscles, ligaments, and tendons, opens to the eyes and is manifest in the nails. Many of its excessive Yang and Fire symptoms stem from restrained Liver Qi, deficient Blood, or Yin and become manifest in the excessive symptoms in the Gall Bladder meridian, or are seen in the Spleen and Stomach meridian when the Liver Fire invades them. Dysharmony in the Liver results in dry and brittle nails, dry eyes or blurred vision, stiffness in the muscles and joints, muscular spasm and twitches, tremors, and irregular, spotty, or absent menstruation. Internalized anger is an important cause of constrained Liver Qi, which causes explosive anger, tightness of the lateral chest muscles, and often migraines or occipital headaches. Disturbance of Liver Blood control causes insomnia. Structurally, the Liver controls the foot, medial knee, medial thigh, external genitalia, and hypochondrial area. Liver Fire is often expressed on the skin as rashes, urticaria, hives, eczema, or herpes. Dense organ problems involve the full spectrum of Liver and Gall Bladder problems from jaundice to hepatitis.

**Anatomical Course:** The Liver meridian starts at the Yang nail angle of the hallux (LR-1) and travels across the web between the first and second toes (LR-2), courses up between the first and second metatarsals to where they meet on the dorsum of the foot (LR-3), courses medially over the medial malleolus (LR-4), ascends the medial or Yin aspect of the lower leg along the posterior surface of the tibia (LR-5 and LR-6) to the medial knee (LR-7 and LR-8). It continues from the knee on the medial surface of the thigh along the sartorius and adductor magnus muscles (LR-9 to LR-11) to the inguinal ligament (LR-12). It then traverses the abdomen obliquely to the tip of the 11th rib in the mid-axillary line (LR-13), and ends in a hole situated in the sixth intercostal space in the mid-clavicular line (LR-14).

## Acupuncture Points of the Liver (LR)

Number of Points: 14
Related organ: Gall Bladder (GB)
Element: Wood
Sense organ: Eye
Active Time: 1-3 A.M.
Alarm — Mu Point: LR-14
Shu Point: BL-18 (T-9)

1. **LR-1 (Dadun)**
   **Location:** Lateral nail angle of the great toe.
   **Clinical:** Jing-Well (Ting) point. Wood point on Wood meridian. Horary point. Departure point for Liver TMM Yin of leg which gathers at CV-2. Removes obstruction of Liver Qi in the lower abdomen. Used in acute emergencies in metabolic disturbances. Also used for prolapse of uterus, menorrhagia, and enuresis.
2. **LR-2 (Xingjian)**
   **Location:** Between first and second phalanges, 1/2 inch proximal to web margin. Associated with the dorsal venous network of the foot and where the dorsal digital nerves split off from the deep peroneal nerve.
   **Clinical:** Ying point. Fire point on Wood meridian. Son point, sedation point. A very powerful sedation and Fire draining point (disperses Liver Heat and Liver Yang) for the whole body. Used clinically for anger, insomnia, dry throat, agitation, and palpitations. Used for the eyes in redness, swelling, itching and tearing. Also used for hypertension and night sweats.
3. **LR-3 (Taichong)**
   **Location:** In the distal depression of the interosseus space between the first and second metatarsals. Related to the dorsal venous network of the foot, the first dorsal metatarsal artery, and a branch of the deep peroneal nerve.
   **Clinical:** Shu point. Earth point on Wood meridian. Yuan point — receives Luo vessel from GB-40. Used for all Liver and Gall Bladder disorders. It is equivalent to LI-4 in the hand and is one of the four great energy points of the body (LR-3, SP-6, ST-36, and LI-4). Excellent for activating Jue Yin energy when coupled with LR-8 or LR-14. Used for sedating Liver Fire (with LR-2) and Yang together with HT-3 (anxiety and insomnia). Good point for all foot pain, all eye problems, nasal congestion, and all allergy. Good for all menstrual disorders, muscular spasms, hypertension, and all metabolic, e.g., hypoglycemia, and endocrine disorders.
4. **LR-4 (Zhongfeng)**
   **Location:** In the depression anterior to the medial malleolus, medial to the tendon of the anterior tibial muscle.
   **Clinical:** Jing point. Metal point on Wood meridian. Local ankle problems.
5. **LR-5 (Ligou)**
   **Location:** In a depression, five inches above the tip of the medial malleolus on the posterior border of the tibia.

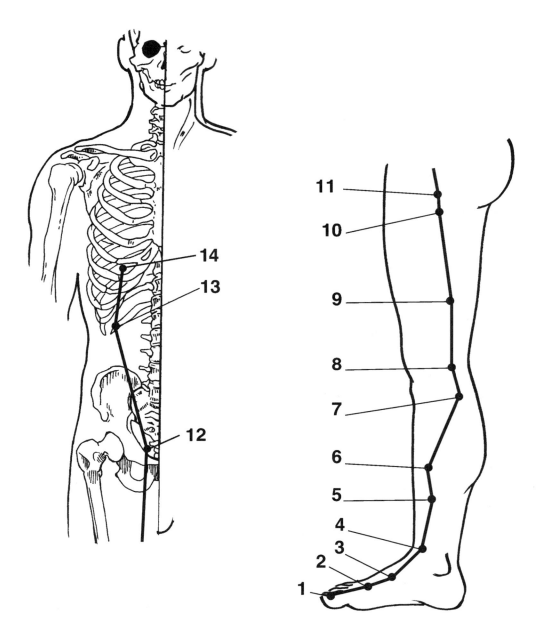

**FIGURE 7.12** Liver Meridian (LR).

    **Clinical:** Luo point — sends vessel to Yuan point, GB-40. Lower Heater energy blockage. External genital problems and dysmenorrhea.

6. **LR-6 (Zhongdu)**
    **Location:** At the midpoint of the tibial shaft, on its posterior border.
    **Clinical:** Tsri or Xi-Cleft point. Additional alarm point for the Liver and will be tender if needled. Used for anesthesia of external genitalia and lower abdominal pain.

7. **LR-8 (Ququan)**

**Location:** On the medial side of the knee joint, in the transverse crease of the popliteal fossa, at the medial border of the semimembranosus tendon. Pinch the fat pad of the medial knee — LR-8 is situated at the highest point of the pad. Related to the saphenous vein anteriorly and the saphenous nerve.

**Clinical:** He point. Water point on Wood meridian. Mother point, tonification point. Clears Damp–Heat and drains Liver Fire. Good point for tonification of Liver organ or meridian when used with LR-3 or LR-14. Good for local knee and leg pain. Specific point for treatment of impotence. Good for diarrhea and UTIs.

8. **LR-9 (Yinbao)**

**Location:** Four inches above the medial epicondyle of the femur, in a hole between vastus medialis and sartorius.

**Clinical:** The importance of this point is that it sends a branch to encircle the external genitalia. Used for any problem relating to the penis, scrotum, testicles, vulva, and vagina. Also used for inflammation in this area, including herpes genitalis, rashes, and urethritis. Use for coccydinia together with CV-1 and CV-2.

9. **LR-12 (Jimai)**

**Location:** On a level with the pubic symphysis, 2.5 inches lateral to the midline, just superior to the inguinal ligament.

**Clinical:** Access point to Liver–Gall Bladder distinct meridian. Used for its connection to the distinct meridian to treat hepatobiliary problems. Also used for gential problems and inguinal hernia.

10. **LR-13 (Zhangmen)**

**Location:** Below the anterior tip of the 11th rib in the mid-axillary line. Where the tip of the elbow touches the lateral chest.

**Clinical:** Mu point of the Spleen. Roe, Hui, or influentual point for the 5 Zang Viscera (LU, HT, SP, KI, LR). Used mostly as the Mu point for Spleen together with CV-12. Mainly digestive problems, diarrhea, abdominal bloating, and vomiting.

11. **LR-14 (Qimen)**

**Location:** In a hole, on the midclavicular line in the sixth intercostal space.

**Clinical:** Mu point for Liver. Used for all Liver disorders and for the Liver cerebral circulation. Harmonizes the Liver and the Spleen. From LR-14, the Yin vital energy (Qi) flows onto LU-1 at about 3:00 A.M., thus reestablishing the cycle of the flow of energy.

## The Yang Ming Energy Subcircuit

*Yang Ming* is the least Yang of all the Yangs, connecting to Tai Yin, the most Yin of the Yins. Most of the problems in this subcircuit are centered around the gut and its connected functions. The two constituent meridians are Large Intestine, LI (in the arm), and Stomach, ST (in the body and leg). Most of the emotional issues relate to food, eating, and being the life of the party. Patients tend to be epicures and bon vivants. Channel structural problems relate first to the external pathways that will include pain and inflammation of the thumb, wrist, elbow, shoulders, and lateral neck; facial neuralgias, external genital pain, knee, lateral anterior compartment and ankle pain; second to the internal pathways that include anosmia, rhinitis, sinusitis, dental problems, throat, esophageal, and stomach; large intestinal disturbances, and eating disorders.

### Large Instestine (LI)

The Large Intestine meridian has both physiological and pathological issues more related to the Spleen than the associated Lung. Its actions and organ problems are similar to those of the large intestine in regular medicine, but it is not usually used for those disorders — the Spleen is used.

Its structural meridian influence is closely attatched to pain syndromes of the lateral arm and shoulder, the throat and thyroid, and the maxillary sinuses and nose.

**Anatomical Course:** The Large Intestine starts at the radial nail angle of the second or index finger (LI-1), goes up the radial side of the index finger to a point distal to the metacarpophalngeal joint (LI-2), to just proximal to the head of the second metacarpal bone (LI-3), to the web space between the thumb and index finger (LI-4), and to the anatomical snuff box (LI-5). It travels along the radial border of extensor digitorum (LI-6 to LI-10) to the radial end of the tranverse cubital crease (LI-11), traverses the lateral head of triceps (LI-13), across the lateral insertion of deltoid (LI-14) to the acromion (LI-15). From the acromion it travels across the anterior shoulder of the supraclavicular fossa (LI-16), to the posterior border of sternocleidomastoid (LI-17), to the mid-belly of sternocleidomastoid level with the superior border of the thyroid cartilage (LI-18). It then crosses the mandible to the area just below the lateral margin of the nostril (LI-19), across the philtrum to the opposite side of the face, half an inch lateral to the nostril in the nasolabial fold (LI-20).

## Acupuncture Points of the Large Intestine (LI)

Number of Points: 20
Related organ: Lung (LU)
Element: Metal
Sense organ: Nose, sense of smell
Active Time: 5 to 7 A.M.
Alarm — Mu Point: ST-25 (2 inches lateral to navel)
Shu Point: BL-25 (L-4)

1. **LI-1 (Shangyang)**
   **Location:** Radial nail angle of index finger.
   **Clinical:** Jing-Well (Ting) point. Metal point on Metal meridian. Horary point. Access point for Yang TMM of leg gathering at GB-13. Dispells wind-Heat. Good point for toothache, tonsillitis, and sore and inflammed throat. Also used in emergencies of fainting and collapse with GV-26.

2. **LI-2 (Erjian)**
   **Location:** On the red–white border on the radial side of the index finger, distal to the metacarpophalangeal joint.
   **Clinical:** Ying point. Water point on Metal meridian. Son point, sedation point. Used for constipation, toothache, and throat problems.

3. **LI-3 (Sanjian)**
   **Location:** On the radial side of the index finger, in a depression proximal to the head of the second metacarpal bone.
   **Clinical:** Shu point. Wood point on metal meridian. Disperses pathogenic Heat. Good for any mucous membrane problem in the channel: cold sores, cracked lips, and throat pain. Also used for toothache, sinusitis, and acne of the face. For acupuncture anesthesia of the teeth and face.

4. **LI-4 (Hegu)**
   **Location:** In the center of the web space between the first and second metacarpal bones, slightly closer to the second metacarpal.
   **Clinical:** The *Major Point of Acupuncture*. Yuan point — receives Luo channel from LU-9. Major energy point with ST-36. Constitutes the "Four Gates" treatment with LR-3 for all pain in the body. Used for any problem in the head and neck. Good sedation point for endorphin release with low frequency (2 to 10 Hz) electroacupuncture. The most important pain point in the body. Used for all anesthesia. Brings on menses. Tonify with ST-36 and LU-7 to strengthen Wei Qi. When in doubt, use it!

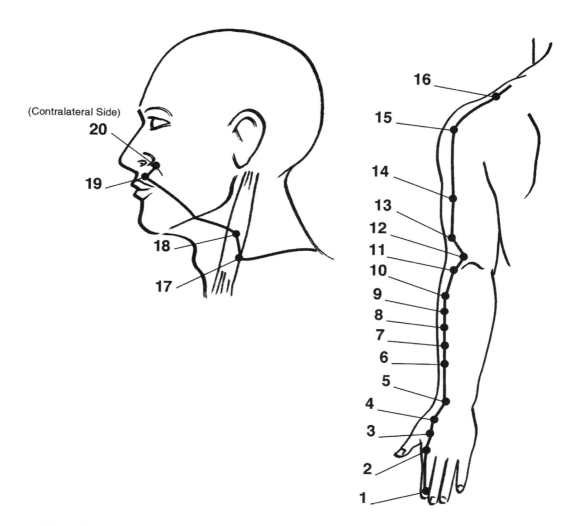

**FIGURE 7.13** Large Instestine Meridian (LI).

5. **LI-5 (Yangxi)**

   **Location:** On the radial side of the wrist in the anatomical snuff box.

   **Clinical:** Jing point. Fire point on Metal meridian. Used for skin disorders such as urticaria, pruritis, and eczema.

6. **LI-6 (Pianli)**

   **Location:** Three inches above the wrist on the radial border of extensor digitorum.

   **Clinical:** Luo point — sends branch to Yuan point Lu-9. Elbow and wrist pain.

7. **LI-7 (Wenliu)**

   **Location:** On the posteriolateral border of the radius three inches up the arm in the same line as LI-6.

   **Clinical:** Tsri or Xi-Cleft point. Used to unblock any energy blockage on the LI meridian — usually problems of excess: toothache, headache, sore throat, acute abdominal pain, and arm and shoulder pain.

8. **LI-10 (Shousanli)**
   **Location:** In a depression two inches below LI-11.
   **Clinical:** Homologous to ST-36. Yang Ming functional and organ problems: abdominal pain and diarrhea. Good point for shoulder pain and elbow problems with LI-11. Good general tonification point with moxa.

9. **LI-11 (Quchi)**
   **Location:** At the lateral end of the transverse antecubital crease, when the elbow is flexed.
   **Clinical:** He point. Earth point on Metal meridian. Mother point, tonification point. Strong activation point for Yang Ming together with ST-25. Best point for all throat problems. For urticaria and all dermatological problems add SP-10, LI-3, LI-4, and GV-14. For early virus use with GB-20. Good for all shoulder and arm pain. Excellent homeostatic and immune-enhancing point to be used for allergies, infections, fatigue, and circulatory disturbances. Tonify with moxa.

10. **LI-15 (Jianyu)**
    **Location:** In the anterior depression lateral to the tip of the acromion process, with the arm abducted in the depression just anterior to biceps tendon.
    **Clinical:** Access point for the Lung–Large Intestine distinct meridian. Excellent point for frozen shoulder and all problems of the shoulder joint. Used together with TH-14 and SI-9.

11. **LI-18 (Futu)**
    **Location:** In the belly of the sternocleidomastoid, three inches lateral to the superior border of the thyroid cartilage.
    **Clinical:** Window of the Sky point. Exit point for Lung–Large Intestine distinct meridian. Excellent point for all throat and thyroid problems including tonsillitis, laryngitis, thyroiditis, and goiter. Use with LI-11. *Somewhat dangerous point* underlying great vessels, vagus nerve, sympathetic trunks, and ganglia and baroreceptors. *Needle superficially.*

12. **LI-20 (Yingxiang)**
    **Location:** Half an inch lateral to the ala nasi and in the nasolabial groove on the contralateral side of the face.
    **Clinical:** All nasal disorders: obstruction, sinusitis, rhinitis, epistaxis, problems of olfaction, and nasal polyps. Use with LI-5 with skin disorders of the face. Also good for toothache and facial neuralgia.

*Stomach (ST)*

Most Stomach disorders tend to be of an excess nature. Symptoms such as belching, distention, and abdominal pain are common. Rebellious Qi causes nausea, vomiting, and hiccups. Stomach Fire presents with GERD, heartburn, gastric ulcer, constipation, epistaxis, and bleeding gums. Although very closely aligned in function, the Stomach and the Spleen thrive in opposite surroundings: Spleen loves the dry while the Stomach loves the damp. Stomach Qi descends, Spleen Qi ascends.

*Disorders of the channel* include trigeminal neuralgia, toothache, Bell's palsy, sinusitis, chest diseases, breast disease, gastrointestinal and menstrual disorders, lower limb joint pain, and paralysis. The anatomical course includes:

1. **Cephalic Division** — The Stomach begins at the infraorbital notch (ST-1), travels downward on the cheek, makes a U-turn at the mandible and follows the ramus upward to the temple passing the infraorbital foramen (ST-2), to the lower border of ala nasi (ST-3), lateral to corner of the mouth (ST-4), just anterior to angle of mandible at anterior border of masseter muscle (ST-5), to the center of masseter at the angle of the jaw (ST-6), anterior to the mandibular condyle (ST-7) to the temple, then lateral to GB-13 (ST-8). From there it travels from ST-5 down the neck on the anterior border of the sternocleidomastoid muscle passing the thyroid cartilage (ST-9 and ST-10), to the

clavicle (ST-11), and jogging laterally along the superior border of the clavicle to the supraclavicular notch in the mid-clavicular line (ST-12).

2. **Thoraco-Abdominal Division** — From the clavicle it descends over the chest in the nipple line (ST-13 to ST-16), crosses the nipple (ST-17) to directly below the nipple in the fifth intercostal space (ST-18). It now jogs medially to the edge of the costal cartilage two to three inches from the midline (ST-19), descends in a straight line two inches lateral to the midline in the crease of the rectus abdominus muscle (ST-20 to ST-29) passing the umbilicus (ST-25), and on to the inguinal ligament (ST-30).

3. **Lower Extremity Division** — This division descends vertically and laterally along the lateral border of the quadriceps femoris muscle (ST-31 to ST-33) to the patella (ST-34), to the lower border of the patella (ST-35), past the tibial plateau (ST-36) and along the groove between tibialis anterior and extensor digitorum longus (ST-37 to ST-39). At this point it jogs upward and laterally for one inch (ST-40), then continues to the ankle (ST-41) crosses the dorsum of the foot (ST-42 to ST-44), and ends up at the lateral nail angle of the second toe (ST-45).

## Acupuncture Points of the Stomach (ST)

Number of Points: 45
Related organ: Spleen (SP)
Element: Earth
Sense organ: Mouth
Active Time: 7 to 9 A.M.
Alarm — Mu Point: CV-12 (between umbilicus and xiphisternum)
Shu Point: BL-21 (T-12)

1. **ST-1 (Chengqi)**
   Location: Directly below pupil on the infraorbital ridge.
   Clinical: Used as alternate polar point (BL-1) for Spleen–Stomach distinct meridian. Used for all eye disorders.
2. **ST-2 (Sibai)**
   Location: In the depression of the infraorbital foramen.
   Clinical: For all eye disorders and excellent point for all facial neuralgias and paralyses.
3. **ST-3 (Juliao)**
   Location: Directly below the pupil, at the level of the lower border of the ala nasi, on the lateral side of the nasolabial groove.
   Clinical: Facial paralysis, toothache, trigeminal neuralgia, sinusitis, and rhinitis.
4. **ST-4 (Dicang)**
   Location: Lateral to the corner of the mouth, below ST-3.
   Clinical: Facial paralysis, trigeminal neuralgia, cheilosis, speech difficulties, disorders of the upper teeth, ulcers, and lip sores. Used for dental anesthesia of the upper jaw.
5. **ST-5 (Daying)**
   Location: Anterior to the angle of the mandible, on the anterior border of masseter muscle.
   Clinical: Facial paralysis, trigeminal neuralgia, toothache, parotitis, and trismus.
6. **ST-6 (Jiache)**
   Location: At the most prominent point of the masseter with the jaws clenched.
   Clinical: Toothache, jaw pain, TMJ, trismus, spasm of masseter, and parotitis.
7. **ST-7 (Xiaguan)**
   Location: In the depression on the lower border of the zygomatic arch, anterior to the mandibular condyle.
   Clinical: Facial paralysis, trigeminal neuralgia, arthritis of the TMJ.

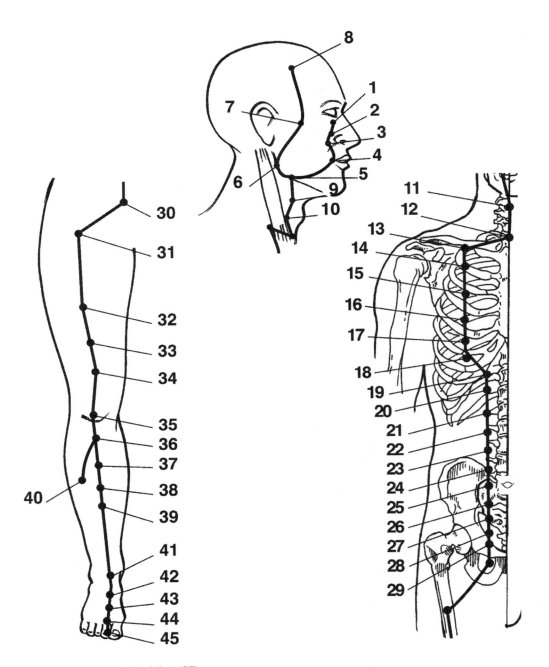

**FIGURE 7.14** Stomach Meridian (ST).

8. **ST-8 (Touwei)**
   **Location:** At the lateral corner of the forehead, 1.5 inches lateral to GB-13.
   **Clinical:** Migraine, ophthalmoplegia, eye pain, and tearing.

9. **ST-9 (Renjung)**
   **Location:** On the anterior border of sternocleidomastoid at the level of the prominence of the thyroid cartilage.

**Clinical:** Window of the Sky point. Use when the energy is unable to rise to the head or to descend to the thorax. Used for pain and swelling of the throat, dysphonia, and vocal cord problems. Used after thyroid surgery to activate the thyroid.

10. **ST-12 (Quepen)**
   **Location:** Center of the supraclavicular notch, on the superior edge of the clavicle.
   **Clinical:** An important intersection and relay point for pulling down Yang Ming energy. Used for angina, chest oppression, asthma, cough, and sore throat. Part of the "scapular belt" of ST-12, GV-14, LI-15, and ST-13.

11. **ST-13 (Qihu)**
   **Location:** Lower border of the clavical in the mid-clavicular line.
   **Clinical:** Meeting point of the distinct meridians of the chest. Used for emphysema, cough, asthma, fullness in the chest, and excessive perspiration of the feet.

12. **ST-17 Forbidden Point** — only used for orientation of other points.

13. **ST-18 (Rugen)**
   **Location:** Directly below the nipple in the fifth intercostal space.
   **Clinical:** Excessive thirst, mastitis, deficient lactation, chest pain, cough dyspnea, and angina.

14. **ST-21 (Liangmen)**
   **Location:** Two inches lateral to CV-12 and KI-19 in rectus abdominus crease.
   **Clinical:** All upper abdominal disorders.

15. **ST-25 (Tianshu)**
   **Location:** Two inches lateral to the umbilicus and CV-8.
   **Clinical:** Mu point of the Large Intestine. Conveys energy to Yang Ming — excellent tonification point together with LI-11. Disperse with ST-36 or ST-43. Excellent point for diarrhea if due to Spleen deficiency — use with ST-36, SP-6, and PC-6. Good for menstrual disorders with KI-5. Used for acute and chronic gastroenteritis, diarrhea, constipation, acute appendicitis, and paralytic ileus.

16. **ST-26 (Wailing)**
   **Location:** Two inches lateral to CV-7, one inch below the umbilicus.
   **Clinical:** Good tonification point for Yang Ming — Large Intestine energy.

17. **ST-30 (Qichong)**
   **Location:** Two inches lateral to CV-2 on the superior border of the pubic bone, superior to the inguinal groove and medial to the femoral artery.
   **Clinical:** Access point for Stomach–Spleen distinct meridian. Major pelvic focal point — all genitourinary and reproductive problems. All pelvic and lower abdominal postoperative problems via distinct meridian. Stimulates labor and delivery.

18. **ST-32 (Futu)**
   **Location:** Center of the anterior aspect of the thigh on the lateral edge of quadriceps femoris, six inches above the upper edge of the patella, on a line connecting the anterior superior iliac spine to the lateral border of the patella.
   **Clinical:** Roe or Hui or influentual point for the veins and arteries of the leg. Opens the vasculature of the legs.

19. **ST-34 (Liangqiu)**
   **Location:** In a depression about two inches above the lateral superior edge of the patella, with the leg straight.
   **Clinical:** Tsri or Xi-Cleft point to unblock Stomach energy. One of the four "knee points" used for knee pain — use with SP-10, LR-8, GB-33 — also add ST-36 and SP-9. Stimulates Blood and QI circulation in Yang Ming. Also good for acute gastrointestinal disorders.

20. **ST-36 (Zusanli)**
    **Location:** One finger breadth lateral to the anterior border of the tibia, about on a level with the tibial crest. An open hand placed palm down on the knee with the finger distal will show the level of the point at the tip of the middle finger.
    **Clinical:** He point. Earth point on Earth meridian. Horary point. Lower uniting He point. One of the two largest and most important tonification and homeostatic points in the body. Use with LI-4 for tonification of Yang energy. Use for homeostasis of all endocrine and metabolic diseases. Used for all pain problems, especially for the abdomen. Use for all abdominal and respiratory problems.

21. **EX-33 (Lanwei)**
    **Location:** Two inches below ST-36.
    **Clinical:** Alarm point for all disease of the vermiform appendix, especially tender in acute appendicitis.

22. **ST-37 (Shangjuxu)**
    **Location:** Three inches below ST-36 in a hollow lateral to the edge of the tibia.
    **Clinical:** Lower uniting He Point of the Large Intestine. Excellent point for dysentery and diarrhea.

23. **ST-38 (Tiaokow)**
    **Location:** Five inches below ST-36.
    **Clinical:** Most important point for frozen shoulder. Stimulate while patient moves shoulder around.

24. **ST-39 (Xiajuxu)**
    **Location:** Three inches distal to ST-37, about halfway down the leg.
    **Clinical:** Lower uniting He point of Small Intestine. Used for all Small Intestine disorders. Disperse excessive Yang in the abdomen and lower extremities. Used for hot swellings, boils, and abscesses.

25. **ST-40 (Fenglong)**
    **Location:** One inch lateral to ST-38 over a muscle mass and in a hole.
    **Clinical:** Luo point — sends branch to Yuan point, SP-3. The Luo shunt to the Spleen is excellent to shunt Yang energy into Yin and to create movement in Stomach and Spleen. Excellent point for Dampness and Phlegm in the whole body.

26. **ST-41 (Jiexi)**
    **Location:** High on the dorsum of the foot between the tendons of extensor digitorum longus and hallicus longus, at the level of the tip of the lateral malleolus with the foot dorsiflexed.
    **Clinical:** Jing point. Fire point on Earth meridian. Mother point, tonification point. Good tonification point for Stomach organ and Yang Ming. Good point for depression. Used for local ankle pain and stiffness, foot drop, and local ulcers.

27. **ST-42 (Chongyang)**
    **Location:** On the highest part of the dorsum of the foot, in the depression between the second and third metatarsals.
    **Clinical:** Yuan point — receives channel from Luo, SP-4. Used for local problems and swollen face.

28. **ST-43 (Xiangu)**
    **Location:** In a depression distal to the junction of the 2nd and 3rd metatarsal bones.
    **Clinical:** Shu point. Wood point on Earth meridian. Strong point to bring excess Yang Ming activity. Especially sedating if used with ST-44. Used for agitation, insomnia, night sweats, and nightmares. Used for headache and redness of face or eyes.

29. **ST-44 (Neiting)**
    **Location:** Between 2nd and 3rd phalanges, half an inch proximal to the web margin.

**Clinical:** Ying point. Water point on Earth meridian. Reduces Heat and inflammation in Yang Ming. Used for toothache, abdominal pain and distention, enteritis, and diarrhea of the hot type. Used in combination with ST-43 for strong Yang Ming sedation. This is the best analgesic point for the lower leg.

30. **ST-45 (Lidui)**
   **Location:** Lateral nail angle of the second toe.
   **Clinical:** Jing-Well (Ting) point. Metal point on Earth meridian. Son point, sedation point. Departure point for Yang TMM of leg, gathering at SI-18. Discharges Yang Ming pathogenic Heat. Used for epistaxis, trismus, tonsillitis, and insomnia. Use with SP-1 in patients who are unable to move in their dreams.

## The Tai Yin Energy Subcircuit

The Tai Yin subcircuit is composed of the two meridians that are most connected with the production of nourishing energy or Rong Qi — the Lung (Metal) and the Spleen (Earth) meridian. Besides bodily Qi, the Spleen is important for containing the Blood in the vessels, controlling bodily water metabolism, and keeping and supporting the organs in their places and the digestive process functioning. The Lung facilitates the supply of moisture to the skin and opens to the nose. Its energy flows downwards to the Kidneys which grasp the Lung Qi. The physical and superficial bodily manifestations are more seen in their Yang pairs — Large Intestine and Stomach.

*Lung (LU)*

Lung is the most delicate of all the organs. It is the one most invaded by Exterior Evils such as virus or bacteria. Channel structural symptoms are minimal and consist of some intercostal pains in the upper chest. Energy-functional symptoms run the full gamut of lung and skin manifestations (skin being classified as the third lung), including sore throats and colds, chronic cough, being short of breath, allergic skin and respiratory problems, canker sores, dry skin, and eczema and psoriasis. More dense organ problems include emphysema, chronic bronchitis, and atelectasis.

**Anatomical Course:** The Lung meridian starts in the area of the first intercostal space below the acromion (LU-1), runs to a depression immediately below the acromion (LU-2), courses over the shoulder and down the arm on the radial aspect of the biceps muscle (LU-3 and LU-4) to the antecubital crease (LU-5). It continues down the forearm along the radial edge of brachioradialis tendon (LU-6), along the radial groove (LU-7 to LU-9), across the thenar eminence (LU-10) to the radial nail angle of the thumb (LU-11).

## Acupuncture Points of the Lungs (LU)

Number of Points: 11
Related organ: Large Intestine (LI)
Element: Metal
Sense organ: Nose, sense of smell
Active Time: 3 to 5 A.M.
Alarm — Mu Point: LU-1
Shu Point: BL-13 (T-3)

1. **LU-1 (Zhongfu)**
   **Location:** In the first intercostal space below the acromial extremety of the clavicle, one inch below LU-2.
   **Clinical:** Mu point. Access point for distinct meridian of the Lung–Large Intestine. The main point for treatment of Lung organ diseases such as cough, dyspnea, bronchitis, pneumonia, asthma, and COPD. Also used for local and shoulder pain if tender. Used for the vocal cords, postoperative intubation trauma. Also used for depression and sadness. Do not needle too deeply — underlying Lung tissue is susceptible to pneumothorax.

2. **LU-2 (Yunmen)**
   **Location:** In the depression immediately below the acromial extremity of the clavicle.
   **Clinical:** Is used interchangably with and is more useful than LU-1.
3. **LU-3 (Tianfu)**
   **Location:** On the upper arm, three inches below the end of the axillary fold, on the radial border of biceps.
   **Clinical:** Window of the Sky point.
4. **LU-5 (Chize)**
   **Location:** On the antecubital crease, on the radial side of the biceps tendon, with arm slightly bent.
   **Clinical:** He point. Water point on Metal meridian. Son point, sedation point. Good Lung energy point for asthma, cough, dyspnea, and sore throat. Used for local elbow pain and anterior shoulder pain. Used for skin disorders.
5. **LU-6 (Kongzui)**
   **Location:** On the palmar aspect of the forearm, on a line joining LU-9 and LU-5, just a little more proximal than midway to LU-5.
   **Clinical:** Tsri or Xi-Cleft point for acute lung problems and blockage along the LU meridian. Good point for homeopuncture of viral and bacterial nosodes in acute viral and bacterial infections. The point will be tender.
6. **LU-7 (Lieque)**
   **Location:** Proximal to the styloid process of the radius, two finger breadths above the wrist crease. When the index fingers and thumbs of both hands are interlocked, the point is under the tip of the upper index finger.
   **Clinical:** Luo point — sends branch to Yuan point, LI-4. Master point of Ren Mo and coupled point of Yin Qiao Mo. Central energy point to tonify Lung and total body energy. Can be used with LU-9 for extra tonification. Also used for occipital headache and stiff neck, pain along back of chest, and all Lung disorders. Because it is the Luo point and shunts energy in to the Large Intestine meridian, it can be used for any problem along the LI line. Used with moxibustion in De Quervain's disease.
7. **LU-8 (Jingqu)**
   **Location:** One inch above the transverse crease of the wrist, in the depression on the radial side of the artery.
   **Clinical:** Jing point. Metal point on Metal meridian. Horary point.
8. **LU-9 (Taiyuan)**
   **Location:** At the transverse crease of the wrist, in the depression on the radial side of the radial artery.
   **Clinical:** Shu point. Earth point on Metal meridian. Mother point, tonification point. Yuan point — receives Luo branch from LI-6. Roe, Hui, or influential point for vascular system including arteriosclerosis, intermittent claudication, and endarteritis. Will settle jumpy and erratic pulses with a simple in and out piqure. Good point for palpatations, systolic hypertension. Strong point to tonify Lung energy. Used for local wrist problems.
9. **LU-10 (Yuji)**
   **Location:** On the thenar prominence at the midpoint of the first metacarpal bone, on the red–white border.
   **Clinical:** Ying point. Fire point on Metal meridian. Good for dispersing Fire in the Lung and anywhere along the Lu line.
10. **LU-11 ( Shaoshang)**
    **Location:** Radial nail angle of the thumb.
    **Clinical:** Jing-Well (Ting) point. Wood point on Metal meridian. Departure point for Yin TMM of arm that gathers at GB-22. Used for all throat disorders. Bleed to create a sweat and break fever or in febrile convulsions.

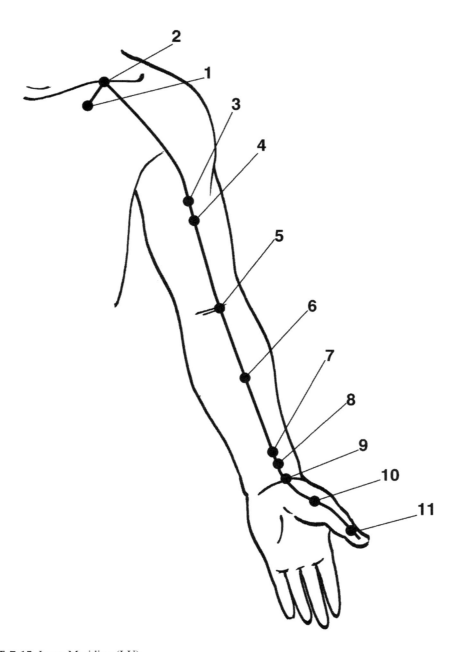

**FIGURE 7.15** Lung Meridian (LU).

*Spleen (SP)*

The Spleen is the most functionally Yin of all the organs. According to tradition, the Spleen functions include those of the pancreas (humeral digestive system) and the reticuloendothelial system of Western medicine. Traditionally, the Spleen is said to regulate Water, Fluid, and Blood metabolism, to influence the skeletal muscles, and to nourish the lips and the tongue. The Spleen keeps the Blood in the vessels, holds up the organs, and prevents them from prolapsing. The Spleen is home of thought and influences concentration and learning.

Most Spleen disorders are deficiency states that manifest as fatigue, lassitude, pale lips and complexion, loss of taste and appetite, abdominal fullness and bloating, abdominal pain, and diarrhea. If there is excess Spleen Damp, then Phlegm will form with chronic catarrh in the nose, sinuses, and Lung. Phlegm can further congeal and form masses, such as fibrocystic disease of the breasts and fibroids. The inability to hold the Blood in the vessels will lead to hemorrhages, petechiae, melena, hematemesis, and menorrhagia. If the supporting function of the Spleen is lacking, then prolapse of any organ can take place. The Spleen is important in metabolism and will show disorders of glucose metabolism if deficient.

Channel–structural symptoms are seen as heavy thighs and calves with extremity edema or knee pain.

**Anatomical Course:** The Spleen meridian starts at the Yin nail angle of the hallux (SP-1), travels along the medial side of the foot from the metatarsophalangeal joint (SP-2), proximal to head of first metatarsal (SP-3), in a depression distal to the base of the first metatarsal (SP-4) to a depression distal and inferior to the medial malleolus (SP-5). From there it courses up the medial side of the leg on the posterior tibial border (SP-6 to SP-8) to the lower border of the medial condyle of the tibia (SP-9). It crosses medial to the knee and ascends the medial aspect of the thigh (SP-10 and SP-11) to the inguinal ligament (SP12). It runs up the anterior abdominal wall four inches lateral to the midline (SP-13 to SP-15) to hit the costal margin (SP-16). It then travels six inches from the midline, lateral to the nipple line (SP-17 to SP-19) to the second intercostal space (SP-20), and descends inferiorly and laterally to a point in the midaxillary line midway between the axilla and the costal margin (SP-21).

**Acpuncture Points of the Spleen (SP)**

Number of Points: 21
Related organ: Stomach (ST)
Element: Earth
Sense organ: Mouth
Active Time: 9 to 11 A.M.
Alarm — Mu Point: LR-13 (11th rib)
Shu Point: BL-20 (T-11)

1. **SP-1 (Yinbai)**
   **Location:** Medial nail angle of the hallux.
   **Clinical:** Jing-Well (Ting) point. Wood point on Earth meridian. Departure point for Yin TMM of the leg gathering at CV-2. Used in acute emergencies such as fainting and collapse; used also in abdominal distention and nausea.
2. **SP-2 (Dadu)**
   **Location:** Medial side of hallux, distal to the first metatarophalangeal joint at the red–white border.
   **Clinical:** Ying point. Fire point on Earth meridian. Mother point, tonification point. Good, but painfull, tonification point used with SP-3. Moves energy of the Spleen. Used for abdominal pain, bloating, and diarrhea. Used for ADHD, inattentive type.
3. **SP-3 (Taibai)**
   **Location:** On the medial side of the foot, proximal and inferior to the head of the first metatarsal bone at the red–white border.
   **Clinical:** Shu point. Earth point on Earth meridian. Horary point. Yuan point — receives Luo branch from ST-40. Used to tonify Spleen together with SP-2 and used clinically for abdominal distention, pain and diarrhea, menstrual disorders, and hemorrhoids.

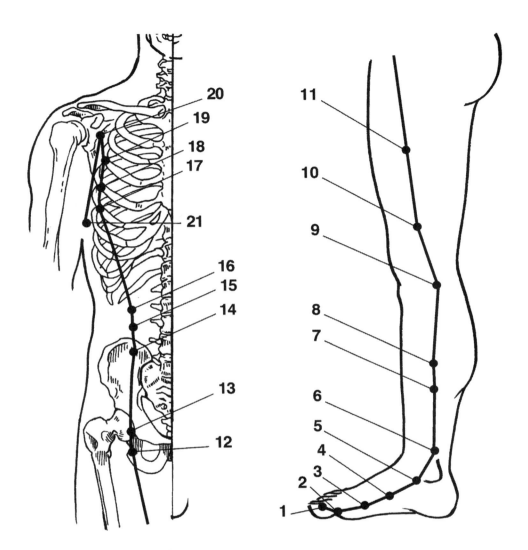

**FIGURE 7.16** Spleen Meridian (SP).

4. **SP-4 (Gongsun)**
   **Location:** On medial side of the foot, in a depression distal to the base of the first metatarsal bone.
   **Clinical:** Luo point — sending branch to Yuan point, ST-42. Master point of Chong Mo and coupled point of Yin Wei Mo. Used for its connection with Chong Mo for endocrine, gynecological, and fertility problems. Also used for disorders of the Stomach, such as dyspepsia and gastritis, because it shunts Spleen energy into the Stomach. Also used for constipation and diarrhea.

5. **SP-5 (Shangqiu)**
   **Location:** At the point of intersection of the two lines drawn tangential to the distal and inferior sides of the medial malleolus.
   **Clinical:** Jing point. Metal point on Earth meridian. Son point, sedation point. Used for local ankle pain and arthritis as well as gastritis, enteritis, diarrhea, and constipation. Good for venous stasis and varicose veins.

6. **SP-6 (Sanyinjiao)**
   **Location:** Three inches directly above the tip of the medial malleolus on the posterior border of the tibia.
   **Clinical:** One of the most important points in the body. All the Yin meridians of the leg meet at this point (SP, KI, LR). This is a major point for Yin tonification in the body. Also used for inside–outside equilibration with GB-38. Used for all menstrual, genital, urinary, reproductive, and gastrointestinal problems. General tonification point for CFIDS and all immunlogical disorders. Major point to induce labor with GB-21. Do not use during pregnancy except to induce labor. Good point for chronic venous stasis ulcers of the leg, which usually are associated with this area.

7. **SP-8 (Di ji)**
   **Location:** Three inches below SP-9 on the posterior border of the tibia.
   **Clinical:** Tsri or Xi-Cleft point. Used for acute disorders due to acute blockage of the digestive system. Used also for menorrhagia, dysmenorrhea, and urinary problems.

8. SP-9 (Yinlingquan)
   **Location:** On the medial side of the leg, in the depression below the lower border of the medial tibial condyle, between the tibia and gastrocnemius.
   **Clinical:** He point. Water point on Earth meridian. Strong Tai-Yin and Spleen tonification point. For all knee pain together with ST-34, ST-36, GB-33, SP-10, and LR-8. Also excellent point for edema, ascites, and swelling of lower extremities.

9. **SP-10 (Xuehai)**
   **Location:** Two inches above the mediolateral border of the patella with the knee flexed, on the highest point of vastus medialis.
   **Clinical:** Excellent immune and allergy point. Used for all allergies, pruritis, menstrual, gynecological, and urinary disorders.

10. **SP-12 (Chongmen)**
    **Location:** On the lateral side of the femoral artery, superior to the inguinal ligament, at the level of the pubic symphysis, 3.5 inches lateral to CV-2.
    **Clinical:** Access point to the Spleen–Stomach distinct meridian. Useful for all postoperative abdominal problems including edema and bloating. Used with electroacupuncture (30 Hz to 100 Hz) for sinus congestion together with ST-30 as lower negative pole to positive upper pole at ST-2/3, LI-20, or BL-2. Also used for local inguinal problems, orchitis, endometriosis, and postpartum hemorrhage.

11. **SP-15 (Daheng)**
    **Location:** Four inches lateral to the umbilicus, on the lateral edge of rectus abdominus.
    **Clinical:** Used for Large Intestine problems together with ST-25.

12. **SP-21 (Dabao)**
    **Location:** On the mid-axillary line six inches below the axillary crease in the sixth intercostal space.
    **Clinical:** Great Luo vessel of the Spleen. Many vessels flow into the sides of the chest from this point and join the Luo vessels of the rest of the body. Used for patient with pain all over the body (disperse the point). Used also for general weakness, respiratory disorders, chest pain, dyspnea, and digestive disorders.

## Extra Acupuncture Points (EX)

These points were discovered or added later than the points of the prinicipal meridians. Only the most important ones will be described.

1. **EX-1 (Yintang) (Du-24.5) (M-HN-3)**
   **Location:** Between the eyebrows at the root of the nose.

Clinical: Access point for Sixth Chakra. Used for sinusitis, rhinitis, and frontal headaches.

2. **EX-2 (Taiyang) (M-HN-9)**
Location: On the temple, in a depression one inch directly posterior to the midpoint of a line connecting the outer point of the eyebrow with the outer canthus of the eye.
Clinical: Headache, migraine (behind the eyes), eye disorders, facial paralysis, trigeminal neuralgia, frontal sinusitis, and toothache.

3. **EX-6 (Sishencong) (M-HN-1)**
Location: These are four points situated like a cross on the vertex, one inch anterior, posterior, and lateral to GV-20.
Clinical: Used with GV-20 in tonification to relieve depression and in dispersion to relieve mania.

4. **EX-17 (Dingchuan) (M-BW-1a)**
Location: Half an inch lateral to GV-14 at level of T-1.
Clinical: Very effective point for calming acute asthma.

5. **EX-21 (Huatuojiaji) (M-BW-35)**
Location: A series of 28 points situated half an inch lateral to the lower border of the spinous processes, on either side of the ligament attaching the transverse processes of the vertebral column from T-1 to L-5.
Clinical: Used to reinforce the Shu point (organ point) at the same level, as well as axial pain and segmental pain radiation. A number of points are used bilaterally at any one time to influence a region of the body:

| | |
|---|---|
| Upper Limbs | T-1 through T-7 |
| Chest | T-3 through T-9 |
| Abdomen | T-5 to L-5 |
| Lower Limbs | T-11 to L-5 |
| Genito Urinary | S-1 to S-4 |

6. **EX-28 (Baxie) (M-UE-22)**
Location: On the back of the hand with the fist clenched, in the midpoints of the finger webs (four in each hand).
Clinical: Circulatory and pain disorders in the hand and fingers.

7. **EX-32 (Xiyan) (M-LE-16)**
Location: The "Eyes of the Knees." Located in the depression medial and lateral to the patellar ligaments. Also called ST-35.
Clinical: Used for knee pain.

8. **EX-33 (Lanwei) (M-LE-13)**
Location: Two inches below ST-26.
Clinical: Mu-Alarm point of the appendix. Used for appendicitis and postoperative appendectomy pain.

9. **EX-35 (Dannang) (M-LE-23)**
Location: One inch distal to GB-34.
Clinical: Mu-Alarm point for the Gall Bladder on the leg.

10. **EX-36 (Bafeng) (M-LE-8)**
Location: The equivalent on the feet of the Baxie points on the hands, with the same indications.
Clinical: Circulatory and pain disorders in the feet and toes.

11. **M-UE-19 (Yaotongdian)**
Location: On the dorsal surface of the hand, between the 2nd, 3rd, 4th, and 5th metacarpal bones, at the last access to the muscle between the bones.
Clinical: Used with GV-26 for calming acute back spasm or neck spasm.

## Ah Shi Points

**Location:** Any area on the body that is spontaneously painful or tender on palpation is called an Ah Shi or "ouch point" and is in need of needling. Most points are not on a channel, but some may be.

**Clinical:** Many of these points over the musculature would be referred to as trigger points and some may even be motor points. If an area is painful, put a needle into it.

### Mu Subsystem of Points

The Shu-Mu subsystem of acupuncture points allows access to both the five Zang, Yin organs (KI, LR, SP, LU, and HT), and the five Fu, Yang organs (BL, GB, ST, LI, and SI). They are very versatile and can be used in many different ways: to focus another acupuncture input on a particular organ or organs; to directly treat the organs themselves and to generally tonify or disperse a functional organ group.

**Back — Shu Points:** The *back Shu points* are *twelve acupuncture points* located on the inner Bladder channel as it runs bilaterally down the back, 1.5 inches lateral to the inferior border of each spinous process, in the erector spinae muscles. These points extend from the level of T-3 (BL-13, GV-12) to S-2 (BL-26, GV-2). Each Shu point represents the entire neurological input and output at that spinal level: the dermatome, myotome, sclerotome (fascia), paravertebral ganglia, neural ganglia and plexi, and the splanchnotome. Each Shu point corresponds to a single Zang or Fu organ (Figure 7.17 and Table 7.1).

The *Shu*, or "transport points," are exquisitely sensitive to any blockage of energy (flow of Qi) going to or from their associated organs. If there is a blockage of Qi, then the Shu point becomes swollen and tender to palaption and causes its local myotome to become irritable and spastic and exhibit allodynia (tenderness over motor points), and the overlying skin to become trophedemic and hyperpathic. The "Peau D'Orange" effect and matchstick test for subcutaneous fluid stagnation may be positive in the affected segment.

The Yin diseases are said to move to the back (Yang), and so the Shu points are more important in influencing the solid, Yin, or Zang organs and are more useful in energy rather than functional problems.

**Front — Alarm — Mu Points:** The 12 Mu points are located on the ventral aspect of the body and are accessed by either the Conception Vessel (6) or by one of the Principal Meridians (3 on their

---

## TABLE 7.1
## Shu-Mu Subsystem

| Shu Point | Vertebral Level | Organ | Mu Point |
|-----------|-----------------|-------|----------|
| BL-13 | T-3 | Lung | LU-1 |
| BL-14 | T-4 | Pericardium | CV-17 |
| BL-15 | T-5 | Heart | CV-14 |
| BL-18 | T-9 | Liver | LR-14 |
| BL-19 | T-10 | Gall Bladder | GB-24 |
| BL-20 | T-11 | Spleen | LR-13 |
| BL-21 | T-12 | Stomach | CV-12 |
| BL-22 | L-1 | Triple Heater | CV-5 |
| BL-23 | L-2 | Kidney | GB-25 |
| BL-25 | L-4 | Large Intestine | ST-25 |
| BL-27 | S-1 | Small Intestine | CV-4 |
| BL-28 | S-2 | Bladder | CV-3 |

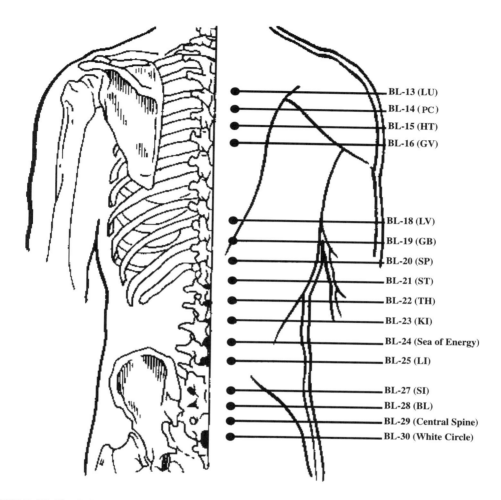

**FIGURE 7.17** Shu Points.

own meridian, 3 on another meridian). As Mu means "to collect," each point represents a concentration of the energy of the associated organ. The Mu points are used more in functional disturbances of the Yang, Fu, or hollow organs. The organs and their Mu points are shown in Figure 7.18..

**Use of the Shu-Mu Subsystem:** Information from the organs travels to and from the Shu-Mu points. Thus, these points will show early signs of organ dysfunction if they are palpated and exhibit tenderness. They can then be used therapeutically to treat that disturbance. They can be used alone, in combination, or as an initial preparatory tonifying treatment, a simultaneous focusing treatment, or a reinforcing treatment. When in doubt, use a Shu point.

Generally you will be tonifying Shu points (Yin deficiency) and dipersing Mu points (Yang excess). Occasionally, you can use the two together to tonify a Yin organ. If this is done, then the electrical hookup is to create the electron flow from Mu point (negative, black lead) to the Shu point (positive, red lead).

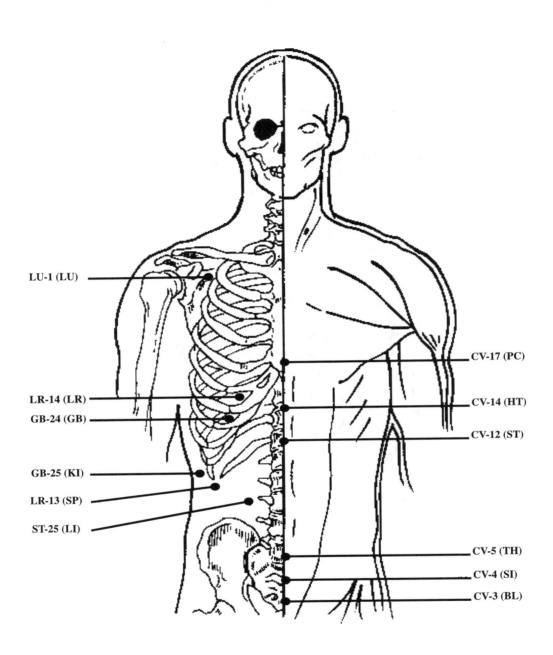

**FIGURE 7.18** Mu Points

In patients with poor resistence, chronic disease, or prolonged fatigue, an excellent treatment is to do a "winterizing" treatment utilizing the Shu points of LR at BL-18 (T-9), KI at BL-23 (L-2), LI at BL-25 (L-4), and SI at BL-27 (S-1). Tonify your input with moxa or use a Heat lamp. This will tonify the Wei Qi of the patient and improve the overall immunity, especially at the change of the seasons. A similar Mu point treatment would utilize CV-4, CV-7, CV-10, CV-12, and CV-13.

## THE DISTINCT MERIDIAN SUBSYSTEM

The *Distinct Meridian (DM) subsystem* is another means to access the organs via acupuncture points on the principal meridians. This access is different from the Shu–Mu system, in that the organs accessed are coupled in Yin–Yang organ pairs and the problems addressed are not those of an energetic or functional nature. The Distinct Meridian pairs are used to influence the course of gross pathological changes in organs. The connection of the Yin channels to the facial area is provided by use of the Distinct meridians, because there are no Yin channels in the head region.

Each Yin and Yang pair starts at the Principal Meridian *access point*, which is usually contiguous to and located near a major joint, and proceeds to its associated organ. There the Yin and Yang energy mingles and exits the organ as a single energy line to be extracted at a superior Yang principal meridian *return point*. The area to be treated is highlighted with local needles or the use of the Shu–Mu system. The direction of energy flow, especially in the Yang energy, will sometimes be counter to the flow of the employed Yang meridian. This is accomplished, as it is in the TMMs, by internal channels. The whole treatment is one of Yin to Yang — from the bottom to the top and from the inside to the outside.

The order of activation of the distinct meridians is: Needle the Yin and Yang access points bilaterally; needle the superior Yang return point bilaterally and; focus the intention of the input by the use of appropriate local needles or use of the Shu-Mu system. One can also needle the TMM gathering point of the involved Yin and Yang organs to reinforce the treatment. This is done on the contralateral side to a single organ and bilaterally to a paired organ.

Although the Distinct Meridian activates both organs in the Yin–Yang pair, it is the general area of activation that is most important, and not which of the two organs needs to be treated. Because most of the uses for this technique relate to dense pathology, the Distinct Meridian can be used prior to or in conjunction with conventional drug therapy or with surgery or, in chronic refractive cases, as an alternate treatment to regular therapy.

Because of the dense material nature of the organ problems addressed, a very intense input is needed to change the dense physical pathology. This usually necessiates the use of eletricity. In electroacupuncture of the Distinct Meridians, the two lower Yin–Yang needles are crossed (they are usually close to each other) and the negative, black lead is attached to them. The positive, red lead is attached either to the focusing local needles or to the focusing local needles and the Yang return point, if that is physically feasible. Energy tonification of the system (chronic problems, even if Yang in nature, and in old or depleted individuals) utilizes low frequencies from 2 to 4 Hz, while acute lesions (spasm, heat, inflammation, or intense pain) need energy movement and utilize high frequency pulses between 70 and 100 Hz. Generally speaking, Yin conditions need electricity, while Yang conditions need a neutral needle technique. Usually, DM treatment should be used only once a week because of the intense stimulation afforded by this treatment.

There are 6 pairs of Distinct Meridians:

1. Kidney–Bladder Distinct Meridians
   **Access Points:** KI-10 + BL-40 (popliteal fossa)
   **Return Point:** BL-10 (nape of neck)
   **Territory of Influence:** Kidneys (BL-23), urinary bladder (BL-28), anorectal region (BL-35, lateral to tip of coccyx), descending colon (BL-25), coccyx (BL-35), uterus and prostate (BL-30), and the anterior surface of the sacrum and vertebral column (Ah Shi points).
   **Clinical:** This couplet is the most effective and versatile of the DMs.
   • *Colon–Rectum–Anus:* Spastic colon, IBS, colitis, diarrhea, internal and external hemorrhoids, and anal fissures.
   • *Urinary Tract:* Pyelonephritis, chronic and interstitial cystitis, nephrolithiasis, urethritis, chronic prostatitis, and incontinence.

- *Uterus and Ovary:* Endometriosis, pelvic adhesions, and posterior wall pelvic pain.
- *Coccyx–Spine:* Coccygeal and deep axial back pain refractory to treatment.

2. Spleen–Stomach Distinct Meridians
   **Access Points:** SP-12 + ST-30 (pubic symphysis and inguinal ligament)
   **Return Point:** ST-1 (under eye) (or BL-1 — patients do not like it!)
   **Territory of Influence:** Pelvic (GB-26, GB-27, and GB-28 — CV-2 and CV-3) and abdominal cavities (CV-4 [SI Mu point], CV-5 [TH Mu point], CV-6, CV-7 [lower Heater], CV-10, CV-12 [Middle Heater and ST Mu point), ST-25 [LI Mu point], LR-13 [SP Mu point]; esophagus (CV-15), tongue, nose, and maxillary (LI-20, ST-2 and ST-3), and frontal (Yin Tang and BL-2) sinuses.
   **Clinical:** Very versatile input for the pelvis, abdomen, and sinuses. It can be activated for any visceral pain in the abdomen.
   - *Uterus–Ovary:* Pelvic adhesions, pelvic cramping and pain, endometriosis, and pelvic floor pain.
   - *GI System:* Abdominal pain and cramps, bloating, postoperative ileus, post abdominal surgery pain, gastritis, gastric or duodenal ulcer pain, esphageal pain from spasm or reflux. Electrical stimulation can be used in the abdomen for sluggish GI function, but when in doubt, start with no electricity in the abdomen, because too vigorous stimulation will aggravate an excess Yang condition.
   - *Sinuses:* Frontal and maxillary sinusitis and congestion after treatment failure with the principal meridians. Most sinus treatments requires high frequency (70 to 100 Hz) electrical stimulation. Cross the SP-12 and ST-30 needles for the negative, black lead and either BL-2, ST-2-3, or LI-20 for the positive, red leads. Turn up the current until the electricity can be felt in the face.

3. Liver–Gall Bladder Distinct Meridians
   **Access Points:** LR-12 (inguinal ligament) + GB-30 (buttocks)
   **Return Point:** GB-1 (lateral canthus of eye)
   **Territory of Influence:** The Liver (LR-14 [LR Mu point]), Gall Bladder (GB-24 [GB Mu point]), (CV-2 — intersection of LR and GB meridian), and the lateral abdominal region.
   **Clinical:** Not used as often, but has good efficacy on the hepato-biliary system. May be used in alternating treatment with the SP–ST DMs, with which there is some abdominal overlap. It may be used unilaterally as it is the only pair where both Yin and Yang organs are only on the right side.
   - *Liver–Gall Bladder:* All Liver disease including acute or chronic hepatitis, acute and chronic cholecystitis, postoperative atonic ileus and pain, especially after cholecystectomy. Electricity is seldom used except for chronic hepatitis where alternating tonification (low frequency 2 to 8 Hz) and movement (high frequency 70 to 100 Hz) should be used.

4. Lung–Large Intestine Distinct Meridians
   **Access Points:** LU-1 (anterior shoulder) + LI-15 (tip of shoulder)
   **Return Point:** LI-18 (lateral throat)
   **Territory of Influence:** The Lung and pleura (CV-16, CV-17, and CV-18; ST-14, ST-15, and ST-16; KI-24, KI-25, KI-26, and KI-27), larynx, vocal cords, and trachea (ST-9 — cross handles with LI-18 in electrical stimulation).
   **Clinical:** The most useful of the three upper torso distinct meridian couplets. having all of its activity directed at the lower respiratory tract and its supporting structures. Activity in this couplet is restricted to the Lung. The Large Intestine is better treated with the KI–BL, SP–ST, and LR–GB DMs.
   - *Lung:* Asthma, pneumonia, chronic bronchitis, COPD. Acute asthma is treated with neutral needle technique; acute bronchitis with a chronic background with electrical movement, while chronic respiratory disease is best tonified with electricity.

- *Pleura:* Pleuritis and rib fractures.
- *Larynx, Vocal Cords, Trachea:* Inflammation, edema and nodules of the vocal cords, laryngitis, postintubation inflammation, and edema of the larynx. Vocal cord and laryngeal problems are best treated with high frequency electrical movement stimulation — positive electrodes on the focusing points in the neck.

5. Heart–Small Intestine Distinct Meridians

    **Access Points:** HT-1 (axilla) + SI-10 (spine of scapula)

    **Return Point:** BL-1 (inner canthus of eye) — substitute ST-1 (under eye)

    **Territory of Influence:** Its range of influence is limited to the heart (CV-17 [PC Mu point] and CV-14 [Heart Mu point]), pericardium, and surroundings. It has no activity on the Small Intestine at all.

    **Clinical:** Do not use electricity; monitor very carefully. Do not leave needles in for more than 5 to 10 minutes, lest you deplete the patient's energy.

    - *Heart–Pericardium:* myocarditis, pericarditis, rhythm disturbances following open or closed cardiac invasive procedures.
    - *Ribs–Chest:* Pain in the ribs or pectoral region unrelated to the Heart.

6. Pericardium–Triple Heater Distinct Meridians

    **Access Points:** PC-1 (lateral chest wall) + TH-16 (below mastoid process)

    **Return Point:** GV-20 (vertex)

    **Territory of Influence:** The entire body. The PC represents the sympathetic nervous system and the TH the parasympathetic nervous system. Their deep pathways influence the body's autonomic and neurovegetative pathways. Focusing points are all the points of the conception vessel.

    **Clinical:** Most poorly defined and least utilized of the DMs. It is indicated in cases of autonomic dysregulation, when chaos reigns supreme in the body, without regulation or coordination. This may be seen as hyperventilation syndromes, somatiform conversion symptoms, chronic fatigue, nervous collapse, vertigo, hypoactive autonomic conditions occuring after anesthesia or illness, or when there is a total breakdown of the integration of the body, mind, and soul. Electricity is not used except if there is an associated depression (with a stable cardiac rhythm).

## SPECIAL POINT GROUPINGS

Some acupuncture points belong to one or more special groups that have a collective function or purpose. The most important of these are the Source–Yuan points, Connecting–Luo points, the Tsri or Cleft–Xi points, the Hui, Roe, or influentual points, points of the cerebral circulation, the lower and upper uniting He points, the Windows of the Sky points, the Horary points, and the five classical Command Shu points.

## LUO-YUAN SHUNTS

The *Source–Yuan and Connecting–Luo points* are extremity acupuncture points on the principal meridians that connect the Yin and Yang channels directly, and enable you to take a short cut and shift the energy from the Yang meridian in a couplet to the Yin meridian or vice versa. The two points are connected by the *Transverse Luo Vessel* which flows from the Luo point on one meridian to the Yuan point on its coupled meridian. This shunt is important for equilibrating the Rong Qi between the two coupled meridians. The Yuan and Luo points each have specific qualities when used individually.

    Yuan Point — The *Yuan or source point* serves as a reservoir of Qi produced in its associated organ. It is the best point to use in energy transfer or equilibration from the meridian to the organ or vice versa. The Yuan point can also tap into the original Yuan Qi from the Kidneys and is an important point to increase the supply of energy to, and to increase the metabolism of, its associated organ. The Yuan point can be acutely tender to palpation in a Yang excess pain, or deeply aching in a Yin deficiency state.

The Yuan point is always the same point on the Yin meridians, that is, the Shu point of the classical command points (Ting-Ying-Shu/Yuan-Jing-He, not the back Shu point). In the Yang meridians it is the point following the Shu point in the classical command points sequence (Ting-Ying-Shu/Yuan-Jing-He). The Yuan point has the same elemental quality as the meridian command point on which it resides: Yin = Earth and Yang = Wood.

Luo Point — The *Luo or connecting point* is important in activating the capillary network of energy vessels that nourishes the tissue between the principal meridians. This network fills out the interstices of the body and these channels are known as the *Luo vessels*. Each Luo point is responsible for activating the Luo channels connected to that particular principal meridian. Although not in a regular position in the command point sequence, the Luo point comes after the Ting and Shu points in the sequence of the command points and, as such, is responsible for stopping perverse outside invaders from entering the Luo capillary network and also from proceeding any more proximal in the principal meridian. Disturbances of the Luo capillary network produce superficial symptoms such as color and temperature changes in the extremities, weakness in the muscles, and stiffness in joints. They are also excellent in any tissue trauma, as is the area they drain.

The activity of the Yuan and Luo points is reinforced when both points on coupled meridians are used together. The *Luo-to-Yuan Shunt* can be used to accelerate energy in the same direction as the principal meridian flow, in the opposite direction, or simultaneously in both directions. If the pain is an excess condition (Yang) and occurs anatomically proximal to the Luo point, then open up the Luo-to-Yuan shunt to transfer the excess to the deficient meridian (Yin) and to drain the excess meridian (Yang). If the pain is anatomically distant to the Luo point, both the Yin and Yang organ Luo-to-Yuan shunts should be opened to allow perfusion of all the distal Luo capillaries through the obstructed area.

## ACCESSORY AND GROUP LUO POINTS

Three additional useful accessory Luo points are described: CV-15, GV-1, and SP-21. Ren Mo (CV) and Du Mo (GV) connect with each other through their CV-15 and GV-1 Luo points

CV-15 is the Luo point for the Conception Vessel, Ren Mo. It activates the Luo capillary network of the abdominal wall and visceral supporting structures.

*GV-1* is the Luo point of the Governor Vessel, Du Mo. It activates the Luo capillary network around the spinal column.

*SP-21* is the great Luo point of the Spleen and activates the Luo capillary network of the lateral and anterior thoracic wall, as well as all the Luo vessels of the body.

There are also a number of Group Luo points that allow Blood and Qi to flow between groups of channels. Each group Luo point connects three Yin and three Yang channels as a group to each other. These points are:

*TH-8* for the upper extremity Yang channels
*PC-5* for the upper extremity Yin channels
*GB-39* for the lower extremity Yang channels
*SP-6* for the lower extremity Yin channels

## TSRI OR XI–CLEFT POINTS

These points are palpated as clefts within the musculature and have no regular position within the Command point sequence. Usually they are in the middle of the leg or forearm. These points are acute indicators of energy (Qi and Blood) blockage in the meridian and will be tender in such instances. They are used to treat acute inflammatory and pain problems in the channel and stubborn organ problems. Because they are often within muscle, they are indicated in musculoskeletal pain problems.

## HUI, ROE, OR INFLUENTIAL POINTS

There are 8 points in the body where the Qi and Jing of 8 different tissues and functions converge. Each point is specific for influencing a single tissue, substance, or body function. They are not connected to any other system or the body's energy, but are used soley to influence their specific component. They may be used singly or in multiples as a single treatment, but usually they are used to reinforce another, more extensive therapeutic input.

The *Eight Influentual Hui or Roe Points* are:

1. *BL-11* for bone (all bones and joints)
2. *BL-17* for Blood — Xue (all Blood flow, menses, etc.)
3. *GB-34* for tendons (muscles and tendons)
4. *GB-39* for marrow (brain and spinal cord, cognitive issues)
5. *LR-13* for solid organs (Zang)
6. *CV-12* for hollow organs (Fu)
7. *LU-9* for system of vessels (all veins and arteries)
8. *CV-17* for energy (Qi)

## THE CEREBRAL CIRCULATION SUBSYSTEM

The three ascending Yin channels from the foot — the Kidney, Liver, and Spleen — continue their influence into the head and affect their associated sense organs and sphere of influence. The cerebral circulations represent focusing subroutines when dealing with disorders of the ear, eyes, and nose. The Kidney cerebral circulation affects the ears and hearing; the Liver cerebral circulation affects the eyes and vision; and the Spleen cerebral circulation affects the nose and olfaction. Access to these cerebral circulations is via points on these Yin meridians and the focusing points are those of their coupled Yang meridians.

1. Kidney Cerebral Circulation
   **Access Point:** KI-27 (sternoclavicular border)
   **Circuit:** K-27 to posterior pharynx, tonsils, optic chiasm (BL-10) — posterior pituitary — inner ear (SI-19).
   **Clinical:** Used as a focusing input, together with a principal meridian program, for all problems of the inner and middle ear and mastoid, including hearing problems, tinnitus, and vertigo. The pathway can also be used to address all acute and chronic viral, bacterial, or inflammatory processes of the ear and mastoid. In these situations, additional focusing points around the auricle include TH-17, TH-18, TH-20, and TH-21. In refractory cases the Kidney meridian can be tonified first with electricity (KI-3 negative lead to KI-27 positive lead) to charge up the meridian, and then you can propel that bolus of energy into the cerebral circulation by electrifying K-27 (negative lead) to SI-19 (positive lead). In all treatments it is important to adhere to the normal N → N+1 circuit in the Kidney–Bladder principal meridian subcircuit. The Kidney cerebral circulation is seldom used for posterior pituitary issues.
2. Liver Cerebral Circulation
   **Access Point:** LR-14 (mid-clavicular line, 6th intercostal space)

**Circuit:** From LR-14 to the optic chiasm — anterior pituitary (GB-20) — globe of the eye (GB-1).

**Clinical:** Influences the structure of the eye and all its problems including: all inflammatory processes; pain from inflammation, trauma, glaucoma, and eye surgery; refractory increased intraocular pressure and decreased intraocular pressure from traumatic puncture. Jue Yin is tonified with depleted Yin-type patients (LR-3 → LR-8), and movement into ShaoYang is done for excess conditions GB-34/GB-38). Preliminary acceleration along the Jue Yin circuit can be accomplished with electricity (LR-3 → LR-14), and then the extra charge can be further accelerated into the cerebral circuit using LR-14 (negative lead) to GB-1 (positive lead). Additional focusing points around the eye include BL-1, BL-2, and ST-1. These points can be used with the Liver cerebral circulation in acute iritis with all needles in neutral. The Liver–Gall Bladder subcircuit should adhere to the aims of the N → N+1 program. The anterior pituitary is only stimulated in a general program for endocrine tonification.

3. Spleen Cerebral Circulation

**Access Point:** SP-20 (second intercostal space, 6 inches lateral to midline).

**Circuit:** SP-20 to oro and nasopharynx — maxillary sinuses (ST-1) — olfactory bulb (BL-1). A third focusing point, ST-9 (over the hyoid bone) is also described. Yin Tang (EX-1) is also a focusing point for both olfactory and sinus problems.

**Clinical:** Used for central and medial sinusitis obstruction and for problems of partial or complete anosmia. The Tai Yin–Yang Ming energy input should not use SP-6 or SP-9 (too wide an influence and related to water movement, respectively). Rather SP-2 or SP-3 with SP-8 should be used on the Yin side and ST-36 and ST-40 on the Yang side for the N → N+1 program.

## UPPER AND LOWER HE POINTS

The *He point* is the most proximal member of the command point sequence on the extremity of each meridian. In addition to their own He points, the three Yang meridians of the arm have a coupled lower He point on the lower extremity. Needling of these two points creates a powerful influence on the hollow Yang Fu organ involved. This input is extremely invaluable for the treatment of gastrointestinal disturbances and can be used as a focusing subset in more comprehensive inputs.

These couplets are used with vigorous tonification, moxa, or electric tonification in intestinal deficiency. The He point couplets are:

*SI-18 and ST-39* for the Small Intestine
*LI-11 and ST-37* for the Large Intestine
*TH-10 and BL-39* for the Triple Heater

## WINDOWS OF THE SKY POINTS

The *Windows of the Sky points* represent 10 points around the head and neck that enable a free flow of Qi between the head and the trunk. If the flow of Qi is blocked in the neck area, as it often is, these points will relieve the blockage, and symptoms of excess in one area (usually head Yang excess) and deficiency in the other (usually body Yin deficiency) will be equalized. The ten points are grouped into major windows and minor windows according to their strength of action.

**Major Window Points:** ST-9, LI-18, LU-3, TH-16, BL-10.
**Minor Window Points:** SI-17, SI-16, CV-22, PC-1, GV-16.
**Clinical:** *ST-9* — deficiency in the head, excess in the body

*LI-18* — disperses excess wind in the head, aphonia, aphasia
*TH-16* — sudden hearing loss of local or central origin
*BL-10* — excess in the head, deficiency in the body
*LU-3* — great thirst and epistaxis, Yang excess

These points will be used mainly for deficient body symptoms: cold extremities, muscle cramps at night, hemorrhoids, variose veins, and weakness of legs and feet; and excess head symptoms: throbbing headache, red eyes, vertigo, tinnitus, insomnia, epistaxis, and anger. Deficiency symptoms in the head consist of mental confusion and lethargy, loss of concentration or memory, and neurological sequelae to cerebrovascular accidents.

## SPECIAL COMMAND POINTS

Four acupucture points have special command and influence over a particular regional area. These points are needled as part of an energetic input or as a reinforcing point. These points are:

LU-7 for the head and back of neck
LI-4 for the face and mouth
ST-36 for the abdomen
BL-40 for the upper and lower back

## POINTS OF THE FOUR SEAS

The twelve Principal meridians are said to flow into the seas. Each sea is a reservoir of either nourishment, Blood, Qi, or marrow. These points are able to balance excess or deficiency of these seas. They may be used alone to influence the seas, or as a focusing or reinforcing point in a more global input.

1. The Sea of Nourishment
   **Points:** ST-30 and ST-36
   **Clinical:**    Deficiency — loss of appetite
                    Excess — abdominal bloating
2. The Sea of Blood
   **Points:** BL-11 (upper body), ST-37, and ST-39 (lower body)
   **Clinical:** Influenced by Chong Mo.
                    Deficiency — general, vague malaise; apathy and emaciation
                    Excess — body feels heavy or expanded.
3. The Sea of Energy
   **Points:** CV-17, ST-9, BL-10, and GV-14.
   **Clinical:** Deficiency — weak, labored voice
                    Excess — pain in chest, dyspnea, and flushed face
4. The Sea of Marrow
   **Points:** Brain, spinal cord, and neurological function — GV-20/16.
   **Clinical:** Deficiency — vertigo, tinnitus, fainting, lassitude, and lower extremity pain
                    Excess — increased energy and sexual desire

## THE HORARY, PHASE, OR NATURAL POINT

These are points on the Principal meridians on the extremities; each has the same elemental designation as the meridian upon which it is located. For example KI-10 is the Water point on the Water meridian. This point brings out the elemental force of its organ and meridian.

**TABLE 7.2**
**Classical Shu points**

| Energy Axis | Meridian | Ting | Ying | Shu | Jing | He | Luo | Yuan | Tsri | Element |
|---|---|---|---|---|---|---|---|---|---|---|
| Tai Yin | LU | 11 | 10 | 9 | 8 | 5 | 7 | 9 | 6 | Metal |
| Yang Ming | LI | 1 | 2 | 3 | 5 | 11 | 6 | 4 | 7 | Metal |
| Yang Ming | ST | 45 | 44 | 43 | 41 | 36 | 40 | 42 | 34 | Earth |
| Tai Yin | SP | 1 | 2 | 3 | 5 | 9 | 4 | 3 | 8 | Earth |
| Shao Tin | HT | 9 | 8 | 7 | 4 | 3 | 5 | 7 | 6 | Fire |
| Tai Yang | SI | 1 | 2 | 3 | 5 | 8 | 7 | 4 | 6 | Fire |
| Tai Yang | BL | 67 | 66 | 65 | 60 | 40 | 58 | 64 | 63 | Water |
| Shao Yin | KI | 1 | 2 | 3 | 7 | 10 | 4 | 3 | 5 | Water |
| Jue Yin | PC | 9 | 8 | 7 | 5 | 3 | 6 | 7 | 4 | Fire |
| Shao Yang | TH | 1 | 2 | 3 | 6 | 10 | 5 | 4 | 7 | Fire |
| Shao Yang | GB | 44 | 43 | 41 | 38 | 34 | 37 | 40 | 36 | Wood |
| Jue Yin | LR | 1 | 2 | 3 | 4 | 8 | 5 | 3 | 6 | Wood |

## THE FIVE CLASSICAL SHU OR COMMAND POINTS

The five classical Command or Shu points are located on the Principal meridians on the extremities distal to the knee and the elbow.

These points are more superficial and, therefore, more easily accessible to acupuncture manipulation. These are the prime points that are used for energy balancing and to move the energy in the channels and their associated organs (Table 7.2).

The word *Shu* means to transport, and these five points relate to water metaphores, as the energy is likened to flowing water, coming from or flowing in:

1. **First Point** — Jing–Well or Ting point; a well. The energy needs to be drawn up to the surface; situated at tips of digits.
   **Element:** Yin meridians — Wood
                 Yang meridians — Metal
   **Clinical:** Used to prevent perverse energy from entering the meridian, hence it is used as access point for the tendinomuscular meridians (TMMs). Also used for acute emergencies.

2. **Second Point** — Ying point; a spring or babbling brook. The energy is shallow with minimal force; situated near the metatarsalphalangeal or metacarpalphalangeal joint.
   **Element:** Yin meridians — Fire
                 Yang meridians — Water
   **Clinical:** Used in energy movement programs, especially in pain problems when the meridian is blocked. It stops external Heat and Cold invasion into the principal meridian.

3. **Third Point** — Shu point; a large stream. Energy is substantial and directed, enough to influence the movement of energy in the whole channel; between the metatarsalphalangeal joint and the ankle or the metacarpalphalangeal joint and the wrist.

**Element:** Yin meridian — Earth

Yang meridian — Wood

**Clinical:** Good for tonifying the meridian energy flow and the organ, if the flow is low or stagnant. Very important point on all Yin channels. Used in combination with the Ting points to activate the tendinomuscular meridians to increase the Wei Qi and prevent the further penetration of perverse energy into the deeper recesses of the principal meridians, once the perverse energy has already invaded the principal meridian.

4. **Fourth Point** — Jing point; a wide deep, slow river. The energy here can influence the tissue surrounding the channel in the entire extremity; located proximal to the ankle or wrist.

**Element:** Yin meridian — Metal

Yang meridian — Fire

**Clinical:** This point is used for structural and channel problems around the point and the limb. It mobilizes obstructed energy in pain problems. Application of moxa on the Yin Jing points dispels Dampness from the muscles, bones, and joints.

5. **Fifth Point** — He point; a delta where the river unites with the sea. The energy goes deep here to influence the organ. The energy is less dynamic and the flow slower than the Jing point; situated at the knee or elbow.

**Element:** Yin meridian — Water

Yang meridian — Earth

**Clinical:** The He point is used to access the organ and influence the territory the meridian passes through getting to the organ. Whatever the origin of the organ problem, from within or without, this point is used to treat the organ.

## ACTIVATION OF THE PRINCIPAL MERIDIANS

The Principal meridians are the structural and energetic fabric that integrate the thought process and therapeutic plan in acupuncture. All the acupuncture subsets, including the Distinct meridians, tendinomuscular meridians, Curious meridians, cerebral circulation and Shu–Mu system, all use points on the Principal meridians to initiate their mode of action and activate their region of influence. However, the Principal meridians also have to be activated to move the Qi around and balance out their Yin–Yang couplets. The most logical therapeutic input that activates the energy flow in the channels of the Principal meridians is called the N → N+1 program (Figure 7.19).

### THE N → N+1 THERAPEUTIC INPUT PROGRAM

This program can be used on any Principal meridian circuit to accomplish any desired output. There appears to be a somewhat linear input and expected output utilizing this program. That is, the chaotic equilibrium is somewhat limited in the directions in which it can be coaxed.

The amount of stimulation and direction needed to perturb the system, and induce a change, is dependent on the initial state of the system, as we have discussed before. If the system is highly agitated or irritated, then a very small input, such as the insertion of a single needle into a subcircuit, producing local agitation, may be all that is necessary to set the new strange attractor. If there is not enough movement in the system for gentle coaxing, then two needles may be inserted at a distance from each other, one in the Yin arm meridian (LU) and one in the Yin leg meridian (SP) of a synergistic Yin subset such as Tai Yin; or one in the Yang arm meridian (SI) and one in the Yang leg meridian (BL) of a synergistic subset of Tai Yang. This may bring about enough local equilibrated agitation for the body to assume a new configuration. A similar input with two needles can be accomplished with one needle in the Yin meridian and one in the Yang meridian of a Yin–Yang couplet such as Liver and Gall Bladder. However, most of the time both of the above inputs do not encourage enough movement in the Principal meridians or the Qi is blocked along the meridian, and a more powerful and directed input is needed. In this dynamic input, called

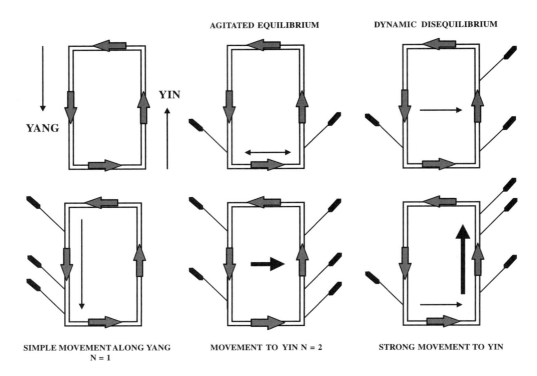

**FIGURE 7.19** N → N+1

N→ N+1, an odd number of needles is used to create a dynamic disequilibrium and to direct the flow downstream to the additional needle. N represents the number of needles used in a balanced input on each side of the equation, and then an additional needle is added to one side or the other (the +1) to direct and encourage flow along the meridian in the direction of the odd needle. The odd needle is placed downstream from the normal flow of the meridian. The two sides of the equation can be a Yin meridian of the leg and a Yin meridian of the arm, a Yang meridian of the leg and a Yang meridian of the arm, a Yin and Yang pair of the upper extremities, or a Yin and Yang pair of the lower extremities. One can even cross sides and do a Yin meridian of the arm on one side and a Yang meridian of the leg on the other side of the body.

The N → N+1 needle input stimulates Qi and Blood to circulate in the Principal meridians through obstructed areas caused by pathological changes. In addition to channel structural problems, the N → N+1 input can be used to address dense organ and energy-functional problems. Increasing the Blood and Qi into the region of influence and to the organ itself may be enough to afford a new equilibrium and for healing to ensue. Additional therapeutic intent is managed by the number and placement choice of the "N" needles. The art of acupuncture resides in selecting the most appropriate number and positioning of needles for the patient and the problem. Many different issues are raised with the selection of acupuncture points, and these will be addressed in the section under patient evaluation and acupuncture treatment.

## THE FIVE ELEMENTS OR PHASES PARADIGM

In the discussion of how to diagnose in TCM, one of the ways of looking at a patient was termed the *Five Elements*. This concept, which ruled supreme at one time in China, is important because it allows an understanding of the psycho-energetic-physiological interface and the integrational nature of TCM. Although the Principal meridians and the associated subcircuits and special points will deal with most common clinical problems, the more complex and layered cases require a more nonlinear, fractal construct to solve the therapeutic problem. The Five Element paradigm is an excellent fractal structure in which to place these complex and difficult patients. One can take the clustered information of the Six Axes and place it in the Five Phases or Elements without much difficulty.

The *Five Element paradigm* takes man, nature, and the cosmos and organizes them in an integrated sense into five organizing biological "poles" or recognizable clusters of behavioral energy that form naturally in the processes of biological generation and destruction. Each of the five organizing poles or phases clusters a collection of correspondences that are particular for each pole. The correspondences include, but are not limited to: cardinal directions, seasons, solid and hollow organs, sensory functions, characteristics of voice, seasons, odors, flavors, colors, emotions, electrolytes, neurotransmittors, and immunoglobulins. The interaction among the organizing poles is a model of nonlinear dynamics, within which each pole has elements of every other pole, much as a Water Principal meridian (KI) has Wood, Fire, Earth, and Metal elements as points within its Shu command points. Thus, the fractal nature of this system of self-repeating elements is revealed and its integrated relationships understood. The Five Elements, the most important identifiers of the correspondences, are Wood, Fire, Earth, Metal, and Water. Each of these elements embodies a cluster of symptoms, likes and dislikes, good and bad emotions, hand shape, body morphology, and other patient characteristics that enable the physician to more or less pigeonhole the patient to a position of "imbalance" (his own chaotic choice), in one or at the most two poles of chaotic patterns of existence. These poles of existence are important clinical metaphors for understanding strengths and weaknesses in the patient profile, in order to construct a treatment plan and predict future pathological trends in the patient.

These poles are positioned in a circle with five poles situated around the circumference of a clock face, each indicated by the cardinal point and its element: South — Fire at 12:00, Center — Earth at 12:12, West — Metal at 12:24, North — Water at 12:36, East — Wood at 12:48. Each elemental pole has its unique part of a system of multiple correspondences relating the patient to both the internal and external manifestations and influences that make up the composite biology called man (Table 7.3 and Fig. 7.20).

Because of the integrated nature of human biology these poles have two important fixed relationships, one called the *Sheng* or *generating cycle* and the other called the *Ko* or *control cycle*. These cycles describe the relationship between the elements, and, as seen in the Yin–Yang symbol, each element has representation of the other elements within it as predicted by the laws of fractal geometry.

## The Sheng Cycle

The *Sheng cycle* relates to the flow of Qi from one element to the other in a clockwise direction around the circle. The Chinese have viewed this generating cycle in a metaphorical sense: Fire is fed by Wood; the ashes become Earth; Metal is formed from the Earth; Water springs from the fluidity of Metal; and Water nourishes Wood, thus completing the cycle. In a practical sense, each of the elements is fed Qi by the element immediately preceding it. In fact, it turns out to be more efficacious to tonify the preceding element, the "Mother," in order to tonify any particular element, which is then the "Son" in terms of their energetic relationships. So, Water (KI–BL) is the Mother of Wood (LR–GB) and the Son of Metal (LU–LI) and so on. These elemental qualities were annotated on the Five Command Shu points as well as on each of the Principal meridians, in order to allow selection of these points in N → N+1 input protocols according to the quality of the point and its intention of use and action in the protocol. So, for instance, LR-2 is the Fire and Ying point on the Liver, a Wood meridian. If we inserted a needle in LR-2 and dispersed it, the Fire in the Liver would be weakened, and the Wood of Liver less susceptible to consumption by its son, the Fire element organs Heart, Small Intestine, Triple Heater, and Pericardium. The Sheng cycle

**TABLE 7.3**
**Five Elements Correspondences**

| Correspondence System | | **Five Phases** | | | |
|---|---|---|---|---|---|
| Element | Wood | Fire | Earth | Metal | Water |
| Direction | East | South | Center | West | North |
| Season | Spring | Summer | Harvest | Autumn | Winter |
| Yin Organ | Liver | Heart | Spleen | Lung | Kidney |
| Yang Organ | Bladder | S. Intestine | Stomach | L. Intestine | Bladder |
| Color | Blue/Green | Red | Yellow | White | Black |
| Flavor | Sour | Bitter | Sweet | Spicy | Salty |
| Voice | Shouting | Laughing | Singing | Sobbing | Moaning |
| Emotion | Anger | Joy/Mania | Worry | Grief | Fear |
| TCM | Sun | Shen | Yi | Po | Zhi |
| Sensory | Vision | Taste | Touch | Smell | Hearing |
| Evils | Wind | Heat | Dampness | Dryness | Cold |
| Opens to | Eyes | Tongue | Mouth/Lips | Nose | Ears |
| Fluid | Tears | Sweats | Aliva | Mucus | Urine |
| Indicator | Nails | Pulse | Flesh | Skin/Hair | Scalp Hair |
| Electrolyte | $K^+$ | Ph | $Mg^{++}$ | $Ca^{++}$ | $Na^{++}$ |
| Neurotx | A. Choline | Catechols | Glycine | Serotonin | Gaba |
| Immuno | Ig D | Ig E | Ig M | Ig A | Ig G |

propagates enhancing qualities that are evolutionary in nature. Most excess (acute disease) problems propagate in a clockwise direction, while most deficiency (chronic disease) problems propagate in a counterclockwise direction (reverse Sheng Cycle).

Practically speaking, we see patients with problems clustering around two or possibly three contiguous elements such as Kidney (Water) and Liver (Wood). Now, Kidney is the Mother of the Liver, which in turn is Kidney's Son. When patients show weakness in both organs, then it is better to tonify the Kidney, because it is the root of the problem and will feed energy into the Liver beause of its position in the Sheng cycle. A single tonification of the Kidney root will solve the entire problem.

## Ko Cycle

The *Ko cycle* is the controlling cycle. The rule of interaction in this cycle is that the elemental position two positions ahead of a given position along the clockwise sequence is controlled, or inhibited, by that given position. The controllers connect every other position and create a star pattern on the inside of the circle (Figure 7.20). The Ko cycle represents the balancing force for the Sheng cycle. The Chinese metaphor is again invoked where Wood at the east position controls the Earth by covering it with its forests; Earth controls Water at the north by damming it; Water controls Fire at the south by extinguishing it; and Fire controls Metal at the west by melting it. Pathological properties that are transformational in nature are generally propagated along the Ko sequence. In considering the Five Elements or Phases, each elemental position can generate energy to or control another position further along the circle.

In general, an exaggeration of the energetic activity or manifestation at one position can be propagated along either the Sheng or Ko cycle. Along the Sheng sequence, an energy deficiency propagates as a deficiency to its Son, and an energy excess propagates as an excess to its Son. Along the Ko sequence, an energy deficiency propagates as an energy excess (it cannot inhibit, because it is too weak) in its Grandson (two positions ahead). An energy excess, likewise, will cause an over-control on its Grandson, who will be weakened and show energy deficiency.

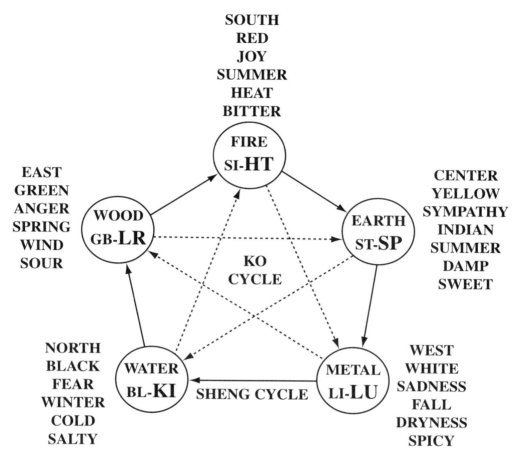

**FIGURE 7.20** Sheng and Ko Cycle.

So, you could needle a Fire point in dispersion (weakening it) to put out the "Fire," or you could needle a Water point in tonification (strengthen it) and let the stronger Water extinguish the Fire, or if very hot, you could do both. Selection of points in any acupunctural input should bear all these elemental qualities and Sheng and Ko relationships in mind.

### The Mother–Son Law

The *Mother–Son (or Child) Sequence* and its relationship to Tonification and Sedation points and Phase–Horary points: In a clockwise sequence, the element before an element is its "Mother" element and the element after the same element is its "Son" or "Child" element. For example, when considering the element Wood, Water is its "Mother" and Fire is its "Son" or "Child." Each Principal meridian and its attatched organ has an attached elemental quality — LR–GB are wood, TH/PC–HT/SI are Fire, SP–ST are Earth, LU–LI are Metal, and KI–BL are Water. When you want to use these elements as an acupunctural input, you usually use the Yin organ of the Yin–Yang meridian pair as the "operator" meridian (point to acupuncture) for both paired meridians. In the meridians, each of the five command–Shu points has an elemental designation. In the Yang meridians the Ting points are Metal and follow the circle around to designate the other elemental qualities to the remaining four points; in Yin meridians the Ting point is Wood and likewise the ensuing points follow the cycle around the circle. The point that is associated with the element that is the

"Mother" of that organ is, by definition of the "Mother–Son Law," the *tonification point* for that organ, for example, the Water point on the Liver meridian. The point that is associated with the element that is "Son" or "Child" to the element of a given meridian is considered the *sedation point* of that meridian. For example, the Fire point on the Liver meridian is its *sedation point*. In treatments, if the organ is deficient, tonify the "Mother"; if the organ is in excess, sedate the "Son" or "Child." You can accomplish either activity by treating the actual preceding or next organ, or by using the "Mother" point and "Son" point in the affected organ.

The *Phase point*, or natural point, or *Horary point* on a meridian is the point whose elemental designation is the same as that of the meridian on which it is located. The Fire point on a Fire meridian will accentuate the Fire quality of the acupuncture input.

### Four Needle Technique

A very sophisticated regulatory acupunctural input utilizing both Sheng and Ko cycles is called the *Four Needle Technique*. This input can be used as an initial input when the patient is strongly centered around one elemental pole and is showing clear excess or deficiency in that pole, or it can be used to attend to a single organ in a sequence of inputs or organ treatments. Always treat the most dysharmonious organ first. The golden rule of acupuncture holds true: "Tonify Yin and the Yang will follow." All excess comes out of a deficiency. So, even if you disperse an excess Yang organ, you will always end up tonifying a deficient Yin organ, so go to the root first and save yourself and your patient time and possible aggravation.

To tonify a deficient Yin or Yang organ of an element:

1. Tonify the Mother element (horary or phase point) of the organ that is the Mother to the affected element.
2. Tonify the Mother element (tonification point) of the organ of the affected element.
3. Sedate the controlling element (horary or phase point) of the organ that is the controlling element of the affected organ.
4. Sedate the controlling element (grandmother point) of the organ of the affected element.

To sedate an excess Yin or Yang organ of an element:

1. Sedate the Son element (sedation point) of the organ of the affected element.
2. Sedate the Son element (horary or phase point) of the organ that is the Son element to the affected element.
3. Tonify the controlling element (horary or phase point) of the organ that is the controlling element of the affected element.
4. Tonify the controlling element (grandmother point) of the organ of the affected element.

## THE CLINICAL PRACTICE OF ACUPUNCTURE

Acupuncture is the practice of inserting small needles into the human body to ellicit a change in balance or nudge the body into the right chaotic direction. All you have to do is insert the needles in the correct place for the right reason.

### THE NEEDLE

Preferences as to what type, gauge, and length of needle depends solely on practitioner preference and the clinical situation at hand. The needle is usually made with a shaft and pointed end of stainless steel (use of gold or silver needles is only for esoteric acupuncture) and a handle of dissimilar material to induce an electron shift into the body, much as a thermocouple, when the shaft is warmer and the handle cooler. Needle thickness is from 40 gauge (0.16 mm) to 26 gauge

(0.45 mm). Length varies from 0.5 inches (13 mm) to 6.0 inches (150 mm). All the needles that I use are disposable. Some practitioners give the patient his/her own needles to reuse every time the patient is seen, and some more elaborate and expensive needles are sterilized and resharpened. Disposable needles have more patient acceptance and safety. Small needles are used in the ear and scalp (0.5 inches, 32 gauge), intermediate needles used on the face and hands (1 inch, 30 gauge), large needles are used on the body (1.5 to 2.0 inches, 30 gauge), and extra-large needles (3.0 to 6.0 inches, 30 or 28 gauge) are used on obese and heavily muscled patients, especially around the buttocks (GB-30). Korean Hand Acupuncture has its own tiny needles and insertion device: a single needle inserter and one with a magazine of needles. Indwelling tacks covered with tape may be used on the ears. Indwelling body needles are not advised. Three-edged, bleeding needles are used to puncture and prick areas to encourage bleeding as a treatment. The *Plum Blossom Needle* is a little hammer with multiple small needles (5 or 7) on the hammer face that can be used either to fricasee hard and fibrosed muscles together with cupping or, in children or the weak, to tap the skin at acupuncture points.

Most practitioners use needles within a *guide tube* for easy insertion. The guide tube mouth, containing the needle point, is placed tight against the acupuncture point on the skin, and the top of the protruding needle is tapped sharply, which pushes the needle point painlessly into the skin to a depth of 2 mm. Additional manipulation or deeper needling is done manually with the guide tube removed. Aggressive, twirling insertions and vigorous manipulations are unneccessary. Needles are inserted in various manners and depths for different therapeutic purposes:

1. **Superficial Needling** — A small filiform needle is placed subcutaneously and energy is moved along the meridian by intent as used in Japanese Meridian Channel Therapy, or a small needle is used to peck in different directions over an irritable muscle group as in the Mark Seem superficial dispersion technique. Needles also may be threaded under the skin for a short distance when trying to influence more than one point, or if the anatomy demands more superficial needling, e.g., BL-1. Needling through the arm, for example, at PC-6/TH-5 is to be discouraged.

   Needling in tonification (for deficiency problems)
   • Use a gold needle.
   • Use thin needles.
   • Insert during inspiration.
   • Needle is angled in the direction of meridian energy flow.
   • Advance needle slowly into tissue after insertion.
   • Turn needle in a slow firm clockwise direction, not too deep.
   • Remove needle quickly and cover hole with finger.
   • Massage area to draw Qi up to the surface.
   • Use of electrical stimulation or moxa.

   Needling in dispersion (for excess problems)
   • Use a silver needle.
   • Use a thick needle.
   • Insert during expiration.
   • Needle is angled against the meridian energy flow.
   • Advance needle quickly and deeply after insertion.
   • Turn needle in a rapid counter-clockwise direction.
   • Needle is withdrawn slowly and the hole left open.

Practically speaking, if you are going to leave the needles in the patient for some time, and want to tonify the point, insert the needle, work it a little by lifting and thrusting with rotation in a pecking motion for 10 to 15 seconds and then leave the needle in for 10 minutes. The needle may be further worked for 10 seconds prior to extraction. If you want to disperse the point, insert the needle and leave it in for 30 minutes without touching it.

The needle is always advanced until you or the patient experiences that sensation of De Qi, or the arrival of Qi. This means that you have contacted the energy of the meridian and are now beginning to move it. I feel it as a sensation of completion of insertion — you may have other sensations. The patient usually appreciates it as a dull aching visceral, numbing, heavy, distending, or electrical sensation depending on the anatomy of the point, the patient involved, and the blockage of energy at the point. Radiation of this feeling may go down the involved meridian. It is not necessary to go any deeper than this depth of insertion.

Needles are always inserted in and taken out in a logical sequence. In Principal meridian use, the foot Yin to hand Yin, then hand Yang to Foot Yang are inserted. Focusing points are always added after any primary input has been inserted. The needles are taken out top to bottom, to prevent excess energy accumulating in the head and causing agitation. It is good practice to indicate the number of needles inserted, so that your assistant can be sure to have removed all inserted needles.

Needles should be left in longer than 30 minutes in acute excess presentations if the peri-needle erythema is still present. Difficulty in removing needles from spastic muscles can be solved by inserting an additional needle close to the retracted needle. This will usually relax the muscle and both needles can be removed. Bleeding from acupuncture points is easily stopped with firm cotton ball pressure to the points, even in patients on aspirin and anticoagulants at therapeutic levels. The prolonged bleeder has too much anticoagulant in his or her system and needs to have medications assessed.

All needles should be disposed of in a legal and acceptable manner, and all assistants need to be gloved when removing needles.

## The Patient

The patient should have an *adequate informed consent* and agree to undergo acupuncture. If the patient is very negative to the thought of acupuncture, the chances of success are poor. Acupuncture is not a mechanical modality of electrical modulation. It is an integrated input into the spiritual–mental–emotional and physical body.

Drugs that interfere with or decrease the efficacy of acupuncture include steroids, phenytoin, carbamazapine, marijuana, and alcohol. Patients should be advised of these interferences and whether it is still advisable to continue with acupuncture. The use of antidepressants in a pain therapy protocol does not seem to defuse acupuncture treatments. Absolute contraindications include pregnancy and severely debilitated patients. In hypertensives and diabetics, acupuncture may result in acute hypotension, and in hypoglycemia in sensitive patients, and they should be monitored carefully.

The patient should be adequately exposed for the circuit that is being contemplated. Pushing up sweaters and pants often makes for bad treatment. The preparation of the patient should be done by a nursing professional and not the doctor. This is done for both legal and ethical reasons. The room should be quiet and warm with some soothing sound, such as a miniature fountain or serene background music. The patient should be comfortable in the acupuncture position, whether sitting, supine, prone, or on the sides, as he or she is going to be in that position for some time. Commercial foam forms are available for use to expose and flex the cervicle area (also allowing the patient to breathe lying face-down), and to afford some flexion to the spine of a prone patient. A light with a dimmer should be turned down after the needles have been inserted to soothe the patient, especially in patients with migraine. If the patient is lying down, cover the patient after needle insertion to create a sense of safety and to avoid chilling. The use of infrared heating lamps is to be encouraged as a way of tonifying a whole area, as well as for comfort. A bell or intercomm device should be within reach of the patient so that help may be summoned if needed.

After acupuncture, most patients are very relaxed and still under the influence of their own endorphins, especially if you have used electroacupuncture. Your assistant should always ascertain if the patient is alert enough to drive or carry on the next activity. If not, the patient should wait a while in the office until fit. Patients should take it easy and not participate in any heavy-duty exercise or physical activity that day. They may feel exhausted or exhilarated after acupuncture, or in some cases, they may become aggravated before resolving their problem.

## COMPLICATIONS FROM ACUPUNCTURE

The most common complication is a *vasovagal syncope or needle shock* in first-time, apprehensive, and nervous patients of both sexes. I was once acupuncturing the knees of a 380-pound ex-Oakland Raider who refused to lie down on the first treatment. I was the immediate "wide receiver" of all 380 pounds of him as he lurched forward off the table after the first needle was inserted. This problem can be prevented by needling first-time, apprehensive patients in a recumbent position, after adequate instruction, and sometimes not allowing them to see the needles. If patients do faint, the needles should be immediately removed and the patient put into the recumbant position with the feet raised above the level of the head. Administer a few drops of "Rescue Remedy" under the tongue. If starting to convulse, the patient should be turned onto his or her stomach, head to the side, the airway kept clear, and regurgitation and aspiration should be avoided. Most patients will recover with reassurance as to the normal nature of this process in 5 to 10 minutes. If the patient is light headed and the needles were in the upper body, ST-36 may be lightly tonified. If needles were in the lower body, LI-4 could be lightly tonified to accomplish homeostasis. If the patient proceeds to unconsciousness, the acupuncture point GV-26 may be stimulated, along with KI-1 if only GV-26 does not work. The patient's airway and vital signs must be monitored and 911 called if appropriate.

Other complications include active bleeding, usually easily stopped with a cotton ball and firm pressure; later bruising or hematomata, mostly on the face or in repeatedly acupunctured points. Infected points and pneumothorax are extremely rare if you are using thin disposable needles and good clinical sense.

## PATIENT RESULTS

In the first week after acupuncture, one of six scenarios can be expected:

1. Total disappearance of the symptoms, without relapse.
2. Gradual and progressive improvement.
3. Marked amelioration and then gradual return to normal.
4. Marked exacerbation and then return to normal.
5. Marked exacerbation and worsening of symptoms.
6. No change at all.

The first four results are considered favorable, with the fifth representing overtreatment and a rebound phenomenon. This usually occurs in sensitive patients, with too vigorous tonification or if electroacupuncture has been used. The last two points are bad prognosticators and mean that you are dealing with either a serious structural problem, malignancy, or a patient who is going to hang onto his disease whatever you may do. In these cases it is reasonable to try one more treatment, and if the same result still applies, this patient should be referred for appropriate investigation and therapy. I once had an HIV-positive patient, whom I knew well, who presented with headache of one week's duration. I acupunctured him twice over the period of one week, with no resolution of the pain. I immediately ordered an MRI, which demonstrated a cerebellar lymphoma. Do not hold on to the worsening patient. There is always a reason for this response, and you may not have the answer.

## SELECTION OF ACUPUNCTURE PROGRAMS

The selection of points is done after the patient and the disease have been assessed (see The Integrated Patient Exam). In general terms, after taking a history, the patient is palpated along the Principal meridians and Shu–Mu system and a thermal reading of the abdominal Heaters is taken to evaluate the depth, anatomical coverage (above and below — ventral, lateral, or dorsal), and organ systems involved. Intense pain suggests an acute lesion, while a dull ache suggests a chronic problem.

Selection of points is also predicated on what symptoms are manifested and at what level.

### Pain Problems

1. Recent superficial tissue problem — use the Tendinomuscular meridians.
2. Deeper musculoskeletal pain problem — use the Principal meridians.
3. Focal acute muscular spasm and myofacial pain — use Ah Shi and trigger point deactivation.
4. Regional complex pain — use Curious meridians with N→ N+1 input.
5. Refractory or intermediate pain problems — use Yamamoto New Scalp Acupuncture.
6. Refractory and malignant pain — use percutaneous electrical nerve stimulation.
7. Bone and malignant pain — use periosteal bone stimulation.

### Organ Dysfunctions

1. Mixed organ and functional disturbances — use Principal meridian N→ N+1 and Five Phases Operators.
2. General endocrine and complex functional disturbances — use Curious meridians.
3. Focal ENT and cerebral problems — use cerebral circulation.
4. Organ problems — use the Shu-Mu system and He points on Principal meridians.
5. Dense organ degenerative problems — use Distinct meridian subsystem.

### Ventral, Lateral, and Dorsal Treatment Programs

One of the easier ways to start a program is to do one of Mark Seem's ventral, lateral, or dorsal treatment protocols.[45] Each protocol is opened up by activating the primary area of influence with a Curious meridian or major point acupunctural input. Then the area is carefully palpated to find Ah-Shi, Kori, or trigger points, and these are treated with insertion of a small thin gauge needle with superficial pecking in all directions around the identified point, until a superficial skin response is appreciated and the area is dispersed.

1. **Ventral Treatment Protocol** (ST and LI Somatic Zone)
   • Open up the zone with Chong Mo (SP-4 and PC-6) or Ren Mo (LU-7 and KI-6′).
   • Open key large points (LI-4, LI-20, ST-2, ST-25, ST-36, CV-7, CV-12, and CV-17).
   • Needle tender points on KI-11 to KI-27.
   • Disperse trigger points in the ventral zone.
   • Tonify and support Tai Yin (SP-6 and LU-9).
2. **Lateral Treatment Protocol** (GB and TH Somatic Zone)
   • Open up the zone with Dai Mo (TH-5 and GB-41).
   • Open key large points (GB-2, GB-20, GB-21, GB-24, TH-15, and TH-23).
   • Disperse trigger points in the zone.
   • Tonify and support Jue Yin (LR-2, LR-3, LI-14, PC-6, PC-7, and PC-8).
3. **Dorsal Treatment Protocol** (SI and BL Somatic Zone)
   • Open up the zone with Du Mo (SI-3 and BL-62′).
   • Open key large points (SI-8, SI-12, BL-10, BL-23, and BL-40).

- Disperse trigger points in the zone.
- Tonify and support Shao Yin (KI-3, KI-6′, KI-10, and HT-7).

Once you have completed these protocols, where applicable, the patient's energy flow will be much improved and quite a few of the symptoms will have lessened.

## AURICULAR ACUPUNCTURE

Acupuncture of the ear has been practiced by the Chinese for centuries. In the early 1950s Paul Nogier of France standardized the practice by systematically mapping the ear and elucidated the underlying neuroanatomy and physiology of auriculotherapy. His interest was piqued by the observation of ear cautery for sciatica in Algerians working in Southern France. The ear represents one of the more useful reflex somatotopic systems that we will deal with in acupuncture. The other two important ones are Korean Hand Acupuncture and Yamamoto New Scalp Acupuncture.

### EMBRYOLOGY, ANATOMY, AND NEUROPHYSIOLOGY OF THE AURICLE

The external ear develops from the embryonic gill plates and contains within it elements of all **three embryonic layers:**

1. **Ectoderm** — the helix and the lobe. Greater auricular nerve of superior cervical plexus (C1, C2 and C3).
2. **Mesoderm** — the pinna. Auriculotemporal branch of the anterior superior trigeminal nerve (cranial V).
3. **Endoderm** — the conchae. The auricular branch of the vagus nerve, which allows access to the parasympathetic nervous system.

There is insignificant innervation from the cranial nerves V, VII, and IX.

The *auricular somatotopic system* coverges its neural input and output at the level of the reticular formation, which in turn has a direct effect on the peripheral body by way of thalamocortical circuits and cranial and spinal motor centers. The auricle reflects all the somatic, organic, and functional activities of the body.

The *auricular reflex microsystem* operates as an inverted homunculus with the body parts distributed around the auricle, showing the following topographical representations: (Figure 7.21)

1. **Internal Organs** — superior and inferior conchae.
2. **Vertebral Column** — along the antihelix, bottom to top.
3. **Musculoskeletal System** — between the inferior and superior crura of the antihelix and the triangular and scaphoid fossa.

### LESIONAL AND MASTER POINTS

Acupuncture points are selected on the basis of:

1. Observed pathological changes of the surface skin, such as redness or discoloration, flaking, scars, pitting, or superficial capillaries. These are called *lesional points*.
2. Point tenderness, elicited by probing with a blunt or rounded instrument. A painful point usually indicates an acute Yang process.
3. Areas of lowered electrical resistance elicited with a handheld, battery-operated point location device. A point with high electrical conduction indicates a disturbed area, either recent or old. Old lesions show electrical changes without point tenderness.

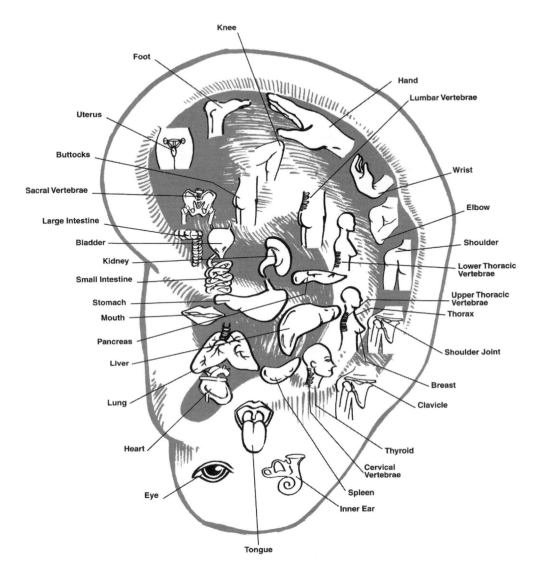

**FIGURE 7.21** The Ear Homunculus.

Master points are a collection of 11 important general points that are used in combination with other points for their particular physiological input. Most of these points are active in every patient (Figure 7.22).

1. **Point Zero**
   **Location:** Between the superior and inferior conchae in a notch at the beginning of the root of the helix.
   **Clinical:** Used for homeostatic balance, including energy, hormones, and brain activity. It controls the visceral organs through the autonomic ganglia.
2. **Shen Men (Divine or Spirit Gate)**
   **Location:** Slightly superior, between the root and the center of the triangular fossa.

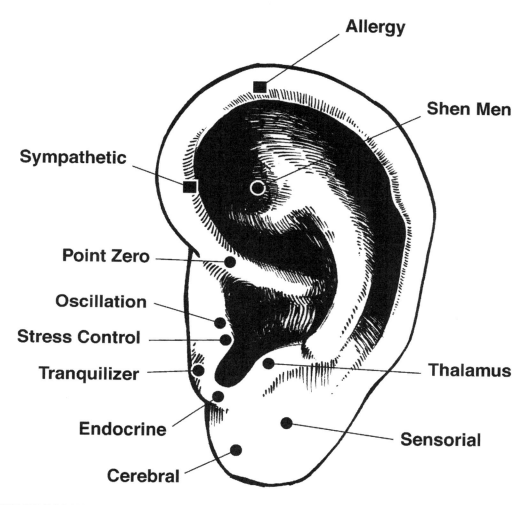

**FIGURE 7.22** The Ear Master Points.

Clinical: Alleviates stress, pain, tension, insomnia, depression, and anxiety. It induces endorphin release. It is active in most patients, is the most used auricular point, and supports the function of all other points.

3. **Sympathetic Point (Autonomic Point)**
Location: At the junction of the internal helix and the inferior crus. It is covered by the brim of the helix root above it.
Clinical: Balances the activity of the autonomic nervous system. It induces blood circulation by producing general vasodilation. It is used in stress-related health disorders.

4. **Thalamus Point (Pain Control–Subcortex)**
Location: Found at the base of the conchae wall behind the antitragus.
Clinical: This point has many nervous connections to the cerebral cortex. It acts as a down regulator of nervous excitement. It decreases chronic pain by activating the thalamic gating system, and also affects the hypothalamic regulation of the autonomic nerves.

5. **Endocrine Point (Internal Secretion, Pituitary Gland)**
Location: Found on the wall of the intertragic notch.

**Clinical:** This point brings all endocrine glands into balance, including their secretions, by activating the pituitary.

6. **Stress Control Point (Adrenal)**
   **Location:** On the external side of the inferior knob of the tragus.
   **Clinical:** It stimulates the adrenal gland to accommodate acute and chronic stress.

7. **Tranquilizer Point (Hypertension–Valium Point)**
   **Location:** Found on the inferior tragus as it joins the face.
   **Clinical:** Produces a general sedating affect, lowers blood pressure, and relieves chronic stress and muscle tension.

8. **Master Sensorial Point (Eye Point)**
   **Location:** Found in the middle of the lobe on the eye point.
   **Clinical:** It reduces distorted perception in the five senses by controlling the cerebral sensory cortex areas of the parietal lobe, temporal lobe, and occipital lobe.

9. **Master Cerebral Point (Omega–Psychosomatic)**
   **Location:** Where the lobe meets the face.
   **Clinical:** Represents the prefrontal lobe of the brain that is involved in decision making and conscious action. It is used for treating nervous anxiety, fear, worry, OCD, psychosomatic disorders, and the negativism that accompanies chronic pain.

10. **Master Oscillilation (Laterality–Switching Point)**
    **Location:** Found on the subtragus rim, internal to the inferior tragus protrusion.
    **Clinical:** This points balances the left and right cerebral hemispheres. The point is active in patients who are left handed or who have mixed dominance. Most patients (80%) show ipsilateral representation of their body organs, while 20% show contralateral representation. This latter group is felt to be "switched" or "oscillators." This is important in auricular therapy and muscle testing, where these patients will give opposite or incorrect results, and need to be switched by stimulation of this point before treatment or testing. This point also corrects problems of laterality such as dyslexia, learning disabilities, and attention deficit disorder. Patients who are inordinately sensitive or allergic to medications, are often "switched."

11. **Allergy Point**
    **Location:** Found on the internal side of the apex.
    **Clinical:** Reduces inflammatory reactions related to allergy, rheumatoid arthritis, and asthma. Can be used for anaphylactic shock — where it is usually bled.

The Master Points are used if they are active or seem to be clinically appropriate. Shen Men, Sympathetic, Thalamus and Stress Control are usually used for pain control. In psychosomatic problems, Point Zero, Shen Men, Stress Control, and Master Cerebral are used.

## CLINICAL USE OF AURICULOTHERAPY

Nogier has developed a very sophisticated and complete multiphasic system for treating the whole body. What follows is a more practical and simplified version that relates to everyday use in the clinic.

Because the ear represents all body structures, organs, and functions, it can be used as a stand-alone modality for a therapeutic input for all levels of dysfunction and pathological manifestation. However, ear acupuncture is usually used as a reinforcing adjunct to a major therapeutic program, pain conditions, and substance abuse management. The ear on the ipsilateral side of the problem is preferred. Patients with scurfy ears, local eczema, psorrhiasis, or possible basal cell carcinomas of the ear should probably not receive ear acupuncture. I have never cleaned the ear (or any body point for that matter) with alcohol prior to needling and have not experienced any local infection to my knowledge.

The points are selected from the patient history in pain and internal medicine problems, and then inspected for activation. Points may also be selected in a TCM sense — the Lung point for eczema or rhinitis (Lung controls the skin and nose) or the Bladder point for low back pain because the back is on the Bladder line. Points may also be selected based on the organs of the Five Elements.

If the points are activated, they are needled with a short (1/2 inch) 30-gauge needle, taking care not to go right through the cartilage. Multiple needles can be used, but the size of the ear usually limits the number to five needles or fewer. Active lesional points and master points are used together. If the correct points are needled, the ear will show a sudden, vascular, red erythema, much as one can appreciate around a body needle. Needles are left in the same amount of time as the main acupunctural program or, if trying to disperse an acute Yang condition, the ear needles can be left in for 30 to 60 minutes longer. The needles can be tonified with electricity, using the same frequency rules as apply to body acupuncture. Polarity of the leads is unimportant, but I usually put the positive (red) lead on Shen Men if it is used. I do not use more than one electrical lead (with a positive and negative), but it is permissable to cross two or more needles and connect them to either pole. After the needles are removed, the points often bleed profusely because of the rich vasculature of the auricular tissue. This is a good sign and should be easily stopped with firm pressure of a cotton ball.

Patients will feel sleepy or a little "high" after electrical stimulation of Shen Men, and should be evaluated as to their ability to drive before they leave the office. Repeat auriculotherapy can take place two to three times a week, but it is necessary to alternate the ears on each visit in order not to create a traumatized area in the ear.

## INDWELLING TACKS, SEEDS, MAGNETS, AND LASERS

One may use an *indwelling tack or seed* to accomplish ongoing stimulation in acute cases or addictive therapy. In this case, the ear is usually swabbed and a more sterile technique used. These devices may be left in place for 3 to 5 days, but should be removed if any pain or inflammation ensues. They usually extrude at six or seven days by themselves.

*Magnet therapy* is also useful, with the north or negative pole used for sedating and the south or positive pole used for tonification.

*Lasers* may be used on the ear, especially in children. *Electrical stimulating devices* are available for diagnosis and therapy, but take time to use and are somewhat uncomfortable.

## SUBSTANCE ABUSE MANAGEMENT

Auricular acupuncture is very successful in the treatment of withdrawal and detoxification issues in persons addicted to habituating substances such as tobacco, alcohol, analgesics, narcotics, and stimulants.

The general protocol is the use of five bilateral ear points simultaneously for 30 to 60 minutes, two to three times a week. The points are: Kidney and Liver at the superior and inferolateral regions of the superior conchae, Lung in the middle of the inferior conchae, Shen Men in the lateral aspect of the triangular fossa, and Sympathetic on the inferior crus of the antihelix, under the root of the helix. The number of treatments varies from individual to individual, but treatments should start out at three times a week for 1 to 2 weeks, then decrease to 1 to 2 times a week for 2 weeks, then to weekly for 4 weeks, or as needed. The ears may have to be alternated if used often. The master control points may also be used concurrently for appropriate symptomatology. These patients should also be treated with homeopathy for emotional issues, Chinese herbs for withdrawal symptoms, and psychotherapy.

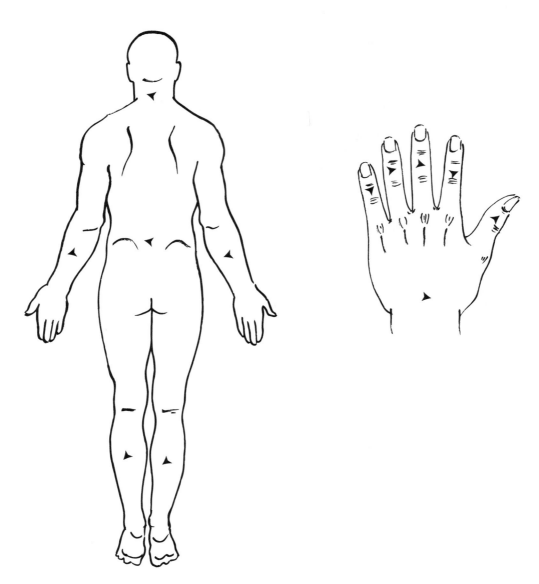

**FIGURE 7.23**  KHA Correspondence Points.

## KOREAN HAND ACUPUNCTURE (KHA)

*Korean Hand Acupuncture* (KHA) was envisioned by Dr. Tae-Woo Yoo as he suffered from a headache one autumn night in 1971. He had an instantaneous revelation that the point on the back of his middle finger corresponded to the pain in his head at GB-20. He found a tender point on the nail angle of his middle finger and inserted a needle. The pain instantaneously disappeared. He visualized the tip of his middle finger as representing the head of the human body, and the rest of his hand as the remainder of the body — the thumb and little finger, the legs; the index and ring finger, the arms. Further experiments revealed these correspondences to be true, and so Koryo Sooji Chim was born.

There are several levels or stages of therapy in KHA. The entire system is:

1.  **Correspondence Therapy** — This therapy utilizes the somatotopic mapping principle as seen in auricular therapy. Holding your own right hand in front of your face and looking at the back of your hand, with the palm facing forward, the hand is seen as the whole body. The back of the hand is the back of the body, the front of the hand is the front of the body. The little finger is the right leg, the thumb the left leg. The ring finger, the right arm and the index finger the left arm. The middle finger represents the head, cervical, and thoracic vertebrae to the tip of the scapular. The remainder of the dorsal hand represents the remaining thoracic, lumbar, and sacral vertebrae. The palmar aspect of the middle finger represents the face, anterior neck, chest, abdomen, and genitalia. All the organs are represented on the palmar aspect. The joints of the hands represent the corresponding joints of the body. Distal interphalangeal joints are the wrists and ankles, proximal interphalangeal joints are the elbows and knees, and the metacarpal-phalangeal joints are the shoulders and hips. If one uses the left hand, then the little finger is the left leg, the thumb, the right leg; the index finger the right arm and the ring finger the left arm (Figure 7.23). In correspondence therapy the tender point on the hand, corresponding to the pain or organ point is either needled, massaged, or stimulated with an ion beam or magnet. This treatment can be done as a stand alone therapy or with auriculotherapy and a body input (Figure 7.22).

2.  **Basic Therapy** — The correspondence treatment can be strengthened and will last longer by also giving a pretreatment of the associated Heater, abdominal, neural, and lumbar basic prescription. One has to learn all the positions of the meridians in KHA, which is beyond the scope of this book. The KHA meridians, while being somewhat similar to the Principal meridians, have more points and different names and trajectories that are, because of the hand, somewhat complex.

3.  **Organ Therapy (Ki Mek)** — The third level of treatment relates to the TCM diagnosis of the Zang Fu organs and their patterns of disharmony. The KHA meridian system is used very much as you would use the Principal meridians for similar patterns of disharmony, but you need to use the meridian point system of KHA, which is different.
    a.  Micromeridian simple stimulation — Simple selection of meridian points according to picture.
    b.  Micromeridian tonification/sedation — Identification of excess or deficient syndromes is accomplished by abdominal palpation with analysis of the *three constitutional types of KHA*, which are: Excess Yang Syndrome — Yin and Yang type (tender at ST-25), Excess Kidney Syndrome — Yin and Yang type (tender in midline at CV-4 and CV-5), and Excess Yin Syndrome — Yin and Yang type (tender at SP-15). These distinctions are accomplished by abdominal palpation (tender points indicate the predominant syndrome) and comparing the strength of the radial (if stronger = Yin type) and carotid pulses (if stronger = Yang type). Patients may have combinations of these constitutions.
        Another method of determining excess or deficiency in an organ is by the use of metal rings. The fingers of the hand each have an elemental designation: the thumb is Wood (LR), the index finger is Fire (HT/PC), the middle finger is Earth (SP), the ring finger is Metal (LU), and the little finger is Water (KI). Placement of a gold ring on the suspect deficient organ will change the reflex area on the abdomen from tender to nontender and normalize the discrepancy between the radial and carotid pulses. Gold or colored rings will tonify the organ, and silver or colorless rings will sedate the organ on each element.
    c.  Five Element Treatment Patterns

d. Five Element Hot/Cold Treatment Patterns

A fifth level of treatment relates the use of the Five Elements relationships to the diseased organ or pole of the body. This allows for: tonification (Jung Bang), sedation (Sung Bang), removal of Cold (Han Bang), and removal of Heat (Yol Bang) The *Four Needle Technique* appears to be the best method for treatment in these syndromes.

4. **Curious meridian KHA meridian therapy** — The Curious meridians can be used to treat the three constitutional syndromes of KHA. The following correspondences seem to work well:

Yang Excess Syndrome — Yang Type: Yang Qiao Mo
Yang Excess Syndrome — Yin Type: Yin Wei Mo
Kidney Excess Syndrome -Yang Type: Yang Wei Mo or Du Mo
Kidney Excess Syndrome — Yin Type: Ren Mo or Chong Mo
Yin Excess Syndrome — Yang Type: Dai Mo
Yin Excess Syndrome — Yin Type: Yin Qiao Mo

5. **Pulse Diagnosis** and **Constitutional/Biorythmic Therapy** — These two topics are beyond the scope of this book, please refer to the Koryo Sooji Chim Institute for more details and training.

### Advantages of KHA

This is a major complete acupuncture system. Most of the acupuncture techniques and circuits used in regular acupuncture can be used in KHA. No undressing is needed, and patients can walk around during treatment. Treatment is relatively painless; patients do not mind the small needles and can even do self-treatment at home.

### Clinical Applications of KHA

KHA can be used as a stand-alone or as an adjunct to other acupunctural systems. It is a very sophisticated system and utilizes multiple means of acupoint stimulation: any mechanical pressure, small needles that need an inserter, magnets, seeds, pellets, ion beam, hand massage rollers, and self-inserting hand pins. For best results, treatments are repeated daily — usually by the patient at home. It is great for children in whom tape-on magnets or acupressure pellets can be used.

## YAMAMOTO NEW SCALP ACUPUNCTURE

Another useful neuroanatomical somatotopic approach to acupuncture is the New Scalp Acupuncture (YNSA) developed by Dr. Toshikatsu Yamamoto of Japan in 1973. This approach utilizes corresponding reflex points on the scalp to influence the underlying central neural processing of pain. It is a complete interactive and diagnostic treatment system for pain relief. It can be used as a stand-alone or as an adjunctive treatment, together with other acupunctural programs.

The treatment is based on acupuncture stimulation of reflex points on the forehead and scalp that follow the micromap of a hunched over homunculus projected onto the fronto-temporal scalp (Yin) and parietooccipital scalp (Yang). Dr. Yamamoto has described a number of clinically useful areas that correspond to anatomical regions. These point groupings are: *basic points, sensory points, brain points,* and *ypsilon points* (Figure 7.24).

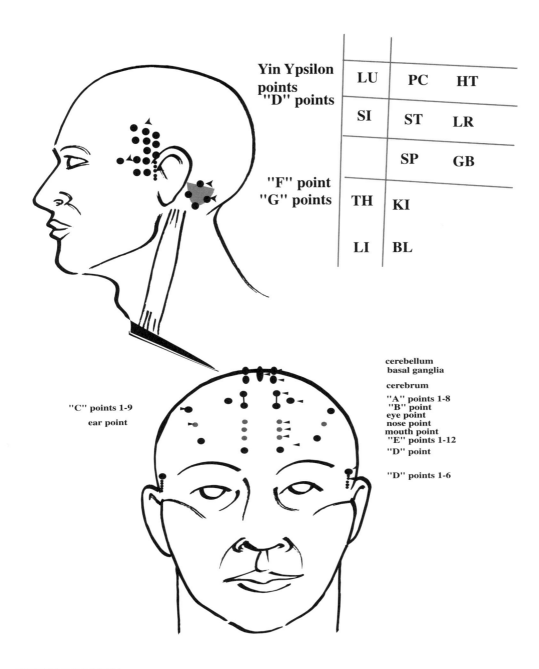

| Yin Ypsilon points "D" points | LU | PC | HT |
|---|---|---|---|
| | SI | ST | LR |
| | | SP | GB |
| "F" point "G" points | TH | KI | |
| | LI | BL | |

"C" points 1-9
ear point

cerebellum
basal ganglia

cerebrum

"A" points 1-8
"B" point
eye point
nose point
mouth point
"E" points 1-12
"D" point

"D" points 1-6

**FIGURE 7.24** YNSA.

## YNSA Acupuncture Points

### YNSA Basic Points (A–I)

1. **"A" Points**
   **Location:** Yin — Located 1 cm bilateral to the midline, at the hairline.
   Yang — Straddles the lambdoidal suture, 1 cm from midline.

**Clinical:** There are eight points on the line representing the head and cervical spine. Used for pain relief post trauma and surgery, headaches and migraines, whiplash, vertigo, any neuralgia, toothache, cerebral disturbances, Bell's palsy.

2. **"B" Point**

   **Location:** Yin — 1 cm lateral to A Point, or 2 cm lateral to midline, at the hairline.

   Yang — Straddles the lamboidal suture, 2 cm from midline.

   **Clinical:** This point represents the shoulder, clavicular region, and shoulder joint. Used for neck–shoulder–arm syndrome.

3. **"C" Points**

   **Location:** Yin — 2.5 cm lateral to B Point, or 4.5 to 5.0 cm lateral to midline. It runs along an imaginary line of 45 degrees from the root of the nose to the border of the frontalis and temporalis muscle, over an area of 2.0 cm.

   Yang — 1 cm lower over the lambdoidal suture.

   **Clinical:** There are six points representing the shoulder joint, upper arm, elbow, lower arm, wrist, hand and fingers. The line is divided into 9 parts, the shoulder being lateral and high, the thumb being medial and low. Used for all pain, inflammation, and tendonitis of the shoulder, the arm, and hand.

4. **"D" Points**

   **Location:** Yin — The divisions of the D point (D1– D6) are located in a verticle line, 1 cm posterior to the main D Point, just in front of the upper root of the ear.

   Yang — The D1–D6 points, however, are in a curvilinear line, starting from the apex of the ear and stretching back and downward for 1 cm on the sphenoid bone.

   **Clinical:** There are six points representing the lumbosacral spine and lower extremities. The D points are in the same order as their anatomical position D1–D5 representing the lumbar vertebra and D6 the coccyx. Used for lumbago, circulatory disturbances of the legs, neuralgia, arthritis, sciatica, muscle cramps, hemiplegia, MS, fractures and sprains, gout, and benign prostatic hypertrophy (BPH).

5. **Big "D" Point**

   **Location:** Yin — The main D point is located in the temporal region at the hairline, 1 cm above the zygomatic arch, 2 cm in front of the ear, over temporalis.

   Yang — The main D point is in exactly the same position, but posterior to the upper root of the ear.

   **Clinical:** Used for all lower back and lower extremity pain.

6. **"E" Points**

   **Location:** Yin — Located over the eyebrow, starting 1 cm lateral to the midline and following a 15 degree oblique line laterally. It is about 2 cm long.

   Yang — Present in a similar position over the occipital bone.

   **Clinical:** There are 12 points along the line representing the chest and thoracic spine. E1 is most superior and represents T-1.

7. **"F" Point**

   **Location:** Only Yang — Located in the retroauricular area, over the highest point of the mastoid process.

   **Clinical:** This point represents the sciatic nerve.

8. **"G" Points**

   **Location:** Located around the bottom edge of the mastoid process.

   **Clinical:** Three points representing the medial (G1), frontal (G2), and lateral (G3) knee. Used for bursitis, arthritis, fracture of patella, chrondromalacia.

9. **"H" and "I" Points**

   **Location:** The H Point is directly caudal to the B Point. The I Point is 1 cm caudal to the C Point.

## YNSA Sensory Points (1 -4)

All, except the ear, are in a vertical line below the A point at 1 cm intervals.

1. **Eye Point**
   **Location:** Yin — 1 cm below the A point.
      Yang — Same.
   **Clinical:** Used for all eye disorders.
2. **Nose Point**
   **Location:** Yin — 2 cm below the A point.
      Yang — Same.
   **Clinical:** Used for all nose and sinus disorders.
3. **Mouth Point**
   **Location:** Yin — 3 cm below the A point.
      Yang — Same.
   **Clinical:** Used for all oral problems.
4. **Ear Point**
   **Location:** Yin — About 1.5 cm from the basic C point on a 45 degree line between the C point and the root of the nose.
      Yang — Same area on occiput.
   **Clinical:** Used for all ear problems.

## YNSA Brain Points

**Clinically,** All these points are used for any neurological disorder: all motor disturbances, hemiplegia and paraplegia, migraine and trigeminal neuralgia, Parkinson's, MS, endocrine disturbances, vertigo, disturbed vision, tinnitus, aphasia, dementia, Alzheimer's, epilepsy, insomnia, depression, psychological disturbances, and stroke.

1. **Basal Ganglia Point**
   **Location:** Yin — Between the cerebral and cerebellar points.
      Yang — Same.
2. **Cerebrum Point**
   **Location:** Yin — Located 1 cm lateral to midline just posterior to the last A point.
      Yang — Same, but anterior.
3. **Cerebellum Point**
   **Location:** Yin — Just posterior to the cerebrum point.
      Yang — Just anterior to the cerebrum point.

## YNSA Ypsilon Points

The Ypsilon Points represent all the Zang–Fu organs of the body. There 12 points Yin and 12 points Yang, all clustered around the anterior and posterior ear area. The indications for using any of the organ points is both clinical and also by using of neck and abdominal reflex analysis.

## YNSA ABDOMINAL DIAGNOSTIC ZONES

Dr. Yamamoto has delineated an abdominal map that is used for selection of ypsilon points for acupuncture. The abdomen is palpated and the tender areas are noted according to the map of the Zang–Fu organs projected onto the abdomen. If an organ area is tender, then the ypsilon point is needled. Once needled the abdominal tenderness should abate.

## YNSA Neck Diagnostic Zone

There is a similar palpatory diagnostic zone for the Zang–Fu Organs on the lateral neck incorporating the anterior and posterior triangles of the neck and the sternocleidomastoid muscle. Clinically, this is a somewhat difficult palpation, but can be done without undressing the patient. Similarly, the tender point will indicate which ypsilon point needs needling, and the tender zone will lose its tender quality after needling of the point.

## YNSA Clinical Practice

YNSA is a very immediate and potent modality for pain relief. The reflex map of the head and scalp has both a Yin and Yang presentation. In 90% of the cases, needling of the Yin point is effective, but if not, the Yang point should be needled. Usually the contralateral side to the pain should be needled, but laterality, if the required ypsilon point is ascertained by squeezing the LI-4 point of the hands and asking the patient which side is more tender. The more tender side is used for mapping and needling. The acupuncture points in the hair and along the hairline are quite difficult to feel, usually as a little grain or bump. They are about 1 mm in diameter, and it is imperative that you hit the point exactly. Upon needling the exact point, the patient should jump, as the point is quite painful. If the patient does not experience this acute pain, then you do not have the point, and you should withdraw the needle slightly and, while it is still under the skin, reposition the needle to obtain pain. You can use the blunt end of the needle handle to probe around an unsuccessful point until the patient indicates a more tender spot for needling.

The needles are left in for 10 to 20 minutes without manipulation, although you can electrify the needles in chronic cases. Treatment can be done every day to every other day, or 1 to 2 times per week depending on the case and the time constraints involved. When all other pain techniques fail, this is the one that will be successful.

# NEUROANATOMICAL ACUPUNCTURE

## Percutaneous Nerve Stimulation (PENS)

This was developed as a form of pain control alternative to classical acupuncture by William Craig, M.D. of Texas. In PENS, the neuroanatomical spinal segments are used as the landmarks for needle insertion and electrical stimulation of these segments is used in sequentially increasing frequencies until pain relief occurs. This technique is very useful with patients who have chronic pain, have failed regular acupuncture, or are suffering from pain caused by malignancies.

Pain can involve any of the four divisions of the spinal segment: dermatomal sensory, myotomal sensorimotor, sclerotomal sensory and sympathetic, and splanchnotomal autonomic. The peripheral and central release of individual pain-controlling neurotransmitters is elicited by different stimulating frequencies. These frequencies are:

| FREQUENCY | NEUROTRANSMITTER | REGION |
|---|---|---|
| Low-Frequency | β-Endorphin | Hypothalamus |
| 2–4 Hz | Met-encephalin | Midbrain |
| Mid-Frequency | Dynorphin B | Spinal Cord |
| 10–30 Hz | Met-encephalin | Spinal Cord |
| High-Frequency | Dynorphin A | Spinal Cord |
| 70+ Hz | | |

The sympathetic innervation is somewhat diffuse and anatomically ill-defined. However, the following table will give some indication of what spinal segment needs to be stimulated:

| T-1 | Head |
| T-2, T-3 | Neck |
| T-3, T-4 | Shoulder and Arm |
| T-4 to T-6 | Thorax |
| T-7 to T-11 | Abdomen |
| T-10 | Lumbar Region |
| T-10, T-11 | Gluteal Region |
| T-12 to L-2 | Leg |

Because of the generous overlap of segmental innervation and the numerous radiating pathways of pain, one has to use a generous band of segmental stimulation in order to completely cover the total innervation of the painful anatomic area. In practical terms, one has to stimulate 2 to 3 segments above the nerve root and 1 to 2 below. The stimulation is divided into central and peripheral modules. The *central module* is used first and consists of bilateral needling of the Principal Bladder meridian line in the selected segments. This usually requires between 6 to 12 needles, 3 or 6 on each side. The needles are deeply imbedded, 3 to 7 cm and angled at 45 degrees toward the transverse processes. Initially, 2 Hz stimulation of the needles is used in an alternating pattern from needle to needle (either across the midline at the top and bottom needle pair, or proceeding from top to bottom) of alternating negative to positive electrodes in a continuous circle of current. A positive lead is attached to the most superior paravertebral needle on the side of the pain. The other leads are connected to the ipsilateral paravertebral needles, alternating negative and positive in a descending direction along the spine. At the bottom of the central module, the spine is crossed and the alternating continues in an ascending direction on the contralateral side (Figure 7.25). One may cross handles and clip adjacent needles together, if the number of needles does not match the number of stimulators available. Low-frequency stimulation has a cumulative effect with each treatment, and one should always have at least one needle pair in low-frequency stimulation to continue building on its effects. In a second treatment, if the first was not successful, the stimulatory frequency may be raised to 4 Hz. If nothing happens at that frequency, then you may go in one of two directions:

1. The central module is split in half into a superior and inferior module, and the inferior module is now stimulated at a higher frequency, or
2. Add a peripheral module of needles progressing centrifugally from the Bladder line outward along the shoulder and arm, or the hip girdle and leg. The points selected for one or two peripheral modules may include neuromuscular motor points, trigger points, painful points, strongly active acupuncture points around the joints, or any barrier or Shu command point.

As the treatment protocol becomes more complicated, always remember to keep the superior module in the low-frequency range and to have your highest frequencies in a stepwise increase from the center to the periphery. Reasonable stepwise increases are 2, 4, 10, 15, 30, 80, or 90 and then 100 to 200 Hz. Always try the first treatment with unstimulated plain acupuncture. Using PENS on the first treatment will often leave you with an aggravated patient and a bad first acupuncture experience. There are no other rules except to see what happens. Patients may often aggravate for 2 to 3 days following an intense input, but you should allow everything to calm down and evaluate the pain relief at that time before instituting any more electrical therapy. Treatments may be done as close together as three times a week, initially, but as soon as the "magic" module that changes the pain is found, the treatments can be spread out to weekly, monthly, or even a yearly "tune-up." In recalcitrant cases, periosteal stimulation can be tried, as long as the periosteal needles are connected to the negative leads and have the highest frequencies.

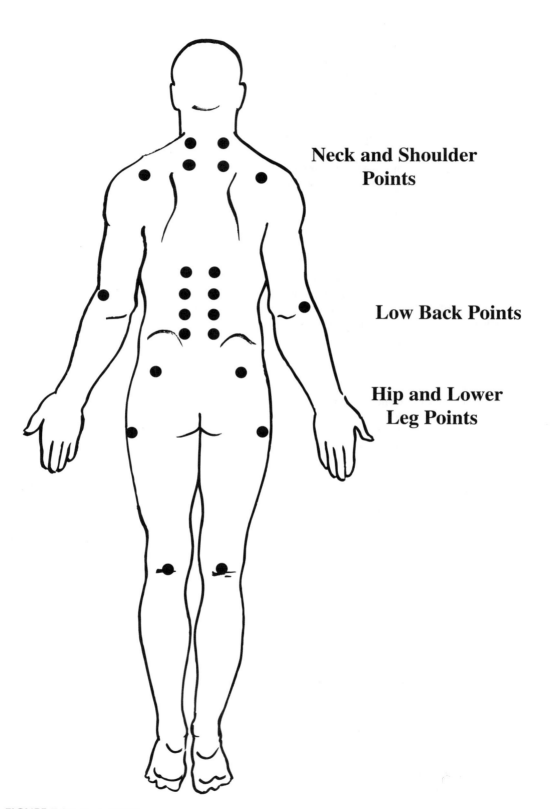

**FIGURE 7.25** Craig PENS.

## PERIOSTEAL ACUPUNCTURE STIMULATION

Periosteal acupuncture was developed in the United States by Ronald M. Lawrence, M.D. for the treatment of deep and chronic pain associated with traumatic or degenerative changes in the bone and body. It relies on the stimulation of the sympathetic fibers around the periostium, which in turn increases local blood flow and modifies vascular sympathetic, segmental nerve responses, and soft tissue inflammation and edema. It can be used for stubborn pain problems, the pain of peripheral vascular disease, and peripheral neuropathy.

The technique is most effective as a local focusing technique of a more general pain relieving input. Selection of the site is based on local bony tenderness, anatomical considerations, and local nerve supply.

## BONY PROMINENCES FOR OSTEOPUNCTURE

| Condition | Puncture Site |
|---|---|
| Headache, frontal | Frontal boss |
| Headache, occipital | Occipital ridge 1 in. medial to medial edge of mastoid process |
| Trigeminal neuralgia | Maxillary os and mental foramen |
| T–M joint | Mandibular condyle and styloid process |
| Dental neuralgia | Alveolar ridge |
| Neck pain | Spinous processes of all cervical vertebrae and the transverse process of C-7 |
| Shoulder pain | Acromion, superior central portion, and coracoid process |
| Shoulder tendonitis | Humeral bicipital groove |
| Sternal pain | CV-17 |
| Intercostal neuritis | Angle of involved rib |
| Discogenic disease | Spinous process of vertebrae — treat above and below the level of the involved disc |
| Epicondylitis — medial | Medial epicondyle |
| Tennis elbow | Lateral epicondyle |
| Pronator terres sd. | Lateral epicondyle |
| Thumb pain | Carpo-radial junction |
| Wrist pain | Lateral and superior radial head, ulnar |
| Arthritis — fingers | Heberden's nodes |
| Low back pain | P.S.I.S, superior dorsal sacrum, and spinous process of L-5 |
| Hip pain | Greater trochanter (lateral approach) and head of femur for deep hip pain |
| Coccydynia | Tip of coccyx |
| Knee pain | Head of fibula, medial tibial plateau, and four corners of the patella |
| Ankle pain | Medial and lateral malleolus and inferior anterior tibia |
| Bunion | Right through the bunion to the underlying bone |
| Heel pain | Plantar surface of os calcis |
| Foot or toe pain | Heberden's nodes or interphalangeal joint |

Several bony prominences within the local area of influence are punctured to the level of the deep periostium with long, thick needles (± 22 gauge). The overlying skin should be swabbed with iodine and alcohol and allowed to dry. The patient will feel the needle as it hits the periostium, and then no more needle manipulation is needed. The electrical stimulation consists of connecting the negative leads to the periosteal needles and the positive leads to selected adjacent involved muscle groups. The frequency used is usually 90 to 150 Hz and can be left on for 15 to 20 minutes. The stimulator may have to be turned higher during the treatment as patients quickly accommodate to high frequencies. Treatments are repeated weekly for 10 to 12 treatments. Some patients may need to be detoxified from their analgesics before the treatment can be adequately accessed. If this course of treatment does not get any results, you are dealing with a deeper, more ominous visceral pain and need to investigate the patient in more detail.

## OTHER REFLEX ACUPUNCTURE SYSTEMS

There are other reflex acupunctural systems that rely on abdominal palpation or the pulses for diagnosis and treatment. The two most important representatives, both described and developed by Dr. Yoshio Manaka, a Japanese surgeon, are use of the "Hara" or abdomen for diagnosis and then treatment with *ion pumping cords* as a constitutional treatment, and *Japanese meridian channel therapy*, utilizing pulse diagnosis as an indicator for "root" treatment, prior to any therapeutic acupuncture input. Both of these methods, while being quite powerful and clinically valid, are beyond the scope of this book.

## OTHER ENERGETIC ACUPUNCTURE SYSTEMS

The French School of Advanced Acupuncture Studies has developed an energetic understanding of all living systems in relation to energy, matter, and the universe. This body of thought utilizes the mathematical order encoded into the trigrams, hexagrams, and sequential energetic graphs to define the process and movement of life into an understandable and useful acupunctural paradigm. This is a very advanced and sophisticated acupunctural treatise and is beyond the scope of this book. I refer you to the work of Maurice Mussat, M.D.[52] and part three of *Acupuncture Energetics* by Joseph Helms, M.D.[44]

A more down-to-earth electrical approach was formulated by Dr. Yoshio Nakatani of Japan in 1950. This technique, called *Ryodoraku*, is an electrostimulatory diagnostic and therapeutic technique based on many observations of electric current recordings made over acupuncture points on the wrists and feet. It offers a means of objectively recording a traditional Zang-Fu diagnosis. Dr. Nakatani worked out an easy numbering system so that he could teach the method to practitioners who had no knowledge of acupuncture. The technique involves electrical measurements on peripheral points on the wrists and feet, interpretation of the pattern, and then balancing of the autonomic nervous system that induced the pattern using a fixed electrical input at particular points. Remeasurement should show a new balanced pattern together with clinical improvement of the patient. Further information and training is available from Hiroshi Nakazawa, M.D.[53]

## ELECTROACUPUNCTURE

The application of electricity to the body, and through acupuncture needles in particular, has been poorly taught because of a lack of fundamental understanding of the physics and physiology involved. I have, therefore, decided to give a somewhat expanded section dealing with this subject. I am indebted to John Stebbins, O.M.D. L.Ac., of Denver, for much of the technical information, which he presented at the 1996 CAAOM meeting.

The use of electricity is not a recent phenomenon. Subtle electrical therapy probably began with the application of loadstones to acupuncture points. These were made of magnetite, which is a naturally occurring magnetic material, and were believed to have a potent life force because they moved by themselves.

The following is a short but interesting history of attempts at electrotherapy:

**First century** A.D. — Scribonius Largus, a physician in Nero's army, treated gout and headaches with an electric eel.

1764 — Gennai Hiraga of Envo, Japan reportedly used electrostimulation with acupuncture.

1757 — Benjamin Franklin used an electrical device to treat frozen shoulder and post-CVA paralysis. He referred to it as being "electricized." He had good results but they were short term, lasting only a few days.

1812 — John Birch, an English physician, used electric shocks to treat nonunion tibial fractures.

**1816** — French physician Louis Berlioz applied DC current to acupuncture needles. The French had been using acupuncture since its introduction by monks who had visited China in the late 1770s.

**1825** — Chevalier Sarlandiere, another French physician, enhanced acupuncture with electrical currents from Leyden jars. He treated gout and rheumatism with this method.

**1860** — Arthur Garret, a Boston physician, published a textbook on electrotherapy. He also applied DC currents to acupuncture needles to treat nonunion fracture of bones.

**1875** — Dr. L. H. Cohen, in the United States, used electrostimulation and acupuncture as anesthesia for removal of a glandular tumor.

**1882** — French surgeon Professor Apostoli treated cancer of the cervix and uterus by inserting a positive electrode into the tumor and passing milliamperage current though it.

**1886** — Dr. Franklin Martin, an American surgeon, followed in Apostoli's footsteps, confirmed Apostoli's results, and received considerable notoriety in the United States.

**1910** — The Flexnor Report (sponsored by the AMA) stated there was no scientific evidence for the use of electromedicine therapies.

**1952** — Chinese began using electroacupuncture for surgery.

**1973** — Dr. Wen of Hong Kong used electrical stimulation of the ear to successfully treat heroin addiction.

Bjorn Nordenstrom, M.D. used microcurrents to treat end-stage cancer patients, with some apparent success in tumor reduction. He pioneered the development of the needle biopsy in the 1950s. Robert Becker, M.D., author of *Cross Currents* and *The Body Electric*,[28,29] is an orthopedic surgeon (retired) who spent thirty years investigating the electrical activity involved in the regrowth of amputated limbs of amphibians. Based on his research he developed treatment techniques for applying microcurrents to nonhealing fractures.

## THE PHYSIOLOGY OF NEEDLE INSERTION

The surface of everyone's body carries an electric charge. Bjorn Nordenstrom suggests that when we insert a needle there is a (subtle) electrical potential difference between the subcutis of the patient and the acupuncturist's fingers. This causes a current flow to allow for equalization of potential differences. Depending on the relative difference between practitioner and patient, current may flow from the patient or to the patient. If there is an insulator (rubber gloves, plastic handle, etc.), an equalization will occur between the charge on the skin surface and the charge in the subcutis of the patient. Factors that may affect this process include relative humidity, skin moisture, interstitial electrolyte balance, and the length of time the needle is in place.

Becker takes a slightly different view. He feels needle insertion produces a very small electrical current. This occurs because the needle produces a local current of injury and the metal reacts with the ionic solution of the body. Manipulating the needle may produce a pulsing current at a very low frequency. Becker believes acupoints act as electrical amplifiers, or boosters, for the tiny DC currents flowing along the meridians.[28,29] The insertion of a needle in close proximity would affect the electrical current there.

## ELECTRIC PARAMETERS OF ACUPOINTS

The two main characteristics of an acupoint to be measured are its *electrical resistance* — the amount of resistance the point offers against an electrical current — and its *electrical conductivity* — the ability of the point to conduct an electrical current.

There is an inverse relationship between these two factors, which are two ways of measuring the same phenomenon. As a point's resistance increases, its conductivity decreases. As a point's resistance decreases, its conductivity increases.

## Basic Electricity

Everything electrical results from the phenomenon of charge which is what we call polarity. It is a fundamental property of matter that exists in two opposite forms (polar opposites), which we arbitrarily refer to as positive and negative: protons + (Yin); electrons − (Yang).

We need to define a few electrical terms in order to speak the same language.

**Circuit:** A complete or partial path over which electrical current may flow. There are complete circuits and incomplete circuits. For any electrical current to flow, a complete circuit must be established, that is, a connection between the two poles.

**Current:** Electrical current can be defined as the flow of electrons between two poles. Electrons are forced to leave their parent atoms to move along specific pathways. Current is measured in *amperes*. Anything that connects the two poles (− and +) and that conducts the current is called a *conductor* or *conductive medium* (e.g., the body). *Conductance* is the ability of a system to transport charge or the ability of a substance to conduct current. The positive (+) pole is called an *anode*. The negative (−) pole is called a *cathode*. When referring to a DC current, the electrons would move from the negative pole (cathode) to the positive pole (anode).

**Amperage (micro vs. milli):** Amperage is the amount of current allowed to escape; the higher the amperage, the greater the current. It can be likened to the amount of water flow available through a faucet or hose (your faucet or nozzle controls how much water you allow to escape, yet the water pressure remains the same). Most medical electronic equipment has the ability to control this, usually measured by *intensity*. As you increase the intensity, you increase the amperage (flow) at the site of treatment.

The relative size of current is important: a milliamp equals 1/1,000 of one amp, a microamp equals 1/1,000,000 of one amp or 1/1,000 of a milliamp.

**Voltage:** The electromotive force or *push* behind the current can be likened to the water pressure available in a faucet or hose. Voltage is used to measure electrical charge or potential. This is built in to most stimulating machines.

**Hertz:** A hertz is a measurement of the *frequency of a cycle* over a given time. A cycle is one complete oscillation of polarization and depolarization, or one complete movement relative to the baseline. With AC current, it is diagramatically represented by a full sine wave (a rise above the baseline followed by an symetrical fall below the baseline). This all occurs over a given time period, generally one second. For example 1 hertz (Hz) = 1 cycle per second and 20 Hz equals 20 cycles per second.

Several types of frequency selections are available in stimulation units:
- *Continuous* — pulses continue at a preset rate throughout treatment.
- *Interupted* — baseline rate that is active for a number of seconds, then turned off for a number of seconds.
- *Dense Disperse* — baseline rate for a few seconds, immediately followed by an increased rate for a few seconds. This does not allow the body to compensate or get too accustomed to the current and is useful for both acute and chronic pain conditions. This type of stimulation is especially good for stagnation, as it does not allow the body to compensate.

**AC vs. DC Current:** A *direct current (DC)* is a more or less even flow of electrons (like a slow flow of water through a hose), as opposed to the back and forth flow of *alternating current (AC)*, which powers most of our appliances (more like a pulsing sprinkler system). *In vivo* direct current is the only type naturally flowing in tissue.

## BODY ELECTRICITY

According to Robert Becker,[28,29] it appears that injured tissues lose some of their electrical potentials (leaking ions from damaged cells) and thereby become electrically undercharged. This creates metabolic sluggishness. By feeding the body normal charges, we promote the correct electrical potentials and support healthy cellular function. Regarding electromedicne, Dr. Becker states: "We're tapping into the most potent force in all biology."

# CELL MEMBRANE ELECTRONICS

There are voltage potentials across all cellular membranes (which means current is allowed to flow if a circuit is completed). Different tissues have different electrical characteristics:
- Muscle, bone — decreased resistance / increased conductivity.
- Fatty tissue — increased resistance / decreased conductivity.
- Nerve trunks, acupoints, motor nerve points — more conductive than surrounding tissues.

In the last two decades nearly all tissues have been proven to produce or carry various electrical charges.

An interesting bioelectrical phenomenon occurs within the body. If batteries are placed together in series, their voltage potentials are combined. Since the human body has trillions of cells, each having small voltage potentials across their membranes, when placed side by side in the formation of tissues, they essentially act "in series" to create much greater voltage potentials throughout.

We are capable of reading and to some extent interpreting some of the electrical information within the body, e.g., with EKGs, EEGs, and EMGs. Various wave forms are seen in the different phases of sleep and arousal:

- Delta waves (0.5 to 3 cycles per second) — deep sleep
- Theta waves (4 to 8 cycles per second) — trance, light sleep
- Alpha waves (8 to 14 cycles per second) — relaxed wakefulness
- Beta waves (14 to 35 cycles per second) — normal consciousness

Acupuncture stimulates alpha wave activity or relaxed wakefulness. Because the blood is filled with charged particles and moves (flows) within the Earth's magnetic field, we are continually generating electricity, and the faster the Blood flows, the more electricity we generate.

Other cosmic frequency issues seem to impact us. For example, the Earth's magnetic field pulses at 10 Hz. The fact that this is the most dominant frequency in animals is evidence that we are connected to the Earth. This frequency must be supplied to astronauts in space.

Subtle electric signals within the body can function as information carriers. This system is important not only in communicating injury to the rest of the body, but also for maintaining overall homeostasis.

Evidence for the importance of electricty within the body comes from multiple and diverse sources. Two Japanese researchers, Yoshio Nagahama, M.D. and Hiroshi Motoyama, Ph.D., have independently concluded that the meridian system lies in the superficial fascia. Motoyama has also demonstrated that what we call Qi energy is not simply the drift of ions through tissue, but rather the flow of electrons. Bjorn Nordenstrom discovered that an electrical system operates through the circulatory system, and Rheinhard Voll discovered that electrostimulation is capable of increasing the circulation of lymphatic fluid.

## THE ELECTRONICS OF CELL INJURY

Becker discovered that all injuries produce a "current of injury." Injured tissues lose some of their electrical potential and thereby become electrically undercharged. This creates metabolic sluggishness. By feeding the body normal charges we promote the correct electrical potentials and support healthy cellular function.

The increased blood flow and inflammation often associated with injuries also provide an area of reduced electrical resistance. This is caused by an increase in sodium chloride, which provides a greater conductive medium for electrical currents. With this decreased resistance, the electrical currents naturally proceed to these areas.

The pathophysiology of injuries is, in part, based on disruption of the bioelectrical potential gradients of the cells involved. That is, interference with the sodium ion pump mechanism within the cells reduces their capacity to process ATP (Adenosine Triphosphate — the cells' fuel).

This eventually degrades the membrane transport mechanism responsible for bringing nutrients into the cell, as well as for removing metabolic wastes. The result is decreased nutrition to and increased wastes within the cells, thereby resulting in accompanying electrical aberrations, as well as decreased cellular efficiency. When the permeability of membranes is increased, the transfer of fluids and nutrient factors into the cells is enhanced. By applying microcurrents to an injured area, we may be able to nudge the body back into efficient operation.

## ELECTRONIC HEALING

According to Becker, healing takes place by means of a continuous direct current (DC) electrical system sending its signals through the perineural cells. He believes that acupuncture points may be amplifiers within this system, used to increase signal strength. The perineural cells seem to conduct very minute direct currents, which are responsible for regeneration.

Becker's research colleague, A. A. Pilla,[28,29] feels that any change in the environment of the cell that causes changes in electrical potential across membranes of the cell will alter cell function. He also feels that a cell can be "stimulated, inhibited, or exhibit passive response depending upon the frequencies and amplitudes of signals employed." Becker has stipulated that the strength of the current passing through the tissue is a factor in determining the tissue's response. Additionally, it seems that different tissues respond to different frequencies and amplitudes. This has been called the "window effect."

Becker,[28,29] Nordenstrom,[30] Bassett,[28,29] and Starish[28,29] all believe there is definite regenerative activity in tissue when provided with the correct electrical environment.

## ELECTROTHERAPEUTIC TECHNIQUES

There are many different ways to energetically impact the body:

1. Techniques in which no external energy is administered to the body include hypnosis and visualization. These treatments only attempt to activate preexisting energetic control systems.
2. Techniques in which external energies are administered to the body, but in amounts similar to those that the body itself uses in its energetic control systems include acupuncture, homeopathy, and pacemakers.
3. Techniques in which energy is administered to the body in amounts greater than those that naturally occur include Milliamperage/TENS, electroshock therapy, and defibrillation.

## PHYSIOLOGICAL RESPONSES TO ELECTRICAL STIMULATION

Electrical stimulation occurs on four basic levels:

1. **Systemic** — Endorphin/enkephalin production (hypothalamus). This is usually in response to pain, but the body can be fooled with nonpainful electrical stimulation.

2. **Segmental** — Nerve roots/anesthesia. The "Gate Theory" where there is some modification in the interpretation of afferent signals.
3. **Tissue** — Local treatment/pain and swelling. Tissue responses include:
   a. Muscles are stimulated to contract or relax.
   - Relaxation of muscle spasm is induced through fatigue or simple electromuscular stimulation.
   - Controlled muscle contraction simulate active exercise.
   b. Reticuloendothelial response to clear waste is enhanced.
   c. Bone is stimulated to enhance growth.
   d. Blood circulaton in general improves in tissues that are stimulated.
   e. The acupuncture point system is stimulated.
4. **Cellular** — ATP, mitochondria, ionic transfers, membrane permeability.

Additional uses of electrostimulation include trigger point therapy, Golgi tendon organ treatment, enhancement of muscle reeducation, and repair and detoxification.

## ELECTRICAL FREQUENCIES USED IN TREATMENT

Electroacupuncture effects are dependent upon the frequency of applied electrical impulses. Generally speaking, the lower the frequency (tonification), the more time it takes to produce some of the beneficial effects of acupuncture and the longer the beneficial effects last. Conversely, the higher the frequency (dispersion), the shorter the time required to obtain the beneficial effects of acupuncture, but the effects do not last as long.

TENS pads need milliamperage and a fast-rising wave to penetrate the stratum corneum, otherwise the charge is too diffuse.

Yoshiaki Omura observed the following electrical peculiarities in 1975:

1. Low frequency electrical impulses (~ 5 Hz)
   - Longer time required for benefits to appear.
   - Longer time required to reach maximum pain threshold.
   - Beneficial effects lasted longer.
   - Penetrated more deeply into the tissue.
2. Medium frequency electrical impulses (20 to 200 Hz)
   Note: most patients derive maximum comfort and beneficial effects in the 40 to 80 Hz range. Use alternating 30 to 100 Hz.
   - Pain threshold reached rather quickly.
   - Benefits receded quickly.
   - Often vasoconstriction occurred between the two electrodes.
3. High frequency electrical impulses (> 10 kHz)
   - Pain often disappeared immediately.
   - Maximum pain threshold can be reached immediately.
   - Pain returned almost immediately.
   - Very superficial penetration.

Note: When in doubt as to what frequency to use, 8 Hz will balance and regulate.

## MILLI- VS. MICROAMPERAGE ACUPUNCTURE

For treatment of pain we can "kill the messenger" (Gate Theory), or we can heal the source of the problem, that is, the irritated or aberrant cells or tissues. The Arndt–Schultz Law (early 1900s) states that small, weak stimulations will enhance the organ's ability, while larger stronger stimulation will interfere or inhibit organic activity.[54] Becker states: "One of the main lessons of electromagnetism so far is that less is more."[28,29]

## Celluar Effects of Microcurrents

Microcurrents first gained popularity as effective therapy for burns, wounds, and ulcerations (they accelerated healing, as well as suppressed bacterial growth), nonunion fractures, and bone implants. Many researchers have looked into the issue of current strength and the effects of small currents in biology — another example of small inputs, with the right initial conditions, producing large changes.

Lerner and Kirsch compared microcurrent stimulation to placebo treatment and found 37% greater short-term relief and 75% longer-term relief from the microcurrents. [ACA Journal of Chiropractic, November 1981]. Cheng et al. showed that microcurrents increased tissue ATP levels threefold to fivefold, and enhanced the cellular membrane transport mechanism and protein synthesis by 30% to 40%. Both factors are critical to tissue repair and healing. [*Clinical Orthopedics and Related Research*, #171 Nov.-Dec.,1982]. Cheng et al. also determined that currents exceeding 1000 microamps (one milliamp or above) actually inhibited protein synthesis, as well as amino acid transport, by as much as 50%. Also, electrolysis, the breakdown of the needle metal as well as the surrounding tissue, becomes more evident with milliamperage currents.[55]

Alvarez et al. studied the effects of microamperage DC stimulation on rat skin *in vitro* and reported a significant increase in collagen synthesis after 5 days. [Journal of Investigative Dermatology, Vol. 81, No. 2 (81:144-148, 1983)]. Carly et. al. found microcurrents speeded wound healing by 150 to 250%. [Archives of Physical Medicine, vol. 66, July, 1985]. Joseph Nessler M.D. and Daniel Mass, M.D. used DC microamperage to clearly enhance *in vitro* repair of tendon specimens. [Clinical Orthopedics and Related Research, April 1987, number 217]. Wolcott, Wheeler, Hardwicke, and Rowley applied microcurrents to a variety of wounds. Treatment groups showed 20 to 350% faster healing than controls. [Southern Medical Journal, July 1986].[55]

Gault and Gatens applied microcurrents to skin ulcers, which exhibited healing twice as fast as controls. [Physical Therapy, vol.56, #3, March 1976].[55] In a Canadian study, laboratory evidence pointed to increased connective tissue cell multiplication, and therefore enhanced formation of new collagen in injured tendons. Microcurrents also increased tensile strength of the tendons. The Canadian Olympic team decreased healing time by 1/3 using microcurrents. Rheinhard Voll, M.D., discovered that microcurrents can stimulate the flow of lymph. Becker, Nordenstrom, Bassett, and Starish all believe there is definite regenerative activity in tissue when using the correct electrical environment.

Although initially developed for treating burns and nonunion fractures, microcurrent therapy has also been used for treating acupoints "without needles" (using handheld probes). However, it turns out that applying electricity to acupuncture needles is better than electrode application to the area. When applying microcurrent stimulation directly to traditional needle acupuncture, we can precisely direct the healing currents to the desired area.

## Techniques and Applications of Electroacupuncture

*Contraindications to electroacupuncture* include sinus arrythmias, pacemakers, pregnancy, cancer or tumors near the vagus nerve, and epilepsy. Never use milliamperage stimulation across the neck or head. Microamperage is acceptable in this area.

**Tonification vs. dispersion** — The predominant frequency in mammals is 10 Hz. This should be viewed as the median or the normal frequency to nuture. In humans the predominant frequency is 7.86 Hz (8 Hz). Therefore, in humans 7 to 8 Hz should be the frequency we wish to reinforce or nurture. If in doubt, use 7 to 8 Hz to regulate.

If 7 to 8 Hz is the predominant frequency, then a higher frequency would be more oriented toward dispersion. With a faster stimulation, as we move toward 20 Hz we are moving toward more of a dispersion (sedation) mode. According to literature and clinical experience, greater than 40 Hz is a dispersive frequency. An extreme example of dispersion is acupuncture anesthesia, which is often initiated above 200 Hz (can be painful). In acupuncture anesthesia you use only one continuous current.

As we move below 8 to 10 Hz, we begin to tonify. Research indicates that 0.3 to 0.5 Hz can help the healing process of injured tendons (microcurrents). This would support the premise that these frequencies were more tonifying. When in doubt, use 8 Hz which will regulate and balance.

For acute problems, treat a microsystem first.

## ELECTRICAL AURICULOTHERAPY

Some points to note include:

- Using the ear greatly enhances treatment.
- We use the same side as the injury 80% of the time.
- For maximum benefit, use both sides.
- Combining ear points and body points can be useful in some cases. Always remember, the ear is usually more sensitive, so electricity may be painful.
- Use one ear point contralaterally with an appropriate body point.
- It is not recommended that you connect one ear with the other electrically. However, this technique has been shown to be useful with microcurrents, especially for addiction withdrawal.

### Ear Points

For chronic body problems, treat the painful side contralaterally, because of neurological crossover. The following points (see Figure 7.22) are used:

1. **Shenmen and Subcortex** — sedative points.
2. **Triple Heater** — point for swelling.
3. **Shenmen** — good for pain/spasm/tranquilizer point, above tragus apex 1/3 distance along superior helix crus.
4. **Heart point** — best for sports injuries; dilates Blood vessels, moves stagnation, decreases swelling, increases tissue resorption; use with Shenmen for acute trauma.
5. **Point Zero** — General balancing point; relieves spasms, stops bleeding and vomiting.
6. **Subcortex** — on inside of antitragus; regulates cerebral cortex; tranquilizes, relieves memory loss, nervousness; almost as good as Shenmen for pain relief; needle toward endocrine; do not needle toward brainstem as it will keep patients awake.
7. **Adrenal gland** — anti-inflammatory, reduces swelling, good for anything allergic, balance with Shenmen, good for smoking cessation.
8. **Apex** — good for relieving pain and swelling especially associated with head and face; bleed for fever.
9. **Spleen Point** — controls the extremities, therefore good for sports injuries; muscle relaxation point, helps circulation, tonifies Spleen and Qi; a very useful point; along lateral border of cavum concha; along antihelix.

## Clinical Uses

**Musculoskeletal** — For limb pain have patient hold limb in painful position, and stimulate corresponding ear point. Range of motion movement may be helpful as well.

**Tendinitis** — This comes in many different manifestations. Chronic cases of one year or more duration may not respond to anything, in part due to the mineral deposits that occur at sites of chronic inflammation. More acute cases can be affected by microcurrent stimulation. A good technique for tendinitis is called "Threading the Tendon." Closely insert your acupuncture needles parallel along both sides of the tendon to be treated. Run 80 Hz for 8 to10 minutes, then 0.3 to 0.5 Hz for 5 to 10 minutes. This should help reduce inflammation. The patient may need five to six treatments. If there are no results by the 6th treatment, microcurrents probably will not help. Make sure you properly address all the muscles involved that may influence the site. This includes the muscle to which the tendon is attached as well as the opposing muscles on the opposite side of the limb (e.g., extensors and flexors). Ergonomic changes may have to be addressed as well.

**Tennis elbow (lateral epicondylitis)** — There is an extra point which will likely benefit the condition. The point is called "Yin Shang Xue" and is located 1.5 cun (one inch) above Yin Ling Quan (SP-3) posterior to the medial eye of the knee. Use this point on the same side, alone, before any other treatment. You may then use local needling in the area of the elbow and connect a circuit between this extra point and the local point. Use for thirty minutes with microstim at 8 Hz.

**Arthritis** — Initially, we need to mildly disperse (high frequency) the area involved. Then we follow with mild tonification (low frequency). Place your needles on both sides of the affected joint. Try to insert them somewhat inside the joint, if possible. Run 80 Hz for about 3 minutes, followed by 8 Hz for about 10 minutes, and ending with 0.3 Hz for 1 to 3 minutes. One treatment should last for several weeks, depending on the severity. Herbal and homeopathic remedies should also be incorporated to move Qi and Blood, warm Cold Bi Syndrome, or expel Damp. Proper nutrition is critical here also. Familiarize yourself with the benefits of glucosamine and chondroitin sulfate, MSM, and SAMe for cartilage degeneration.

**Scar Tissue** — Scar tissue can profoundly impede the circulation of Qi in the channels. This can sometimes account for why a patient does not improve. Make sure you are aware of any surgeries the patient may have had (especially abdominal). Scars can be very tricky to treat. They are often deep, and there is no way of knowing how much scar tissue is present. To treat scars, needle along the perimeter of the lesion and run currents across the scar. Begin at the disperse setting of 80 Hz. Use this current for about 10 minutes and follow with several minutes of 0.3 to 0.5 Hz. This should open some the scar tissue to the flow of Qi. With sufficient use, it may actually help diminish the scar size. To treat deep scars, use perpendicular or oblique needle insertions. To treat superficial scars, use oblique or horizontal insertions. You may even "thread" your needle along the side of the scar. Topical herbal salves made with Radix Lithospermum (Zi Cao), or injected mixtures of lidocaine and homeopathic thuja and silica may be helpful.

## GENERAL GUIDELINES FOR USING ELECTROACUPUNCTURE

When treating a local region, set up your circuit locally, relative to the lesion, in order for your current to proceed through that area. For example, when treating a internal knee injury, your circuit should be established so that the currents pass from one side of the knee through the center to the opposite side.

When using milliamperage for dispersing an area, use a dense-disperse setting, if possible. An alternative, if your machine does not have dense-disperse, is a discontinuous setting. This setting changes the frequency of the stimulation at regular intervals to prevent the body from accommodating. Of course, for dispersion, we must use a slightly higher frequency.

Optimal frequencies for treatment of acupoints are between 7 Hz and 40 Hz. The maximum frequency that can be used is 1000 Hz. The maximal refractory period of a cell's action potential is one millisecond. Therefore, a frequency greater than 1000 Hz will not generally have the maximum separation between the positive and negative electrodes, within a given treatment protocol. This will prevent the current from flowing between the poles in a superficial manner. This is especially important when using pads.

When stimulating distal acupoints on the extremeties, the electrodes from the same output may be placed over the needles bilaterally. This allows the current to travel deeper through the body. This should not affect the patient's heart.

When treating two sets of distal points bilaterally, such as the Four Gates (LI-4 and LR-3), you may prefer to place your electrodes contralaterally on one acupoint from each set. Clinically, this is less complicated and seems to work as well as using electrodes on all four points. This simplifies the treatment and does not overload the patient's nervous system. Too many accupuncturists overtreat their patients with electricity. This overloads their nervous systems and may, on some level, interfere with the proper energy balance we are seeking.

When using auricular points with electrical stimulation, do not always set up a circuit using two electrodes on the same ear. It is preferable either to use ear points bilaterally or to establish a circuit between one ear point and one body point. This ear–body connection may be unilateral or contralateral.

Do not run a milliamperage current directly across the spinal cord. This may interfere with the neural transmissions and effectively paralyze the patient for some time. I have never heard of this actually happening, but it pays to be conservative here. The FDA prohibits electricity from being sent through the brain; therefore, do not establish a circuit where milliamperage may be used across the head.

Never use two different frequencies at the same time in one area, unless it is interferential. Never use milliamperage and microamperage stimulation at the same time.

Never use electrical stimulation on patients with abnormal heart rhythms, pacemakers, pregnancy, cancerous tumors, or epilepsy, or in the area of the vagus nerve. Do not apply current directly over or through the heart region. It is also recommended that you do not use electricity across a nonunion fracture or recent scar.

The amount of sensation associated with electrical stimulation should never reach the painful level, because vasoconstriction will occur and the smooth flow of Qi will be disrupted.

## ACUPUNCTURE CIRCUITS FOR ELECTROSTIMULATION

The negative, black lead is attached to the start of the electron flow, and the positive, red lead is attached to the needle where the flow is to which directed or terminated. Circuits can be of almost any construct, depending on the clinical effect required. Yin energy moves upward, while Yang energy moves downward. Frequencies in general are 0.1 to 4 Hz for tonification and 30 to 150 Hz for movement or dispersion. So, the following sequences are possible:

1. Yin point (low in the foot or leg) to Yin point higher in leg (SP-6 [-] to SP-9 [+]); or to synergistic Yin meridian point in the arm (SP-9 [-] to LU-7 [+]).
2. Yang point (in hand or arm) to Yang point lower in arm or shoulder (SI-3 {-} to SI-9 [+]); or to lower synergistic Yang meridian point (SI-3 [-] to BL-62' [+]).
3. Yin point to Mu-Shu or CV point for focusing.
4. Mu–Shu tonification, Mu negative to Shu positive (from Yin to Yang).
5. Electrical tonification in TMMs (Ting points negative and gathering points positive) and Distinct meridians (access points negative and superior return Yang points positive).
6. Ear points.
7. Scalp acupuncture points.

1. Tai Yang Electroacupuncture (SI-BL)
   **Upper Points:** SI-3 and SI-4 (negative, black lead).
   **Lower Points:** BL-60 or BL-62' and all Shu Bladder points on the back.

**Clinical:** Used mostly for arm, shoulder, and back, or dorsal muscle spasm and pain. Start with a high frequency to break through the blockage, and then use lower frequency if the pain is chronic.

2. Shao Yin Electroacupucnture (KI-HT)
   **Lower Points:** KI-3 and KI-5 (negative, black lead).
   **Upper Points:** KI-7 or KI-10 or Kidney Shu point BL-23 (positive, red lead).
   **Clinical:** Used to tonify Kidney Yin energy, low back pain, Kidney deficient chest pain and asthma, tinnitus, and vertigo, always using a low frequency. The Heart meridian is never tonified. The Pericardium meridian is used.

3. Shao Yang Electroacupuncture (TH-GB)
   **Upper Points:** TH-5 and TH-8 (negative, black lead).
   **Lower Points:** GB-34 and GB-38 (positive, red lead).
   **Clinical:** Used for excess Yang symptoms in the head such as TMJ, migraines, headaches, red eyes, muscular spasm in the neck and shoulder, and pain problems in the lateral chest, hip, and leg. Because the symptoms are all in excess, a high dispersing frequency is used to break through the meridian blockage and tonification is not used.

4. Jue Yang Electroacupuncture (LR-PC/MH)
   **Lower Points:** LR-3 and PC-6 (negative, black lead).
   **Upper Points:** LR-8 and LR-14; CV-17 (positive, red lead).
   **Clinical:** Used to tonify the Liver and move stagnated Liver Qi. This will also help excess symptoms in Shao Yang. Tonification of the Heart is accomplished by the circuit PC-6 (−) to CV-17 (+). The Pericardium or Master of the Heart meridian is usually used for a calming effect and is usually dispersed.

5. Yang Ming Electroacupuncure (LI-ST)
   **Upper Points:** LI-4, LI-10, and LI-11 (negative, black lead).
   **Lower Points:** ST-25, ST-26, ST-36, and ST-40 (positive, red lead).
   **Clinical:** This is the one Yang synergistic energy line that is usually tonified. Low frequency is used, especially LI-4 to ST-36 (whose leads need to be crossed over, left LI-4 to right ST-36 and vice versa, because LI subnasally decussates to the opposite side of the body at its termination at LI-20). Used to tonify total body energy (LI-4 to ST-36); LI-10 or LI-11 to ST-25 or ST-26 or ST-40 will activate Yang Ming as a whole and address Stomach or Large Intestine organ problems.

6. Tai Ying Electroacupuncture (SP-LU)
   **Lower Points:** SP: SP-3 and SP-6 (negative, black lead).
        LU: LU-6 and LU-7. (negative, black ead).
   **Upper Points:** SP: SP-9, SP-12, CV-2 and CV-12, LR-13 (positive, red lead).
        LU: LU-1 (positive, red lead).
   **Clinical:** Tonification with low freqency is utilized. Used for Spleen energy (SP-3 to SP-6); fluid movement (SP-6 to SP-9); gynecological problems (SP-6 to SP-12 or CV-2); Spleen energy and organ problems (SP-9 to LR-13 [SP Mu point] or SP-9 to CV-12). Lung energy tonification use LU-6 to LU-1; Tai Yin tonification use SP-6 to LU-6; and Tai Yin-Yang Ming tonification use combined LI-4/LU-7 (−) to ST-36 (+).

## OTHER METHODS OF TONIFICATION

Other methods of tonification are the use of moxibustion, a heat lamp, and friction massage of the skin.

## MOXIBUSTION

*Moxibustion* is an ancient Chinese method of tonifying the energy of the body through the acupuncture points. The acupuncture points or the needles inserted into them are heated with a burning preparation of Artemesia vulgaris or the common Mugwort. Moxibustion can be applied directly to the skin with rolled up cones of the herb until the heat is felt, or by a lit moxa cigar, which is waved around the acupuncture point skin area, or around the needles to be heated for 5 to 10 minutes. Be carefull not to burn the patient with the moxa (although this method of scarification is used in China) by removing the moxa cone in time or by blowing the ash formed on the cigar every now and again, so that it will not fall on the patient's bare skin.

## RADIANT HEAT LAMP

The smell and smoke caused by the moxa seems to permeate the office and is irritating to allergic patients. A better idea is to use a radiant heat lamp source with a liquid moxa spray. The lamp can be positioned safely to heat any area of the body (usually in the prone position with heating of Shu points), and the area in question is sprayed with a liquid moxa, which, under the influence of the radiant heat, seems to do the job. The lamp can be timed and is usually left on for 15 to 20 minutes.

# Section III

*Other Forms of Alternative Medical Treatment*

# 8 Homeopathy

## HISTORY

Homeopathy is a unique system of healing developed by Samuel Hahnemann (1755–1843), and is based on the Law of Similars. Hahnemann's clinical observations and experiments were outlined in his book *The Organon of the Medical Art*, first published in 1810. Five subsequent editions, each one further developing his philosphies, have been published. The sixth edition was completed in 1842, a year before his death. Many disciples of Hahnemann carried his teachings throughout the world, including to the New World. The first American homeopath was Hans Graham who arrived in America in 1825. In 1844 Constantine Hering, who became known as the great American father of homeopathy, helped found the American Institute of Homeopathy, which still exists. Other important American homeopaths include James Tyler Kent (Kent's General Repertory is still used today) and Timothy F. Allen who wrote *The Encyclopedia of Pure Materia Medica*. The contentious relationship between homeopathy and the AMA has already been discussed.

## HOMEOPATHIC CONCEPTS

The prime aim of homeopathy is to restore, to its maximum potential, the "Vital Force" that vivifies the body, and which is disturbed in disease.

### THE LAW OF SIMILARS

*Homeopathy* comes from the Greek *omoios* meaning similar and *pathos* meaning feeling, indicating the use of a reinforcing or similar remedy to aid the body in the direction in which it was already proceeding. Hahnemann[56] called Western style medicine *Allopathy*, using the Greek root *allios* meaning other or opposite, to indicate the method of opposing symptoms with an opposite force. In his experiments from 1790 to 1810, Hahnemann noted that all medicinal substances produced a standard array of signs and symptoms in healthy people and that the medicine whose symptom picture most closely resembled the illness to be cured was the one most likely to initiate a curative response in that patient. Homeopathy, then, was a method of selecting curative remedies from the total picture of the diseased body. The formal description of this process is the *Law of Similars* — let likes be cured by likes — *Similia Similibus Curentur*.

### THE LAW OF THE MINIMUM DOSE

While the Law of Similars can be accepted when noting the similarity between the bases of allergy desentization and immunization (actually the "identical" rather than the similar — a practice known as *isopathy*), the Law of the Minimum Dose is more difficult to comprehend in Western medical terms.

During his experiments on friends and acquaintances, Hahnemann found that if he used a gross material amount of substance on the patient, he usually obtained a healing aggravation, or worsening of the disease, before he got an improvement in the clinical picture. In order to obviate this healing crisis, he started to dilute the remedy to see if he could lessen the aggravations produced by a strong dose. The doses did not seem to work on patients in his office, but did work on patients when he did house calls. The only difference was that the remedies, which he carried with him in the carriage, had been shaken by the wheels of the carriage bumping over the cobblestone roads. So he developed a technique of mixing the diluted remedies by thumping against a family Bible to simulate the bumping in the carriage. This mixing process he termed *succussion*.

He then formulated the *Law of Minimum Dose* which states that one should use the smallest dose and the lowest frequency of repetition to treat a patient. He found by clinical experience that the more you diluted and succussed the remedy, the more biological activity it elicited. He envisioned that the succussing liberated the energy from the healing substance, and that it was this energy that induced healing in the organism. Modern physics has shown a sinusoidal, ever amplifying resonant frequency curve that changes as the remedy is further diluted and succussed. The frequency of the substance is the small input that nudges the chaos within the organism towards a more acceptable pattern.

## THE TOTALITY OF SYMPTOMS

Hahnemann believed that all disease existed on a dynamic or energetic plane before pathophysiological changes could be seen. The body's response to those energetic shifts was to produce a responding shift to balance out the disturbed energy, and to do this, the body produced a pattern of symptoms, or the total picture or totality of symptoms. It is this state of the whole patient that is to be cured, not merely a single presenting symptom, and the remedy is similarly selected based on the total patient picture, not just the presenting major symptom. The most important parts of the total patient picture are the characteristic, or odd, and singular signatures of each individual patient's response to the imbalance. In fact, the patient and not the disease is treated. The great Indian homeopath, Rajan Sankaran recounts his frustration in his early years with prescribing on the major symptoms of the presenting disease, and getting very mediocre results. Then one day a lady patient presented to him with vitiligo and the only other symptoms he could elicit from her was that she was very talkative and humorous, was warm blooded, and liked to walk in the open air. He repertorized (looked up the one remedy that contained all these features) the lady under the rubrics (symptoms): loquacity with jesting, walking in open air ameliorates, and warmth in general aggravates. The remedy found was Kali Iodatum, but it was not mentioned under the patient's main complaint: "skin discoloration, white spots." Nevertheless, he administered the remedy and the vitiligo disappeared. He had treated the dynamic disturbance, or totality of the patient, and not the symptom, and the symptom had resolved.

## THE LAW OF THE SINGLE REMEDY

It follows from the concept of the *Totality of Symptoms*, that only a single remedy could exactly fit the similarity of the patient's total picture. From this concept, the *Law of the Single Remedy* was developed. This law allows the administration of only a single dynamized remedy to the patient at any one time, and then waiting sometimes for months or even years to allow the full effect of the dynamic disturbance, produced by that single administration, to take effect. This law is ignored by homeopaths using composite (mixed) remedies.

## THE LAW OF CURE

Classical homeopaths have traced the order in which symptoms and diseases appear and disappear and have formalized these observations into a general direction in which "cure" is said to take place. The four rules of cure were postulated by Constantine Hering between 1865 and 1875.[16] These four rules of cure relating to symptoms are that symptoms:

1. Move from above downward, from the head toward the feet.
2. Move from inside outward, from interior to exterior.
3. Move from more to less important organs or vital structures.
4. Change from the most recent to the oldest, in the reverse order of appearance in the patient's history.

## HOMEOPATHIC PROVINGS AND THERAPY

Hahnemann, in his search for new remedies to heal his patients, did the first double-blind, placebo-controlled pharmaceutical experiments on more than eighty different substances. The pharmacological activity of any substance in nature, whether animal, vegetable, or mineral, can be elicited by documentation of a healthy volunteer's secondary reaction on exposure to that substance, that is, what kind of reactive chaotic picture is induced in the person with a stable biology (healthy and devoid of manifest disease) when provoked by an external substance (remedy). This picture is called a "proving" of the substance. This *proving* or *remedy picture* forms the basis of the *Materia Medica* or PDR (*Physician's Desk Reference*) of remedies from which the homeopath can select medications for sick patients. The selection of a remedy for any particular symptomatic manifestation is done based on the Law of Similars — the remedy picture should match the disease picture.

For instance, taking into account my local situation in Reno, Nevada, if a gambler from California partakes in one of the numerous cheap buffets at one of the lower echelon casinos, has the misfortune to order a breakfast omelette, and acquires *Salmonella* enteritis with nausea, vomiting, sweating, and a sensation of coldness and impending doom, then, as a homeopath, I need to find that single medication or remedy which, when given to a healthy volunteer, will produce a similar biological response and pathophysiological picture. The single remedy that produces a similar picture, of the many thousands of homeopathic remedies, is homeopathic white arsenic or Arsenicum album. The homeopathic preparation (which is not poisonous) is given to the patient and creates a secondary or competing response with the Salmonella. Because the homeopathic remedy is energetically more powerful than the actual disease, which is more material and less energetic, the body focuses its attention on the artificial homeopathic "disease" and loses its physiological response to the Salmonella (instantaneous decreased susceptibility). Because the homeopathic stimulation is evanescent (short lasting and extinguishes quickly), the manifest symptoms now have nothing to stimulate them any further, are attenuated, or end prematurely. Thus, the duration and acuity of the enteritis is cut short and the patient recovers quickly from the disease. This is the essence of the homeopathic method. Much like a bullfighter (the disease), with his cape, the bull (the patient's response or symptoms) is distracted by the cape (the homeopathic remedy), which, when he charges, is pulled away revealing empty air and no bullfighter (resolution of the disease).

The format of the proving is quite standardized and blinded to both the assessor and the healthy volunteer, or prover. First, the prover is interviewed and his or her health status documented. Then for a period of time, a daily diary is kept by the prover documenting baseline symptomatology and physiology. The homeopathic medicine or a placebo is then administered to groups of provers until symptoms appear. The provers are then followed for a set time, and every day they document new objective and subjective changes in thoughts, feelings, physical sensations, sleep, appetite, cravings, aversions, etc. At the end of the proving period, the lists of changes from the baseline, documented by individual provers, are tabulated and compared with each other. Commonalities among provers are noted as important symptoms for that remedy picture, and less often experienced changes are judged on their merit for inclusion into the proving for that substance.

Information regarding the "picture" of a substance can come from other sources. The texts on toxicology are an important source for drug pictures, as they represent an actual proving on a patient, albeit a toxic proving instead of a harmless homeopathic proving. One can also use the primary pharmacological action of a drug or its side effects as a pseudoproving. I once cured a patient with oral pemphigus utilizing a homeopathic preparation of Captopril, because this symptom was a side effect of the drug. It is often of some help to document the side effects patients have had from the various drugs that they have been taking, or their exaggerated or idiosyncratic reactions to these drugs. For instance, most patients who react adversely to sulfa drugs have a particular susceptibility to Sulphur as a homeopathic remedy.

Another offshoot of drug side effects is the use of homeopathic preparations of drugs that are necessary for some patients, but are causing intolerable side effects. A homeopathic preparation using the drug can be made and administered together with the actual drug, to alleviate the trouble-some side effects without lowering the primary effect of the drug. I have done this numerous times for children on Tegretol, who are made drowsy by the drug, or to protect patients' livers from the side effects of systemic antifungals and the statin HMG-CoA reductase inhibitors. My most gratifying use of this isopathic technique was on a young lady whom I had kept going for five years on high doses of homeopathic Phosphorus for her chemically damaged liver. She had ingested carbon tetrachloride as a youngster and was steadily going into liver failure with cirrhosis. She was eventually transplanted in Minnesota and put on a then new antirejection drug, called FK-506 or Tacrolimus. The Tacrolimus caused her to experience severe body pain, probably of a myofascial origin and severe low back pain associated with her suddenly rising blood urea nitrogen (BUN) and creatinine. Her transplant doctor in San Francisco, where she was being followed, was about to take her off the drug, when I suggested to the patient that we could make an isopathic preparation of the Tacrolimus to decrease the side effects and renal toxicity of the drug. She agreed to a one-week trial and her BUN dropped from 84 mg/dl to 18 mg/dl and her creatinine from 3.6 to 1.0 mg/dl. All her dysphoria and body pain was gone by the end of the week and has never returned as long as she has been on the homeopathic preparation. We did stop the homeopathic after a year to see what would happen, and lab values soared again, only to return to normal within two days once the homeopathic preparation was restored. The disappearance of her raised lab values and lack of dysphoric symptoms were commented on by her hepatologist. The patient explained what we had done, but was told it had nothing to do with her improvement. She showed the physician the two episodes of homeopathic withdrawal and treatment values and was told politely that it was not possible. Even after a lead article in the *New England Journal of Medicine* in October 1994 commented on the 14% failure rate of tacrolimus due to nephrotoxicity, my telephone call to the transplant unit in San Francisco was actually met with cold disdain after I explained the "magical" cure. I have never heard from them despite the fact that my patient is their most successful transplant follow-up patient; has never had a rejection episode, raised liver functions, or any symptoms or signs of liver failure or drug toxicity; and is on 1/4 to 1/2 the usual dose of Tacrolimus. I guess they do not want to be confused by the facts.

## MATERIA MEDICA AND REPERTORY

From all the thousands of provings and clinical experience over the last two hundred years, about 2500 remedies have been indexed. The average homeopath rarely uses more than 200 remedies in everyday practice. The description or picture of some remedies occupies up to 80 pages of text, especially in the older *Materia Medicas*, where almost every prover's experience was detailed. Most Materia Medicas are now computerized and the selection of the remedies to match the patient's disease picture is done far more easily using a computerized cross-referencing *repertory* or listing of symptoms with associated remedies. So, for example if you wanted to know what remedy to give for chronic tonsillitis, you would look for the rubrics or symptoms listed as: **THROAT**, INFLAMMATION, **tonsils**, recurrent. The remedies that are listed under this rubric are: *alumina,* **baryta carbonicum,** *baryta muriaticum, hepar sulphuris,* lachesis, lycopodium, *psorinum, sangui-naria,* sepia*, silica,* and sulphur. You will note that the remedies are printed in three different styles — **bold**, *italic*, and plain. This differential printing indicates the strength of indication seen in the original provings. Almost all the provers experiencing Baryta carbonicum had a chronic sore throat during the entire length of the proving, while fewer provers of the remedies in italics had chronically inflamed throats, and only a few experienced the symptom when proving the remedies in plain type. This does not mean that you always give the remedy in bold type, but that if that symptom is predominant in the patient picture, then it warrants serious consideration. What you are attempting to do is to cover the whole patient picture including the predominant presenting symptom. For example, if the patient with the chronic tonsillitis also experienced inflammation only on the right side of the throat, craved sweets, had bad cracking of the skin on his heels, and was fearful of people, then you would look at all these symptoms and their associated proved remedies and see which remedy is common to them all. This remedy then would cover the patient's whole picture and lead to stability of all these chaotic manifestations or symptoms in the patient. The remedy, by the way, is Lycopodium clavatum (see Figure 8.1).

The first comprehensive repertory still in use was formulated by James Tyler Kent, who was a convert from the Eclectic School of Medicine after his wife was cured by a homeopath. His book of 1423 pages was an unbelievable compilation considering it was done by hand from his notes and readings. There are many newer repertories, mostly from European homeopaths, including the *Synthetic Repertory*, the *Complete Repertory*, *Murphy's Repertory*, and *Synthesis*. There are also competing computer programs including *McRepertory*, *CARA*, and the *Expert System*. All have their proponents and enemies. Homeopathy is a very passionate enterprise, because to be good, you have to devote your entire life to its learning and practice. This kind of devotion is not taken lightly and neither are their likes, dislikes, and ways of its practicing members.

## HOMEOPATHIC SCHOOLS OF PRACTICE

Just as in acupuncture, where there are many schools of thought and practice, the same is true in homeopathy. The five competing approaches that seem to be the most popular are:

### CLASSICAL HOMEOPATHY

In the Classical approach, the initial patient interview can take up to two hours, where every detail of the patient's life, attitudes, and physiology is elicited and examined. The information gathered is then turned into rubrics (symptoms) found in the repertories. The major rubrics are extracted from experience, and the single remedy that includes all the chosen rubrics and represents patient's whole picture, is administered in a single high dose as the only treatment. The patient is then

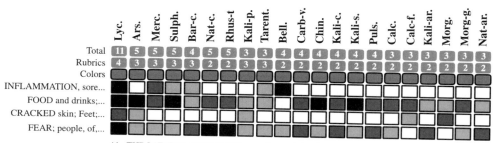

*1. THROAT; INFLAMMATION, şore throat; right: Bell., Lyc., caps., lac-c., merc., merc-i-f., adren...
*2. GENERALITIES; FOOD and drinks; sweets; desires: Arg-n., Ars., Cann-i., Chin., Chin-s...
*3. EXTREMITIES; CRACKED skin; Feet; heel: lyc., morg., syc-co., ars., arund., calc-f., coc-c...
*4. MIND; FEAR; people, of, anthropophobia: Cic., Hyos., Lyc., Nat-c., Rhus-t., acon., anac., anh...

**FIGURE 8.1** Computerized cross-referenced repertory.

followed over a prolonged period watching for changes in the chosen rubrics or the appearance of new rubrics. Once the homeopath is satisfied that the single remedy has run its course (months to years), the same remedy may be repeated if the patient experiences a similar relapse, or a new remedy is selected based on the new symptoms and rubrics elicited. This process is continued until the patient has improved his or her basic health to his or her satisfaction, or the homeopath or patient feels that no further progress is possible. As discussed previously, the main rubrics in contention in the Classical approach relate to the emotional roots and delusions of the presenting pathology.

**Pros:** The major advantages of this approach are the resolution of deep, fixed emotional pathology and healing of the total patient over time. There is no other approach in medicine, with the exception perhaps of Ericsonian hypnosis, that provides such an all-encompassing cure and is able to enhance the health of the individual and enable him or her to manifest full potential.

**Cons:** Modern society always demands the quick fix, and this is not it. It is also difficult to practice Classical homeopathy on a complex, fast-moving, multilayered biology, with so many obstacles to cure. Only the dedicated, introspective patient is going to get full benefit from this practice. The administration of higher potencies and nosodes (homeopathic remedies made from diseased tissue or organisms) is governed by law and is allowed to be dispensed only by a medical doctor.

## COMPLEX HOMEOPATHY

In the Complex approach, championed by the Germans, a mixture of homeopathic remedies are combined to address a single or small complex of symptoms or "Keynotes" such as sore throat, allergic rhinitis, or headache. The concept employed here is not one of the whole patient picture, but of a shotgun approach to a single clinical presentation, where all the remedies in bold type associated with a positive proving for that symptom are collected together in a single complex or mixed remedy and administered to the patient multiple times a day, for as many days as it takes to extinguish the symptoms.

**Pros:** Most over-the-counter medications for home use are of this type and can be readily and easily used by the layperson. In most instances, these remedies afford some relief, do no harm, and are certainly to be preferred to inappropriate antibiotic use, for instance, in otitis media.

**Cons:** The use of mixtures may confuse the patient's picture over time and may be detrimental due to the treatment of superficial symptoms only. Self-medication and the prescribing of these complex homeopathics by health food clerks may lead to a false state of security, especially where symptoms are those of a more serious underlying medical problem.

## FRENCH PLEURALISTIC AND CONSTITUTIONAL THERAPY

Hahnemann moved to Paris in his later years and died there in 1843, where his tomb remains in PereLachaise. He begat many French pupils, who proceeded to develop a new style of homeopathy, peculiar to the French. Beginning in 1912, Leon Vannier, O. A. Julian, and Max Tetau created a new style of homeopathy termed *Biotherapy*. This style was more materially based, and was more interested in the "terrain" of the patient, that is, the constitutional diathesis of the patient or his or her "chronic reactional mode," and in the physiological processes, especially detoxification and drainage, that could be impacted by the homeopathic method.

At the beginning of the 20th century, Nebel, a Swiss from Lausanne, noted that certain patients with specific bodily morphologies often presented specific pathological tendencies that could be cured with "constitutional" remedies. Three basic mineral constitutions were described corresponding to the three skeletal calcium salts — Calcarea carbonicum (Carbonic constitution, short and stocky mesomorphic or endomorphic individuals), Calcarea phosphorica (Phosphoric constitution, tall and thin ectomorphic individuals), and Calcarea fluorica (Fluoric constitution, short and thin with asymmetry).

The French combined these concepts into a low-dose homeopathic system that focused on the gross physiology and pathophysiology and its treatment with newer types of biological substances. The newer substances used included the extensive use of homeopathic preparations of pathological excretions, tissues, and organisms (*nosode therapy*); macerates of fresh buds and other vegetative tissue in the growing stage that promote drainage especially in chronic disease (*gemmotherapy*); diluted and dynamized minerals and rocks used for drainage (*dechelating lithotherapy*); and preparations of single and multiple minerals employed to activate specific enzyme pathways (*oligostim therapy*). Subsequently, ethical type drugs, such as penicillin, cortisone, phenobarbital, chlorpromazine, haloperidol, and others were used in homeopathic preparations.

The French also developed a system of administration that was different from any other. Instead of giving a Classical high dose or a Complex mixed dose, they took the centrist position and gave multiple, different, single doses at different times of the day. Each different remedy addressed a separate element of the case. This was called the *Pleuralistic style*. For example, in a simple case of whooping cough they would prescribe:

- **Symptomatically** — for the barking cough, Drosera 6X and Bryonia 6X, three granules, alternating every 6 hours.
- **Nosode therapy** — for immune stimulation, Pertussin 12X, 3 granules at bedtime.
- **Reactional mode** — for metabolic activation, Sulphur iodatum 12X, alternate with Pertussin, 3 granules at bedtime.
- **Terrain** — for hereditary chest weakness, Tuberculinum 30 X, 5 granules once a week.

The French are forbidden to use high potencies in homeopathy (above 30CH), and so this lower potency and multiplicity of remedies enables them to hit all levels of the individual in an entirely different way.

**Pros:** This system works quite well if you are not too interested in deeper emotional issues and you need a sure therapeutic hit. It also has some benefit in correcting the underlying terrain in which the patient's illness is developing. It is able to cut through the morass of complex layers that one sees in modern day patients, and it is easy to modify one or another level of the input without disturbing other levels. This is important, because each level (symptomatic, nosode, reactional, and constitutional) moves and reacts at its own pace — some fast moving with continual changing of the remedies as symptoms evolve and change, and some slow moving (such as the reactional mode), needing the same remedy for months or even years.

**Cons:** The patients have to be highly compliant with the complicated dosing to make it work. You have to have a large inventory of remedies.

## HOMOTOXICOLOGY BY H. H. RECKEWEG

Homotoxicology is a modernized method of practicing homeopathy developed by Dr. Hans-Heinrich Reckeweg in Baden-Baden, Germany in 1955. Reckeweg utilized the concepts of homeopathy as a base to integrate the basic medical sciences and molecular biology into a unified biological whole. Homotoxicology represents a perspective on cellular disease where the extracellular *Matrix* as described by Pischinger, is the arena in which all biological reactions and regulation take place. He redefined acute disease, and inflammation in particular, as a biological advantageous defensive measure to cleanse the matrix of what he termed *homotoxins* that produce negative biological changes in the host's matrix, regulation, and cellular organs. Homotoxins could be of internal or external origin and could include substances such antigen–antibody complexes; abnormal or excessive products of intermediary metabolism such as free radicals, peroxides, histamine, wild peptides, or false proteins; pesticides, heavy metals, drugs, or invading organisms. Homotoxins can also be thought of as toxic and internalized emotions.

**TABLE 8.1**
**Table of Homotoxicosis (abridged form)**

| Tissue | Recovery | | | Lingering Illness | | |
|---|---|---|---|---|---|---|
| | Humoral Phases/Diseases of Disposition | | | Cellular phases/Constitutional Diseases | | |
| | Excretion phases | Reaction phases | Deposition phases | Impregnation phases | Degeneration phases | Neoplasm phases |
| **1. Ectodermal** | | | | | | |
| a) Epidermal | Perspiration, cerumen, sebum, etc. | Furuncles, erythema, dermatitis, eczema, pyodermia, etc. | Atheroma, warts, keratosis, clavi, etc. | "Tattooing," pigmentation, etc. | Dermatitis, lupus vulgaris leprosy, etc. | Ulcus rodens, basalioma, etc. |
| b) Orodermal | Saliva, coryza, etc. | Stomatitis, rhinitis, aphthous stomatitis, etc. | Nasal polypus, cysts, etc. | Leukoplakia, etc. | Ozaena, atrophic rhinitis, etc. | Cancer of the nasal |
| c) Neurodermal | Neurohormonal secretion of cells, etc. | Poliomyelitis in the pyrexial stage, herpes zoster, etc. | Benign neuromas, neuralgia, etc. | Migraine, tics, etc., virus infections (poliomyelitis) | Paresis, multiple sclerosis, optic atrophy syring omyeliz, etc. | Neuroma, gliosarcoma, etc. |
| d) Sympaticodermal | Neurohormonal secretion of cells, etc. | Neuralgia, herpes zoster, etc. | Benign neuromas, neuralgia, etc | Asthma, ulcus ventr. et duodeni, etc. | Neurofibromatosis, etc. | Gilosarcoma, etc. |
| **2. Entodermal** | | | | | | |
| a) Mucodermal | Gastrointestinal secretions, $CO_2$ stercobilin, etc., toxins with faeces | Pharyngitis, laryngitis, enteritis, colitis, etc. | Polypi of the mucous membranes, constipation, megacolon, etc. | Asthma, hoarseness, ulcus ventr. et duodeni, carcinoid syndr. etc | Tuberculosis of the lung of the intestine, etc. | Cancer of the larynx, stomach, rectum, etc. |
| b) Organodermal | Bile, Pancreatic juice, thyroid hormones, etc. | Parotitis, pneumonia, hepatitis, cholangitis, etc. | Silicosis, goitre, cholelithiasis, etc. | Toxic damage to the liver, pneumonopathy, virus infections, etc. | Cirrhosis of the liver, hyperthyroidism, myxoe.dema, etc. | Cancer of the liver, gall bladder, pancreas, thyroid gland, lungs |
| **3. Mesenchymal** | | | | | | |
| a) Interstitiodermal | Mesenchymal interstitial substance hyaluronic acid, etc. | Abcesses, phlegmons, carbuncles, etc. | Adiposis, gouty tophi, oedema, etc. | Forestages of elephantiasis, etc., influenzal virus infections | Sclerodema, cachexia, velamen vulvae, etc. | Sarcoma of various locations, etc. |
| b) Osteodermal | Haemopoiesis, etc. | Osteomyelitis, etc. | Osteophytosis, etc. | Osteomalacia, etc. | Spondylitis, etc. | Osteosarcomas, etc. |
| c) Haemodermal | Menses, blood and antibody formation | Endocarditis, typhus, sepsis, embolism, etc. | Varicose veins, thrombosis, sclerosis, etc. | Angina pectoris, myocarditis, etc. | Myocardial infarct, panmyelophtisis, pernicious anaemia, etc. | Myeloid leukaemia, angiosarcomas, etc. |
| d) Lymphodermal | Lymph, etc., antibody formation | Angina tonsillaris, appendicitis, etc. | Swelling of the lymph glands, etc. | Lymphatism, etc. | Lumphogranulomatosis, etc. | Lymphatic leukaemia, lymphosarcomas, etc. |
| e) Cavodermal | Fluid, synovia | Polyarthritis, etc. | Dropsy, etc. | Hydrocephalus, etc. | Coxarthritis, etc. | Chondrosarcoma, etc. |
| **4. Mesodermal** | | | | | | |
| a) Nep hrodermal | Urine with catabolites | Cystitis, pyelitis, nephritis, etc. | Hypertrophy of the prostate glands, nephrolithiasis, etc. | Albuminuria, hydronep hrosis, etc. | Nephrosis, contracted kidney, etc. | Renal carcinomas, hypernephroma, etc. |
| b) Serodermal | Secretions of the serous membranes | Pleuritis pericarditis, peritonitis, etc. | Pleural effusions, ascites, etc. | Forestages of tumours, etc. | Tbc. of the serous membrane, etc. | Cancer of the serous membranes, etc. |
| c) Germinodermal | Menses, semen, prostatic fluid, ovulation etc. | Adnexitis, metritis, ovaritis, salpingitis, prostatitis | Myomas, hypertrophy of the prostate gland, hydrocele, cysts, ovarian cysts, etc. | Forestages of tumours, (adnexa, uterus, testicles, etc.) | Impotentia virilis, sterility, etc. | Cancer of the uterus, ovaries, testes, etc. |
| d) Musculodermal | Lactic acid, lactacidogens, etc. | Muscular rheumatism, myositis, etc. | Myogelosis, rheumatism, etc. | Myositis ossificans, etc. | Dystrophis musculorum progressiva, etc. | Myosarcoma, etc. |
| | Excretion principle, enzymes intact, tendency towards a spontaneous cure, favourable prognosis | | | Condensation principle, enzymes damaged, tendency towards deterioration, dubious prognosis | | |

The homotoxic phases are arranged vertically, and the tissues affected by the homotoxins are arranged horizontally. Each phase can be related to practically any other through the vicariation phenomena.

When the body encounters a homotoxin, it initiates a series of reactions mediated by the *greater defense system* (consisting of the RES, adenohypophyseal–adrenocortical system, neural reflex system, detoxification function of the liver, and detoxification within the connective tissue) to eliminate the toxin or to control its effects. The defense reaction against the homotoxins manifests itself as disease and makes up the *Six Phases of Disease* (see Table 8.1). These reactions enable the homotoxin to be neutralized and coupled to form an inert *homotoxone* which can then be physiologicaly excreted from the body (*Excretion phase* — like diarrhea in food poisoning), cause a pathological reaction for excretion, such as pus (*Reaction phase* — like a sinus drainage or vaginal discharge), or be unexcretable and just deposited as a means of limiting its effect (*Deposition phase* — nasal polyps). These first three defense phases of the Six Phases of Disease are termed the *humeral phases*. The humeral phases represent the harmless and appropriate elimination or deposition of the homotoxins, while the next three defense phases are termed the *cellular phases*:

- Impregnation — cell damage from free radicals;
- Degeneration — damage to cell protoplasmic structures, like respiratory enzymes and mitochondria;
- Neoplastic — entails damage to the DNA or genetic mechanism of the cell.

The cellular phases represent a homotoxic injury and are accompanied by the concentration of homotoxins or homotoxones in one of the damaged areas, that now undergo further defensive changes to maintain homeostasis (such as cirrhosis, leukemia, MS, paralysis, and cancer). So, the concept of disease, as defined in scientific and molecular biological terms by Reckeweg, is the body's expression of the defensive actions against internal and external homotoxins (phases 1 through 3); in phases 4 through 6 the diseases are the expression of the damage caused by the deposited or recirculating homotoxins for which the organism tries to compensate. The humeral phases of elimination and inflammation are, in fact, essential to early recovery and should be encouraged with homeopathic remedies, which act as anti-homotoxins, and never suppressed with drugs.

Reckeweg also postulated that the homotoxins, if not dealt with initially, would move from their original tissue entry point to a different tissue, and produce a totally different bodily reaction or different disease manifestation. He was able to track this movement by identifying the germ cell or embryonic layer where the diseased tissue had its origin. He constructed a Table of Homotoxicosis (Tablel 8.1) with the Six Phases of Disease across the top and the tissue germ cell layers along the left side. Within the cells were the body's disease response (diagnosis) to the homotoxin's phase. If the homotoxin moved tissue layers or its phase, then it produced a new disease. Thus, Reckeweg could track a patient's progress in pathological and tissue terms.

Note that the Six Phases of Disease are somewhat similar to the Six Levels of Disease in Traditional Chinese medicine.

One of the interesting outcomes of such tracking is that it reveals certain trends in the patient's progress that have very important prognostic indications. Reckeweg termed this the tissue and phase change of the organism or the *vicariation phenomenon*. If the patient's disease trail is moving to the right or downward in the table, this is a bad prognosis irrespective of how the patient is clinically, and Reckeweg termed this retrogressive trend a *progressive vicariation*. If the patient's disease trail was moving to the left or upward, then the patient was getting better biologically, even if he or she felt worse, and this he termed *regressive vicariation*. You will recognise Hering's Laws of Cure in this scenario. When progressive vicariation (worsening) is caused by suppression of symptoms or repoisoning, usually by the use of suppressive drug therapy, the biological phase is usually shifted across the "biological wall" to the right side of the table (to phases 4 through 6). This produces a bad prognosis and it is almost impossible to return to the left side of the table. This is termed chronic disease.

Reckeweg explains the mechanism of the homeopathic remedy in this process in the following way. The homeopathic, because it is similar to the homotoxin, stimulates a supplementary defense system, which effectively supports the first defense system (called *disease*), and causes accelerated healing. This is very similar to Hahnemann's explanation of the remedy causing a second artificial disease.

The attainment of cure is defined as the attainment of regressive vicariations up to the physiological excretion phase in the ectoderm. Healing is defined as becoming free of all homotoxins and of all damage caused by homotoxins.

Reckeweg was an innovative medical genius and he developed his concept to include the use of nosodes, sarcodes (homeopathic preparations of normal tissue, usually porcine), intermediary metabolic pathways (Krebs Cycle intermediates), homeopathically adjusted Western drugs, vitamins, quinones, and biological catalysts. He documented all his clinical findings in one book, called the *Ordinatio* or Biotherapeutic Index, which I had the arduous job of updating in 1992. In the book he lists Western allopathic diagnoses, gives the phase of disease and tissue layer that it represents, and gives the homeopathic therapy best suited to its resolution.

## ELECTRONIC HOMEOPATHY

Nevada and Utah are unique in the United States for being at the root of what is termed *electronic homeopathy*. In Classical homeopathy the single remedy is chosen based on the symptom picture of the patient. In electronic homeopathy the remedy is chosen based on its bioelectric and biomagnetic resonance with the body. If we consider the whole electromagnetic form of the body to be a composite standing wave hologram representing the chaotic resonance at any one time, then disturbances in the wave form, brought on by any external or internal stressor, will cause a shape, amplitude, or phase shift in the waveform. This, in turn, causes the physical and functional manifestation of the hologram to change, and we appreciate this change as symptoms of disease. If we provoke the distorted hologram with a correcting resonant waveform, we can reestablish the old pattern of harmonic resonance and the symptoms of disease disappears. The selection of the correcting waveform (homeopathic remedy) is accomplished by a technique called *Electro-Acupuncture According to Voll* (EAV), or more recently *Electro-Dermal Testing* (EDT) or *Meridian Stress Assessment* (MSA). EAV, which was invented by Dr. Reinhold Voll in Munich in the early 1950s, is the technical mode of selecting the remedies. In this technique, the electrical characteristics of the acupuncture points on the extremeties are measured using a sophisticated ohm meter. The system has three zones of response to this measurement: balanced (in harmonic resonance), too high (inflamed or irritated), or too low (degenerated or neoplastic). These results are very reminiscent of Reckeweg's Normal, Humeral, and Cellular Phases. After establishing the disharmonious electrical pattern of the Yin and Yang organs, then homeopathic remedies are introduced into the circuit to normalize either a high or low reading. If the homeopathic remedy accomplishes that correction on remeasuring the aberrant acupuncture point, then that remedy is selected for the patient. Not surprisingly, remedies selected in this manner always produce a biological response, because you have already demonstrated that activity by the remedy's normalizing the electrical reading. This technique will be further discussed in the section on Bio-Energetic Medicine.

**Pros:** The homeopath can select mutiple remedies (a harmonic chord) rather than a single remedy (a note) and can test them out electronically together to assure appropriateness and tolerance. There is no guessing. The remedy either balances the point or it does not. The exact dosage can be tested so that aggravations or healing reactions can be minimized. It can be used as a premorbid screening tool, as it will pick up disturbances in the energy field of the organs and body long before positive blood tests or tissue or cellular pathology occurs. It can detect, by resonance with the corresponding nosode, the energetic presence of any environmental pollutant, toxin, organism, drug, allergen, or analyte, which, although not diagnostic, appears to be clinically very relevent in assessing patients.

**Cons:** The FDA has a big problem with the technology because it is such a threat to the medical–industrial complex, and has gone out of its way to harass practitioners using this technology. Not everybody can practice the technique.

# THE HOMEOPATHIC PHARMACY

Homeopathic remedies are lawfully governed by the Homeopathic Pharmacopoeia of the United States (HPCUS) and overseen by the FDA. The HPCUS was grandfathered into the original Food, Drug and Cosmetic Act of 1938, and also written into the Medicare Act of 1965. The preparation of homeopathic remedies is outlined in monographs approved by the HPCUS.

## PREPARATION OF A HOMEOPATHIC MEDICINE

The modern terminology for the process of producing a homeopathic medicine is *Serial Agitated Dilution* (SAD) or better known in the homeopathic literature as *potentization*, the process of making the biological activity of the substance more potent as it is diluted out. In the process of producing a homeopathic remedy, the macerated herb or plant is dissolved in pharmaceutical grade alcohol and a *Mother Tincture* (MT = $\varnothing$ ) is made. From the MT, one part of this solution is mixed with 9 parts (decimal, D, or X) or 99 parts (centesimal, C, or CH) of alcohol diluent and then agitated or, as the homepaths term it, *succussed*. This process of serial dilution from the mixture below it, with subsequent succussion each time, produces the homeopathic remedy at whatever dilution (potency) you require. The dilution of low potencies ranges from 3X to 12X ($10^{-3 \text{ to } -12}$) or 3C to 9C ($10^{-6 \text{ to } -18}$); intermediate potencies in the 12C to 30C ($10^{-24 \text{ to } -60}$) range and high potencies from 200C ($10^{-400}$) to CM ($10^{-100,000}$). Each potency has a specific activity and Wolfgang Ludwig in Germany has shown that, as you go up in dilutions, you produce a shifting sinusoidal curve of infrared absorption. Recent studies have also shown that low potencies tend to stimulate activity, middle potencies balance or regulate activity, and high potencies inhibit activity. Lower potencies tend to affect more recent, material, or dense physical problems, and higher potencies tend to affect more temporal, remote, and emotional issues.

Insoluble substances that cannot be diluted, such as minerals, heavy metals, or insoluble stems, or fibrous parts of plants, are first triturated or ground together in a pestle and mortar with 9 or 99 parts of powdered lactose, and after the sixth trituration are then converted to liquid dilutions. The homeopathic remedy may be taken as the liquid, as lactose pellets that have been sprayed with the solution, or with lactose powder mixed with the solution and then compressed into tablets.

# THE SCIENCE OF HOMEOPATHY

The major criticism of homeopathy is based on the professed biological activity of solutions containing little or none of the original substance in the remedy. Based on Avogadro's number in chemistry [($6.02 \times 10^{23}$), the number of molecules in a mole, or the gram molecular weight of a substance], when solutions dilute out beyond Avogadro's number, no more atoms or molecules of the substance exist in the solution and all that is left is the solvent. This dilution corresponds to 12C or 24X, a level of potency that is often used and does not even address the higher potencies. The clue to the effect is that the succussion provides thermal and kinetic energy to the solute–solvent mixture, which produces energy storage in the bonds of the diluent in the infrared spectrum, that downloads into patterned clathrates or patterned crystalline water. These clathrates are able to reproduce their patterning on further dilution and succussion. The body is able to react to these external patterned inputs, because all of the body's interaction with its exterior is via patterned frequency inputs — light, color, sound, etc. This input is seen as a perturbing force that moves the susceptible chaotic standing wave form (the sick patient) to a new resonant equilibrium (cure).

Of even more interest is the finding that you can induce the pattern and frequency of a homeopathic remedy into a water–alcohol mixture by means of an alternating current magnetic field, inject the mixture into the patient, and get an immediate clinical result. Electronic homeopathy has come of age.

Two important meta-analyses of homeopathic clinical trials are available for review, and each shows that homeopathy works.[57,58]

## THE PRACTICE OF HOMEOPATHY

How do you use 2500 remedies in multiple potencies on a single patient? Practically, you first use complex type, low potency homeopathy to correct the gross pathophysiology of the patient — to detox the liver, improve circulation, and remove pesticides, heavy metals, old viruses etc. You then use pleuralistic style, intermediate potency, regulating, organ–specific remedies to help balance out disordered physiology or foci or energetic blocks in the body. Thereafter, you use classical style, high potency homeopathy to correct the emotional–mental imbalances that are the main cause of disease in the body.

You can also invoke the use of miasmatic nosodes (homeopathic remedies that remove hereditary traits or weaknesses) to eventually restore health to your already balanced patients, or to remove these weaknesses before conception or in the developing embryo.

### POSOLOGY — HOMEOPATHIC DOSING

Homeopathic dosing depends on the clinical picture and the potency being used. The following are general rules:

1. **Acute disease, low potency** — 10 drops or 5 pellets or 2 tablets under the tongue every 15 minutes to one hour apart, decreasing to 3x/day as the symptoms let up. Usual duration is from 1 to 5 days.
2. **Chronic disease, intermediate potency** — dosing is daily, with intercurrent dosing to address all problems. This may last for weeks to months.
3. **Emotional disease, high potency** — a single sublingual dose or three escalating doses over three days only. Wait for at least one month and maybe for years.
4. **LM potencies** — In his last (6th) edition of the *Organon*, Hahnemann departed from using dry doses, that is, doses on lactose, and went entirely to the use of aqueous LM ($10^{-5000}$) potencies. In this prescription, a 1:50,000 dilution was used by taking a single teaspoon of the solution out, diluting it in a glass of pure water, stirring, and then taking a single teaspoon of the water from the glass as the homeopathic dose. The advantage of this method is that you get an ever-escalating dose of the remedy every day, so that the body cannot accommodate to a repetitive input (tachyphylaxis). This method in water is also very gentle, and you will not see any aggravations, which can occur quite often with dry dosing, when the body is too vigorously stimulated.

Contrary to the belief of the Classical homeopaths, Chinese herbs, acupuncture, and a host of other modalities can be used concurrently with homeopathy. Homeopathic remedies, because their activity is based on an electromagnetic (EM) frequency, have to be kept away from external sources of EM energy and radiation that would disturb their patterns. Care must be taken not to expose them to excessive heat, the sunlight or freezing, and all electrical and EM fields, such as TVs, computers, microwaves, and electrical outlets. If this is done, they will last forever and, in fact, one of Hahnemann's original homeopathic preparations was tried recently and worked as expected.

Patients taking homeopathics have to have a clean mouth for the remedy to take effect and should take their homeopathics at least 10 minutes before or after a meal. Homeopathics can be put into creams, oral sprays, and injecting solutions and can also be rubbed on the forearm skin, a technique that is sometimes used in infants. Some substances are said to neutralize the action of the homeopathic remedy after it has been taken. These include coffee, any mint- or camphor-related substance, and some strong odors. A traumatic incident as well as dental work has been seen to cause neutralization of the remedy action. In such cases, redosing of the homeopathic remedies the problem.

It is not possible to teach homeopathy from a book such as this. Anyone with interest, dedication, lots of time, and no commitments should avail themselves of the many courses of at least 3 to 4 years duration that are now available in many parts of the country.

# 9 Anthroposophical Medicine

Rudolf Steiner, the founder of the anthroposophical approach to health and healing, gave us a wider appreciation of man and his relationship to the cosmos. The term *anthroposophical* is derived from the Greek words *antropos*, meaning "man" and *sophos*, meaning "wisdom." Steiner was able to relate the wisdom of man to every facet of his activities and being, including agriculture, education, and medicine.

The anthroposophical approach to medicine views man as being composed of four essential elements (a recapitulation of Arthur M. Young's description of man's ascent from inert matter, in his book, *The Reflexive Universe*[1]):

1. The *physical body* (material or mineral nature),
2. The *vital force* (etheric body or plant nature),
3. The *astral body* (organized feelings and emotions or animal nature),
4. *"I" organization* (individual spirit or human nature).

The concepts of the etheric, astral, and mental body are drawn from esoteric anatomy and find their roots in the study of Eastern philosphies. The aim of medical anthroposophy is to bring all of these parts of man into balance utilizing special homeopathic preparations, the most famous of which is Iscador™, a homeopathic preparation of mistletoe. While these homeopathic preparations show no distinct advantage over conventional homeopathics, Steiner's broader concept of man and his integration with his environment and spiritual aspect should be emulated by any physician wishing to be a real healer. Further information and training may be obtained from the Physicians' Association for Anthroposophical Medicine.

# 10 Neural Therapy

## HISTORY OF NEURAL THERAPY

Neural therapy is a holistic system of treatment for chronic pain and illness. It involves the injection of local anesthetics into the subcutis, autonomic ganglia, peripheral nerves, scars, glands, trigger points, and even organs. It acts by regulating the effect that the "interference field" or "focus" has on the central nervous system, autonomic nervous system, and pituitary–endocrine axis.

In 1905 Einhorn discovered novocaine, and in 1906 G. Spiess discovered that regional infiltration with novocaine hastened wound healing. In 1925 Dr. Ferdinand Huneke mistakenly injected his sister intravenously with an Atophenyl/procaine mixture (an anti-inflammatory for rheumatism) to try and alleviate her migraine headaches. To his surprise, her migraine immediately vanished, as did her depression, and neither symptom ever returned. What he had actually done was to give her a mixture that contained procaine, which was actually meant for intramuscular use. Both Ferdinand and his brother Walter further discovered that they could affect all kinds of problems almost instantaneously by the use of novocaine injections into perivenous and intramuscular sites.

In 1940 Ferdinand made a further startling discovery. He had a woman come to him with capsular arthritis of the right shoulder. The treatment of the day was to remove any structure that might be seeding the affected shoulder, and to this end she had all her teeth and tonsils removed. Then it was thought that the seeding was coming from a 25-year-old area of osteomyelitis in her left tibia, and amputation of the leg was being considered. Ferdinand tried to help her pain by injecting Impletol (Bayer's novocaine with caffeine) around the shoulder, intra-articularly, and into the stellate ganglion. All these injections had no effect, and Ferdinand discharged the woman uncured. A few weeks later the woman returned to point out to him what had happened to the osteomyelitis scar on her left tibia. It had become angry, red, and swollen, and she could now hardly walk. Ferdinand immediately injected the scar and the area around it with novocaine and experienced his first "lightning reaction." The shoulder pain on the right side immediately disappeared and she was able to move her arm with a full range of motion, and the pain in the scar ceased. This was the first proof that a neural interference field could act as a trigger for an illness at a distance from the field. In the United Statees, neural therapy has been championed, developed, and taught by Dietrich Klinghardt, MD, Ph.D, of Seattle.[41]

## NEURAL THERAPY THEORY

### INTERFERENCE FIELDS

In order to start treatment, the abnormal *focus* or *interference field* must first be identified. Any part of the body can become an interference field. The most important areas include the tonsils, teeth, sinuses, scars, appendix, and pelvis. From clinical experience, about 35% to 40% of all patients have an interference field as part of their pathology and ongoing illness. Most commonly, the interference field is one of a number of fields of disturbance, irritation, inflammation, or dysfunctional inputs into the chaotic system causing disharmony. Other stressors that the patient is undergoing, such as emotional stress, may convert an inactive interference field into an active field. In these cases both issues have to be addressed to accomplish healing.

In some patients the concomitant use of certain medications such as steroids, antibiotics, antihistamines, and antidepressants will obviate the effect of neural therapy, acupuncture, and homeopathy.

Indicators that bring an interference field to mind include:

- Unresponsive to other therapies,
- Aggravations by other therapies,
- All problems being gathered on one side of the body,
- Disease developing after an operation, not being well since.

Methods to find the interference field include:

1. **History** — look for last illnesses, surgeries, trauma, dental work.
2. **Systematic search** — do a careful range of motion examination on the painful area; search and treat all scars and repeat ROM to see if it has been affected. In the second session treat the pelvis. In the third session treat the chest.
3. **Empirical approach** — empirical relationships exist clinically between certain problems and certain interference fields. For example: tonsils — knee joint; abdominal scars — large joints and low back; leg scars — sciatica; tonsils and teeth — migraine; prostate, stomach, and sinuses — neck pain; gallbladder scar — shoulder; pelvic scars — PMS, depression, and arthritis. Also remember the acupuncture meridians. If any scar crosses a meridian, it could cause a problem along any part of the meridian. An interesting case comes to mind in this regard. For three months to no avail I had been treating a 65-year-old man with a 12-year history of chronic idiopathic chest pain. Usually you will find Kidney Yin deficiency and sometimes associated Coxsackie B virus as the cause. But not so in this case. I had looked at the Principal Kidney meridian as it coursed up parasternally, but could find no evidence of a scar. My dear wife was passing by and casually remarked, "How about looking at all the energy lines in Tai Yang — Shao Yin." So I searched the entire meridian complex and finally found a 1 mm scar on the acupuncture point HT-9 on the tip of the little finger. I asked him about the scar, which was a thorn prick that had occurred when he had moved residences and was carrying his potted roses, about 12 years ago. Eureka! A single 0.1 ml injection of novocaine into the scar caused an immediate lightning reaction, the first I had ever seen, and immediate and permanent relief of his chest pain.

## THE NERVOUS SYSTEM THEORY

In cases of chronic illness that produces associated changes in the autonomic nervous system, the associated and adjacent autonomic ganglia undergo changes in their membrane potentials. These changes can result in abnormal signals coming from both afferent and efferent connections with the spinal cord and the central nervous system (CNS). The CNS, responding to abnormal information responds inappropriately, and a vicious cycle is set up. The injection of novocaine normalizes the aberrant focus and the nervous informational patterns are restored to normal.

The physiological effect of a novocaine injection is to restore the -80 mV membrane potential to the nerve. This allows for restoration of the nerve's membrane ionic pumping activity, with removal of intracellular waste and toxins, thereby regaining normal function.

## THE FASCIAL CONTINUITY THEORY

The fascia surrounding each muscle and muscle group in the body are interconnected, to the extent that there is continuity of the plantar fascia all the way up to the meninges. An adhesion or scar can affect the fascia by creating tension in it. This tension or tugging of the fascia will be transmitted along the entire myofascial system and cause displacements and torquing of the system at a distance from the scar. Also to be considered are the electrical gradients caused by this tensile and shearing force and the charge in the scar itself, which can range up to 1.5 V as opposed to the normal 80 mV of the body. Injecting the scar allows the abnormally high electrical charge to discharge and the electrical activity of impacted acupuncture meridians to flow.

## THE MATRIX–GROUND SYSTEM THEORY

This is the most popular, but least understood theory, concerning the matrix of the extracellular space as described by Pischinger.[46] The extracellular space is a soup of nerve endings, fibroblasts, arterioles and capillaries, lymphatics and venules, cell membranes, and a sol-gel matrix of glyco-proteins and proteoglycans. This space is where all interaction, whether electrical, ionic, or osmotic is happening. These regulating properties can be changed by manipulation of any of the physical, anatomical, or humeral properites of the space. This ground system has a very interesting property, in that a small change in one area causes a full phase shift in the whole system throughout the body (sounds pretty much like nonlinear dynamics and chaos to me.). The matrix is probably a liquid crystal, with different properties depending on its phase of existence. Injecting novocaine or lidocaine into this matrix at an appropriate focus or point, will cause a phase shift in the entire system, with resolution of the symptoms that the previous phase was causing.

One of the most interesting phenomena that you can actually demonstrate on any patient is the instantaneous return to a balanced electrical reading in Meridian Stress Assessment (MSA) with the injection of an appropriate homeopathic remedy into the associated meridianal acupoint. Before you can get the needle out of the skin, the electrical parameters have changed, and, in the sensitive patient, the symptoms instantaneously disappear.

## THE LYMPHATIC SYSTEM THEORY

Fleckstein, in the 1970s, showed that injections of novocaine into lymph nodes caused dramatic widening of the lymphatic channels and increased transport of lymph. He also showed that chronic lymphatic channel spasm and lymphatic stagnation could be instantaneously opened with intranodal novocaine injection.

Injection into tonsils often will relieve chronic migraine headaches caused by encephalopathic intoxification.

## THE TOOTH — FUSE BOX THEORY

Dr. Voll and others have shown quite clearly that the teeth represent the "fuse box" of the acupunc-tural meridian system. All the acupuncture meridians at some point go through the teeth, and any poor or inappropriate dental work, unerupted teeth, wisdom teeth (unerupted or not), root canals, bone cavities, cysts, nonvital teeth, granulomas, periodontal disease, disease of the tooth socket, or healed or active osteomyelitis of the jaw will cause a major energy problem in the whole meridian that is affected by that tooth. The accompanying chart shows the relationship between the organs and the tooth that affects them (Figure 10.1).

## The energetic relations of teeth (or odontons) with respect to organs and tissue systems.

| Zones | I | IV | III | II | I | | I | II | III | IV | V |
|---|---|---|---|---|---|---|---|---|---|---|---|
| Paranasal Sinuses | | Maxillary Sinus | Ethmoid Cells | | Sphenoidal Sinus / Frontal Sinus | | | Ethmoid Cells | Maxillary Sinus | |
| Endocrine Glands | Anterior pituitary lobe | Para Thy- / Thy- roid | Thy-mus / Post pituit-ary | Inter med. | Pineal Gland | | Post. pituitary | Inter med. / Thy mus | Thy-roid / Para thy-roid | Anterior pituitary lobe |
| Sense Organs | Cavernous Sin | Tongue | Nose | Eye | Nose | | Eye | Nose | Tongue | Cavernous Sin |
| Tonsils yin | Lingual | Laryngeal | Tubal | Pal | Pharyngeal | | Pal | Tubal | Laryngeal | Lingual |
| | Heart | Pancreas | Lung | Liv | Kidney | | Liv | Lung | Spleen | Heart |
| Vertebrae | C2 C1 TM1 C7 Th7 Th6 Th5 S2 S1 | C2 C1 Th12 Th11 L1 | C2 C1 C7C6C5 Th4Th3Th2 L5 L4 | C2 C1 Th8 Th9 Th10 | C2 C1 L3 L2 Co S5 S4 S3 | C1 C2 L2 L3 S3S4S5Co | C1 C2 Th8 Th9 TH10 | C1 C2 C5 C6 C7 Th3 Th4 L4 L5 | C1 C2 Th11 Th12 L1 | C1 C2 C7 TM1 Th5 Th6 Th2 S1 S2 |
| Organs yang | Duodenum Terminal Ileum | Stomach Esophagus | Large Intestine | Gallbladder Biliary Ducts | Urinary bladder Genito-uranary area Rectum Anal Canal | | Biliary Ducts | Large Intestine | Stomach Esophagus | Duodenum Jejunum Ileum |
| Jaw Sections | HE SI CS | SI PA | LI LU | LIV GB | BL IK IK BL | | LIV GB | LU LI | SP ST | HE SI CS |
| right ... left | 1 | 2 3 | 4 5 | 6 | 7 8 9 10 | | 11 | 12 13 | 14 15 | 16 |
| right ... left | 32 | 31 30 | 29 28 | 27 | 26 25 24 23 | | 22 | 21 20 | 19 18 | 17 |
| Jaw Sections yang | HE SI CS | LI LU | ST PA | LIV GB | BL KI KI BL | | LIV GB | SP ST | LU LI | HE SI CS |
| Organs | Terminal Ileum | Large Intestine | Stomach Esophagus | Gallbladder Biliary Duct | Rectum Anal Canal urinary bladder Genito-urinary area | | Biliary Ducts | Stomach Esophagus | Large Intestine | Jejunum Ileum |
| Vertebrae | C2 C1 Th1 C7 Th7 Th6 Th5 S2 S1 | C2 C1 C7 C6 C5 Th4 Th3 L5 L4 | C2 C1 Th12 Th11 L1 | C2 C1 Th8 Th9 Th10 | C2 C1 L3 L2 S5 S4 S3 Co | C1 C2 L2 L3 S3 S4 S5 Co | C1 C2 Th8 Th9 Th10 | C1 C2 Th11 Th12 L1 | C1 C2 C5 C6 C7 Th3 Th4 L4 L5 | C1 C2 C7 Th1 Th5 Th6 Th7 S1 S2 |
| yin | Heart | Lung | Pancreas | Liv | Kidney | | Liv | Spleen | Lung | Heart |
| Tonsils | Lingual | Tubal | Laryngeal | Pal | Pharyngeal | | Pal | Laryngeal | Tubal | Lingual |
| Sense Organs | Ear Tongue | Nose | Tongue | Eye | Nose | | Eye | Tongue | Nose | Ear Tongue |
| Endocrine Glands | | | Gonad | | Adrenal Gland | | Gonad | | | |
| Paranasal Sinuses | | Ethmoid Cells | Maxillary Sinus | | Frontal Sinus / Sphenoidal Sinus | | | Maxillary Sinus | Ethmoid Cells | |

**FIGURE 10.1** The energetic relations of teeth (or odontons) with respect to organs and tissue systems.

I have had two personal experiences with this problem. I have been very susceptible to Coxsackie viral infection all my adult life, and have been hospitalized twice, once with Coxsackie B pleurodynia and bilateral orchitis and on another occasion with Coxsackie B myocarditis and pericarditis. It was only after I had my rotten wisdom teeth attended to that the Coxsackie attacks stopped. The wisdom tooth is attached to the Heart meridian. In another family instance, my wife developed chronic urinary tract infections, of which she had had no history. I later found that they all started after she had had her two front upper incisors capped. The incisors are attached to the Bladder meridian. Removal of the caps stopped the UTIs. The most problematic foci in the teeth, from my clinical experience, are root canals on teeth that should have been pulled. This problem is made doubly ominous by the anecdotal finding of increased breast cancers on the same side as root canals on tooth numbers 4, 5, 12, 13, 20, 21, 28, and 29.

The problems of local galvanic currents due to the use of mixed metals in teeth is also quite clinically apparent when various chronic problems disappear if a single metal (usually gold) is used to replace the dental battery. The issue of metal amalgams and mercury, tin, copper, and nickel toxicity is not as important in my experience as bad root canals, infected tooth sockets, dry sockets, and focal osteomyelitis of the jaw. The recent descriptions of Non-Infected Cavitating Osteonecrosis (NICO) lesions in the periodontal tissue adds fuel to the disturbed energetic fire.

Many patients show quite acute allergic reactions to the restoration materials that are used on their teeth, and a case like this may lead to chronic inflammation and dental focus formation as long as those allergic materials are in the mouth. This problem also applies to the plastics that dentures are made of, in particular those with a pink color. The way to prevent this occurrence is to have a dental test kit on hand or one in your computer library and to test the patient against the proposed materials for compatibility. If there is an absolute requirement for an allergic material, then you can desensitize the patient to the material using the ALR-G-ANSR.

## THE CLINICAL PRACTICE OF NEURAL THERAPY

Neural therapy can be used for almost any symptoms where you suspect an interference field problem. It is mainly used for pain and functional diseases. I use 1% lidocaine, and sometimes some added marcaine for all tissue injections, and preservative-free 1% novocaine for intravenous injections. I rarely use more than 5 ml and I often mix in an equal amount of a specific homeopathic injectable remedy. For intradermal wheals, quaddles, and all face work, I use a 5 ml syringe with a 30-gauge, 1/4 inch needle. For scar infiltration and deeper muscle and ligament work, I use a 28-gauge, 1 to 1.5 inch needle. I do not perform any ganglion, abdominal, or deep pelvic injections or blocks. If I need such a block, I send the patient to an anesthesiologist I work with. You can treat superficial ganglia with penetrating electrical current using an apparatus called the *electroblock*.

Absolute contraindications for the use of neural therapy include:

- malignancy (opens up lymphatics)
- genetic illness
- nutritional deficiencies
- diabetes (may become unstable)
- tuberculosis
- psychiatric illness (except depression)
- too weak a patient with end-stage chronic illness

The techniques used can be divided up into direct and indirect techniques. *Direct techniques* deal directly with the interference field itself and include: infiltration of scar tissue, injections of autonomic ganglia and epidural spaces, surgical removal of scar tissue, and extraction of any tooth that constitutes a dental focus (work together with your biological dentist). Remember, the umbilicus is our first scar — check it first.

*Indirect techniques* are also known as *segmental therapy*. You have to activate the cutanovisceral and periosteovisceral reflexes of the neurological segment that affects the organ. This is accomplished by injecting the overlying skin surface intradermally (quaddles) or injecting into the associated superficial periostium of bone or the associated paravertebral segments (Hua Tuo Jia Ji points). Another indirect technique is the intravenous injection of an extremity with preservative-free novocaine or lidocaine after first applying a tourniquet on the extremity above the injection site. The novocaine is allowed to first work on the perivenular autonomic fibers, thereby affecting the autonomic of the whole arm, and then the tourniquet is released.

Interference fields can be tested by a trial injection of novocaine into the scar, area, or periodontal tissue. This is usually done with an MSA base reading or using biokinesiology (see next chapter on Bioenergetic Medicine). If the patient tests strong after the injection, you have identified the field and a full injection therapy is warranted.

Galvanic currents in teeth, as shown by a weak muscle test localizing to the jaw, can be tested using a tape demagnetizer. Run the instrument in front of the open mouth and retest, the muscle test should be normal. Now wait 15 minutes and have the patient close his mouth and oppose his teeth like a closed circuit breaker causing the galvanic current to flow again and he or she will test weak again.

You know you have hit the right area if you get a lightning reaction of pain disappearance. Other confirming signs include hot flashes in the head after the injection due to release of Yang energy; a sensation of euphoria after the injection; a sudden emotional release, usually in females with pelvic injections; delayed symptom improvement, usually the next day because the pathology takes a day to defervesce; and aggravation where the patient feels worse at first, but improves in 16 to 20 hours.

If improvement lasts only a day, you have hit an area that is anatomically close. Search in the local area for other likely foci. If improvement occurs but is not complete, you have found only one of the foci in a chain of foci, search for the others. If improvement occurs, but a new focus develops, this is called a retrograde phenomenon and is actually one of Hering's Laws of Cure, the patient going back in time to another previous focus.

For further training in neural therapy contact Dietrich Klinghardt, M.D., Ph. D.[41]

# 11 Bioenergetic Medicine

As has been mentioned in the section dealing with the energetic components of medicine, bioenergetic medicine is the most foreign of the alternative modalities to comprehend and appreciate. But it turns out that if we are to make a quantum paradigm change in the way we think of disease and practice medicine, this is the modality where the breakthroughs will occur. In the following sections I outline in a very abbreviated fashion, the history and clinical implications of this part of our physiology and being.

## BIOENERGETIC MEASUREMENTS

In regular medicine we use the patient history, physical exam, laboratory, and other special tests to assess the biological state of the patient. In bioenergetic medicine we use the measurements of bioenergy, that is, electricity, heat, and electromagnetics as our symptomatic baseline, and then we challenge or provoke the system in an algorithmic way to interrogate the body as to the specifics and levels of dysharmony and disease. The body is always aware of its state of being, down to the last biomolecular detail, and all we have to do is find a way of asking the correct question. This statement reminds me of my apprenticeship with Dr. Yuan Tang, a crusty old Harvard-trained mainland Chinese gentleman, who would never tell me anything unless I asked the correct question. So, in this early start to the new millennium, energetic measurements and provocation are one way of interfacing with this bioinformation.

When measuring the energetics of the body, we may do so with conventional direct energetic measurements, or we may use more holistic and global indirect methods. We will discuss both methods.

### THE ELECTRICAL APPROACH

Bioenergetic regulatory techniques all measure electrical activity in meridians, quadrants, or sides of the body. This electrical activity is used as information to evaluate organ function. An integral part of the technique is to stress the biology during testing to bring out hidden or occult energetic disturbances. Bioenergetic stress techniques have a long history in medicine, and the following highlights are significant in its development:

In the European literature, Roger de la Fuye of Paris described the idea of electroacupuncture in the 1940s in his book entitled *Traite d'Acupuncture* (Treatise on Acupuncture).[59] The electroacupuncture was carried out using special electrodes attached to the inserted needles, connected to a diathermy machine, operating at a high frequency to supply the current to the needles. The treatment time was very short, ranging from fractions of a second to the longest treatment time of two seconds.

In 1953, Reinhold Voll, M.D. developed a technique of provoking the acupuncture points with direct current of 10 micro-amps and 1 volt, and measuring the subsequent skin resistance called Electroacupuncture According to Voll (EAV), Electrodermal Testing (EDT), or Meridian Stress Assessment (MSA). The instrument he used for these measurements was the K+F "Diatherapuncteur." The instrument was calibrated from 0 to 100 and was marked with the number 50 at the central position, indicating that the organ, or part of an organ, associated with the acupuncture points was free of pathology (Figure 11.1). He constructed a "pathological anatomic evaluation of measurement values" such that values of:

| | |
|---|---|
| 90–100: | total inflammation = total "itis" |
| 82–90: | partial inflammation = partial "itis" |
| 66–80: | cumulative irritations |
| 52–65: | physiological irritation |
| 50: | normal state, homeostasis |
| 40–48: | incipient degeneration |
| 30–38: | advanced degeneration |
| 20–28: | considerable degeneration |
| < 20: | probable cancer |
| < 10: | premorbid |

The most important electrical finding in EAV was not the inflammatory or degenerative reading, but the so called "Indicator Drop" (ID). The ID is an electrical manifestation of parenchymal cell death and degeneration and is always reproducible. Electrically, it represents an inability of the organ to hold the charge, which leaks out as you measure the resistance at the acupuncture point. The peak value is not maintained, but starts to fall from the peak value to a lower number. The greater the drop, the worse the parenchymal destruction.

Voll also investigated and annotated the relationship between acupuncture points and special extra points representing the anatomical parts of various organs. For example, the radial aspect of the index finger contains the measurement points for the large intestine and the successively more proximal points, starting from the Ting or Jing Well point, are numbered as follows:

**Right Hand:**

AP 1.   Right colon = transverse colon, right part.
AP 2.   Right colon = right colonic flexure.
AP 3.   Right colon = descending colon.
AP 4.   Right colon = cecum.
AP 4a. Right colon = appendix and ileocecal lymph nodes.

**Left Hand:**

AP 1. Left colon = sigmoid.
AP 2. Left colon = descending colon.
AP 3. Left colon = left colonic flexure.
AP 4. Left colon = transverse colon, left part.

Measurements of these and other organ points enables the examiner to elucidate the state of initially energetic dysfunction and later of gross pathology of the associated organs.

The measurement points for pancreas (right-sided Spleen meridian) bear a direct correlation to measurable metabolic problems. For example:

**AP 1** = exocrine protease secretion. If ID present, it indicates intestinal autointoxication and dysbiosis.
**AP 2** = nuclease enzyme and nucleoprotein metabolism. If ID is present, hyperuricemia is always present.

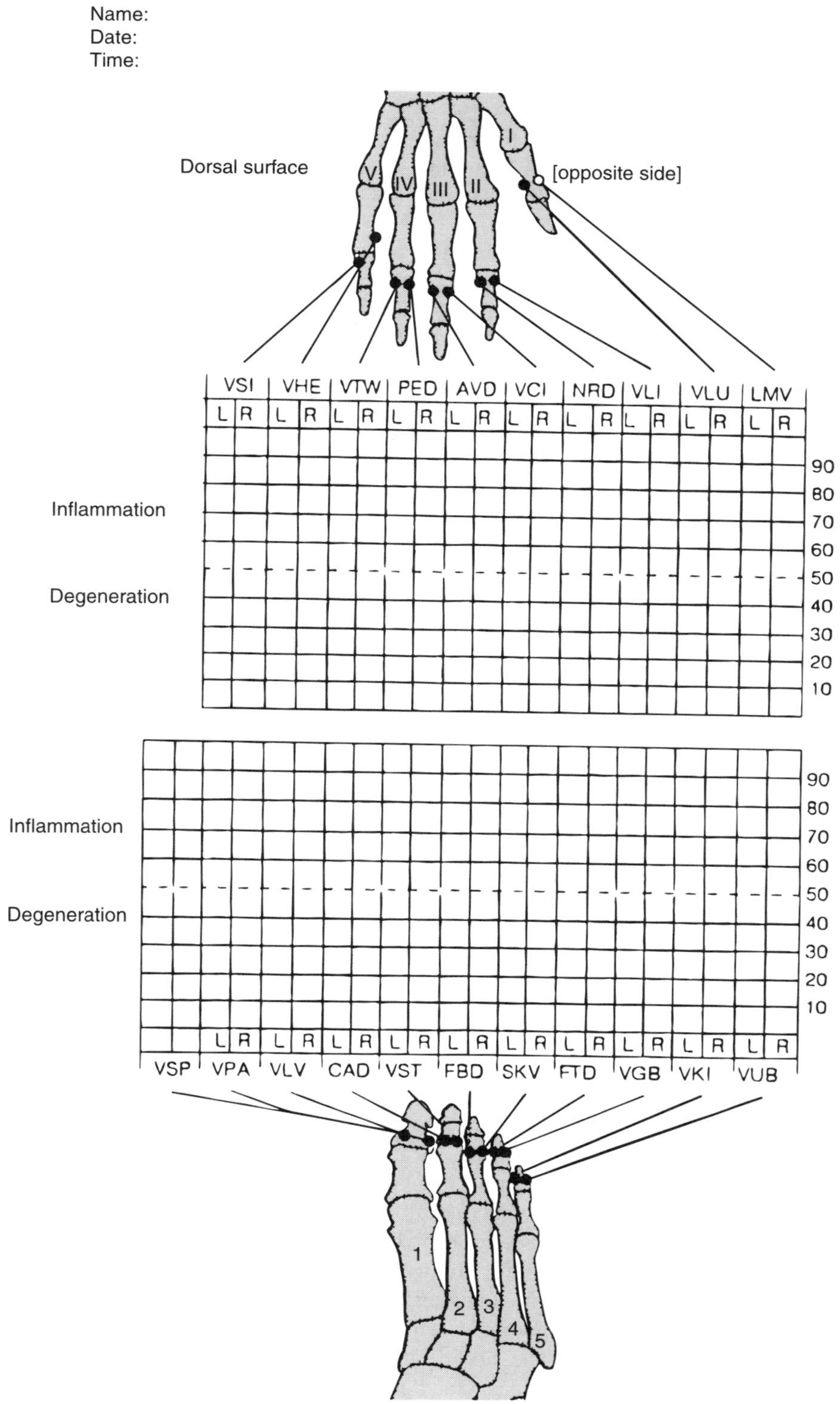

**FIGURE 11.1** Control Measurement Points in MSA.

AP 3 = amylase and maltase production. If ID is present, hyperglycemia is always present.

AP 4 = lipase production. If ID found, hyperlipidemia is always present.

EAV today has more than 800 points, 200 of which constitute new points. EAV, however, has not only found individual new acupuncture points, but has also located new vessels or meridians including the lymph meridian, the nerve meridian, the allergy meridian, the skin meridian, and the fatty, epithelial and parenchymatous, articular and connective tissue degeneration meridians. With these meridians and points it is possible to assess the status of every anatomic part of every organ, blood vessel, nerve plexus, and serosal surface in the body.

Other recently discovered important points that are not known in classical acupuncture are the *control measurement points* (CMPs). These are control points for the whole Organ and can immediately assess whether there is an inflammation, inflammation and degeneration, or a degenerative event taking place in the entire Organ. These findings enable the physician to immediately pinpoint the origin of symptoms and the nature of the pathology (Figure 11.2).

Possibly the most important serendipitous discovery by Voll was the advent of *medicine testing*. Any medicine introduced into the electric circuit when point measurements are being made, will, if the medicine is correctly chosen, change the reading values made at the acupuncture point to a more normal level. This represents an ability to choose a biologically active medicine without first trying it on the patient. The use of homeopathic nosodes (homeopathically diluted out pathological samples, bacteria, viruses, etc.) adds a resonant diagnostic flavor to the medicine readings. For example, if a patient complains of sore throat, plugged ears, and rhinitis, the differential diagnosis includes allergy, viral syndrome, or possible streptococcal pharyngitis, to name the most common possibilities. Testing of the Lymphatic meridian reveals a high reading, indicating inflammation of Waldeyer's ring. Introduction of viral nosodes such as adenovirus, rhinovirus, or coxsackie into the electrical circuit by placing these glass vials on a metal plate in circuit do not change the readings. Measurement of the Allergy meridian is normal. Placing the nosode for streptococcus in circuit while measuring the Lymphatic meridian lowers the high inflammatory reading to a normal level. This is indirect evidence that the energetic resonant clinical problem is streptococcal pharyngitis. Placement of amoxicillin in circuit will also normalize the Lymphatic meridian reading indicating the correct antibiotic choice. Measurement of the Allergy meridian with amoxicillin in circuit does not cause an inflammatory high reading and, therefore, the patient can take amoxicillin without risk of allergic reaction. All this can be accomplished in 5 minutes without any lab testing or inconvenience to the patient.

The one drawback of this kind of testing is the large number of samples and ampoules that must be introduced into and removed from the circuit during medicine testing. This problem was solved by Roy Curtain in Utah utilizing scalar wave technology, with the development of the first computerized Enterro device and software. Subsequent developments have been seen in computerization of the testing libraries of more than 48,000 resonant energy signals in the Listen device, the Avatar, the Acupro from Computronix, Digital Health's Omega Acubase, and most recently and more importantly, the BEST System by Bio Meridian of Draper, Utah. Attempts have also been made to obtain an automated whole body reading utilizing multiple channel biofeedback with multiple energy signal provocation, to form a complete pathological picture of the patient. The first such device, the Eclosion, was not too successful because of personality and technical problems. I have not had the opportunity to assess the second device, the Bodyscan 2010 by Phazx Systems. The Elast Corporation of Las Vegas has a prototype instrument that is able to electronically read the allergy sensitivities of a patient without doing a blood or skin prick test. I have personally been able to manually measure specific blood glucose values by resonant comparison to glucose standards, but it is too time consuming. The most difficult part of reading energetic values off the body is the background noise, which is significant, and getting a clear signal is difficult. Recent improvements in probe technology by Pindi Corporation of Reno have overcome these problems and can

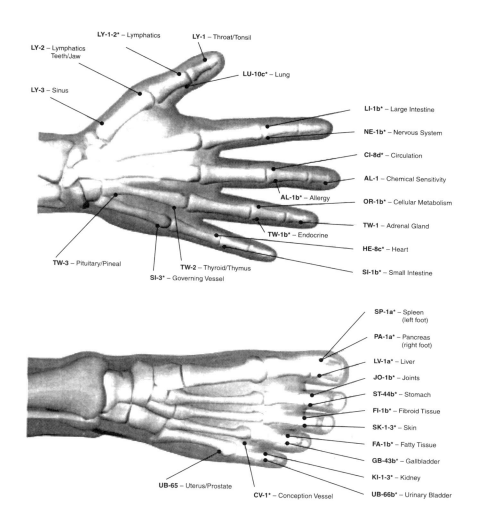

**FIGURE 11.2** MSA Organ Points.

now do a noninvasive glucose test with good reproducibility. The clinical laboratory will be a thing of the past within two to three years.

Helmut Schimmel, a doctor and dentist, took the concept of EAV a couple of steps further by introducing some biologically innovative approaches called *Vega testing*. His first innovation was not to measure each meridian, but to use only one acupuncture point as an electrical window into the body and to inform the body of the desired anatomical measurement point by placing a sarcode ampoule (homeopathic preparation of normal tissues and organs) in circuit, as a resonance filter. The identity of the organ to be measured is represented by the frequency of the organ ampoule and the correct electrical reading is gleaned from the body by harmonic resonance.

Other filters could also be used to pose different questions to the body. Most of these filters were homeopathic remedies that were shown to exhibit resonance with the particular question asked. For instance, if the ampoule Ferrum metallicum 12X is inserted into the circuit with a medicine, it will determine whether it is effective; the use of Manganum metallicum 30X will determine medicinal tolerance. There are many filter sets and hundreds of filters, each of which can pose a specific question to the body.

Schimmel also introduced the concept of *biological stressing* before testing to uncover sequestered biological information. He utilized a piezoelectric sparking device to shock the organism to uncover dysregulation.

The last innovation of Vega testing was the introduction of the concept of *biological age*. A set of homeopathically diluted solutions of mesenchyme were tested against the patient and an approximation of the patient's biological age could be determined. This was compared to the patient's chronological age, and an estimation could be made of the degenerative state of the patient. Readings were taken after treatment to see if the biological age had regressed at all.

The Vega Company of Schiltach/Black Forest in Germany produced a computerized device that stressed eight quadrants of the body with electrical stimulus and took a reading of skin resistance. The *segmental electrograph* (SEG) applies a 13 Hz exploratory voltage over each quadrant in sequence, and the response in terms of change of impedance with time in each quadrant is recorded. The quadrants include: head left and right (quadrants 1+2 forehead to C7); chest left and right (quadrants 3+4 C7 to T4); abdomen left and right (quadrants 5+6 T4 to L3); and pelvis left and right (quadrants 7+8 L3 to S4). Abnormal responses following stressing points to pathology in the organs of the associated segment. These quadrants bear a close parallel to the three heaters of Chinese medicine.

*Mora therapy* was conceived, and the instrument designed by Dr. Morell and an electronic engineer, Erich Rasche. Mora therapy was the first of a series of techniques and instruments designed by the Germans to practice B.E.R., or bioenergetic regulation. In Mora therapy the patient's own electronic frequencies or oscillations are taken off the body by a hand-held electrode, foot pad, or roller electrode, amplified or amplified and inverted, and fed back to the patient by another electrode. The unit also has a number of built-in electronic filters that are able to separate the patient's harmonic and dysharmonic oscillations, amplify and invert the dysharmonic oscillations, and amplify the harmonic oscillations. Another filter can restrict the frequency range of returned oscillations. The concept is that disease produces dysharmonic oscillations, and that by amplifying and inverting these oscillations and returning them to the patient, the "disease" can be canceled out in the patient. Mora seems to be more effective on sensitive patients.

In *Mora color therapy* the unit uses a full spectrum lamp filtered with three color filters (red, yellow, and blue). Combinations of these three primary colors allow the colors violet, orange, and green to be produced. These colors are converted into electromagnetic oscillations by an optoelectric converter, and the electromagnetic output is administered to an acupuncture point or points by an electrode. The Vega company makes a color therapy intrument that allows direct color input into an acupuncture point.

*Indumed therapy* is a magnetic therapy using very low intensity pulsed magnetic fields. The field strength is about 0.4 gauss — close to the Earth's magnetic field strength. The pulse that is used lasts one millisecond and each pulse has a steep rising edge and rapid drop to its stimulating signal, producing harmonic frequencies up to 5 MHz. This broad harmonic content is the key to its biological effect.

Two very sophisticated instruments, the *Bicom* and *Multicom*, were developed by the Hans Brugemann Institute in Gauting, Germany to deliver what they term *Bioresonance Therapy*. Bioresonance and Multiresonance are forms of therapy that chiefly work with ultrafine biological environmental signals.

The human body is a flow system and for its health requires a large number of items of information from the environment, which are stored biophysically in the body. If there are no such signals, or the intensity is too low, then this deficit can lead to illness. However, if these signals are supplied therapeutically in appropriate harmony and intensity, powerful pulses are created that reactivate the endogenous cybernetic control circuits.

The *Bicom* is very similar to the Mora, but it utilizes a magnetic field to pick up the patient's oscillations, thereby acquiring more deep tissue information. The *Multicom* is a multiphasic instrument for multiresonance therapy, that allows the input of electrical and magnetic frequencies, colors, gem frequencies, sound, metals, and Schumann waves into the deficient patient.

Dr. Hiroshi Motoyama has been conducting experiments at the Institute for Religious Psychology in Tokyo since the late 1970s to demonstrate, with clear electrophysiological evidence, the existence of the network of chakras and nadis that form the infrastructure of the subtle energies existing in the pranic and psychic dimensions. These dimensions in turn activate and underlie the physical and material body of man. The *AMI*, or *Apparatus for Measuring the Functional Conditions of Meridians and their Corresponding Internal Organs*, is an instrument designed to measure the initial skin current, in response to DC voltage externally applied at the Jing Well or Ting points of the fingers and toes. The data from these experiments (2,000 patients) has been collated into a set of criteria for the assessment of functional conditions, whether normal or disordered, in terms of excess, deficiency, or imbalance of Qi.

*Ryodoraku therapy* is an electrostimulatory diagnostic and therapeutic technique based on many observations of electric current recordings made over acupuncture points on the wrist and feet. It offers a means of objectively recording a traditional Zang Fu diagnosis. These measurement points of low electrical resistance were discovered by Dr. Yoshio Nakatani working in Kyoto, Japan in 1950. He worked out an easy numbering system so that he could teach the method to practitioners who had no knowledge of acupuncture. It is probable that he was the first to measure and attach diagnostic and therapeutic significance to electrical measurements made over acupuncture points. He was probably the originator of the idea of applying electricity to stimulate acupuncture points. The system is alive and well in Japan and has over 40,000 practitioners. Nakatani is convinced that balancing the meridians causes balance of the autonomic nervous system.

## THE INDIRECT APPROACH

In the indirect approach, the physician interrogates the patient utilizing the patient's, or his or her neuromuscular responses, to confirm the answer. Although this may seem very unscientific, in clinical practice it is indispensable and will save you and your patient time, money, and aggravation, not to mention hastening the therapeutic process.

The first attempt to record a physical change in the body upon introducing homeopathic medications was by Dr. W. E. Boyd, a medical doctor from Glasgow, Scotland, in the early 1920s. He used an instrument called an emanometer, an electrical circuit with an inductance and capacitance in series, upon which a homeopathic remedy was placed. The patient was used as a primary testing mechanism in circuit, using dull or clear notes on percussing over the abdominal wall.

In the 1930s "Chapmans reflexes" were introduced and the neurolymphatic relationships with organs and reflexes were established.

The next evolution came in the 1960s with the development of *applied kinesiology* by Dr. George Goodheart, a Detroit chiropractor. Dr. Goodheart observed in his patients a specific relationship between muscle weakness and physical ailments or weaknesses. He spent years working out a reflex system to diagnose areas of subluxation and to correct these neuromuscular–organ relationships.

Dr. John Diamond is an Australian psychiatrist who held the chair of psychiatry at Mount Sinai Hospital and Medical School in New York City. He developed the science of *Behavioral Kinesiology* in which he showed that patients reacted with muscle weakness to emotions, people, and food stuffs. He used a single muscle to test, usually the deltoid muscle.

Yoshiaki Omura described the Bi-Digital "O" Ring method of muscle testing in his book: *Practice of the Bi-Digital "O" Ring Test*, written in Japanese in 1986. He was able to demonstrate, using the ring formed by approximation of the index finger and the thumb, that the fingers could be pried apart by the examiner when the patient was in resonance with a particular indicated organ or testing ampoule. He was able to show for instance that the Stomach 36 acupuncture point secreted gastrin when stimulated. The scientific basis for this technique has been shown to be suppression of cortical evoked potentials with exposure to noxious agents, indicating that the brain is the sensor for the test process. This technique may be used to select therapeutic acupuncture points or medications in patients. Most of his later data can be found in the many articles published since 1990 in *Acupuncture and Electro-Therapeutics Research*.

In the mid 1980s Dr. Roy Martina combined the concept of filters from Vega testing and utilized the O-ring muscle test of Omura to conceive the technique of *Vega Biokinesiology*. This was much faster and simpler than Vega testing and required no apparatus.

In 1992 Dr. Martina simplified the system still further in a technique he called *INTEGRA*. This technique utilized body reflexes, hand modes, and acupuncture points on the body, which took the places of many vials, ampoules, and filters.

In 1994 Dr. Martina also introduced the *Integrated Bioenergetic Score* (IBS) *Index*. This system measured toxicity, degeneration, and blockages of each organ system, similar in concept to the biological age of the Vega system. The IBS led to the development of the *OMEGA* (O-ring Muscle Evaluation of Geo-bioresonances and Acupoints) technique in 1996. OMEGA uses the IBS scores, organ sarcodes, color filters, and simple causal chaining protocols, cutting testing time and improving therapy.

Since 1986 M. M.Van Benschoten of Reseda, California has developed multiple testing techniques utilizing the bidigital O-ring test. He has developed testing systems including homeopathic dilutions in vials and colors to represent TCM syndromes and states. He also pioneered the *biophoton acupoint measurements*, a sensitive technique to noninvasively assess the compatibility, toxicity or therapeutic potential of any substance.

## THE CLINICAL APPLICATIONS OF BIOKINESIOLOGY

The schema of Vega testing (developed out of electro-dermal screening according to Voll — EAV or MSA) by Dr. Schimmel, was the use of filters and ampoules of homeopathic testing kits to elucidate resonant electrical information from the energetic system of the patient. Muscle testing or applied kinesiology developed by Dr. Goodheart was used to seek information about organ weakness by detecting muscle weakness in corresponding muscles. If you put the two approaches together you get biokinesiology, in which muscle testing of the patient is used together with filters to extract bioresonant information. This system of patient interrogation can result in both diagnostic information and in the selection of treatment modalities, as medicine testing is part of this provocative technique. In this section we will focus on meridian-based diagnosis and treatment using TCM diagnosis, Chinese herbal mixes, and diluted biological response modifiers (homeopathic remedies and filters) to change meridian and organ dynamics and levels of resonant dysharmony.

### BI DIGITTAL O-RING VS. STRAIGHT ARM MUSCLE TESTING

The advantages of using the bidigital O-ring approach, as opposed to straight arm muscle testing is that it is simpler and more reproducible, can be repeated multiple times without the patient or doctor tiring, and allows access to filters and testing kits.

### THE PRACTITIONER

The doctor should be in energetic balance before attempting testing and should remove all electronic items (beeper) and jewelry before testing. Some practitioners wear special antimagnetic belts, while some use protective filters in circuit with the patient.

## Bi-Digital O-Ring Muscle Testing

The test is done by the patient forming an "O" ring with the thumb and index finger of one hand (Figure 11.3). Depending on the strength of the individual, the middle, or ring, or, at last resort, the little finger may be used in very strong individuals. The doctor attempts to open the ring by breaking the ring with his two hands, one hand opening each side of the ring. The opening should not be a quick jerk, but a steady slow pull — it is an opening of the bridge. Exert only enough force to open the ring. It is not a contest of strength. After the initial opening, the doctor lets go of the ring and the patient relaxes. It has to be decided what protocol to use with the O-ring result. I use a weak test (the ring breaks) meaning "Yes — Positive Result," and strong test (the ring is intact) meaning "No — Negative Result." This protocol applies only to a single, direct, yes or no question. The next O-ring test can take place only after 3 seconds have passed. If there is a steady stream of openings, one after the other, the information gained may be false due to phantom information and energy residue remaining from the previous opening.

## Disorder Control

In order to assess whether the patient's ANS and CNS are connected with your testing, you need to differentiate a weak test from a strong test. If the test is strong, the O-ring will not open (negative result). If the test is weak, the O-ring will open (positive result). In order to find out if this will happen, we place a toxic substance in the other hand of the patient (such as a battery or bottle of correction fluid) and test the O-ring — it should weaken. In medication and resonant information testing, provoking the acupuncture point PC-6 (MH-6) is used as a disorder control. The acupuncture point is located and the doctor strokes the point proximally and tests, and then distally and tests. One direction should test strong and the other direction weak with the O-ring. If both are strong (too Yang) or both are weak (too Yin), the patient is not testable and needs correction of this problem. This may be due to multiple issues including heavy metal toxicity, toxic focus (usually teeth or sinus), TMJ, dysbiosis, geopathic stress, psychological trauma, etc. Temporary reconnection may be established by rubbing both KI-27 points and CV-6 vigorously, and retesting. Another way of getting around this problem is to use a piezoelectric sparker on Voll points Allergy 1 and Lymph 1. The zero point in both ears may also be vigorously rubbed. Once the connectiveness of the patient has been established, you can now proceed with a polarity check.

## Polarity Check — Switching

The patient has to be in a sympathetic tone to be testable. If the patient is in a parasympathetic state, the results are not valid and the patient needs to be switched back into a "wakeful" sympathetic state. In order to find out if the patient needs switching, touch the patient's glabella with the back of your hand. This should cause a weakened or positive O-ring. Touch your palm to the glabella and the test should be strong. If both tests are weak or both tests strong the patient has a switching problem, which must be corrected before going forward with testing. A quick way to correct this problem is to massage the zero point of the ear with the tips of your index fingers for 30 seconds and retest. A soft laser can also be used on the zero point for 10 seconds. Usually the atlas is out in chronic switchers. Chronic switchers can have CFIDS, extreme stress, or be chronically exposed to petrochemicals.

## Hand Electrode and Testing Block

A simple brass electrode, copper wire, and aluminum testing block are used to house the testing ampoules, filters, or therapeutic remedies. This enables the doctor easy access to changing the substances while testing. The patient holds the electrode instead of the samples (Figure 11.4).

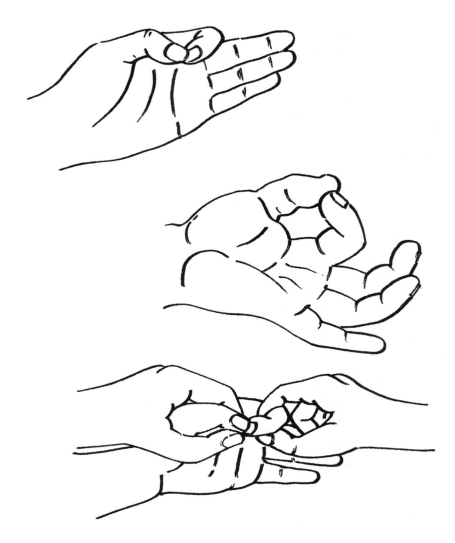

**FIGURE 11.3** Bi-Digital "O" Ring.

## TESTING ENERGETICS

The *meridians and organs* to be tested are identified with the meridian test ampoules. You can test for a paired Yang or Yin channel or for individual meridians and organs. The O-ring test will become weak when an affected meridian test ampoule is placed in the block. Continue testing until all affected meridians and organs have been identified. Usually you can guess which meridians and organs correspond to the patient's problems, and this will shorten the process. It is unusual to have more than 8 individual meridians or organs showing a problem. As we shall see further in the discussion, you do not try and treat all the meridians and organs.

The *Mudra* or *hand mode* represents a particular shape and form of an electromagnetic field that triggers subconscious memory patterns (Figure 11.4). Its action in weakening the O-ring is mediated through the reticular activating system in the brain through autonomic signals. These symbols are transcultural, transgenerational, and imbedded in our memories. The hand modes are used by the

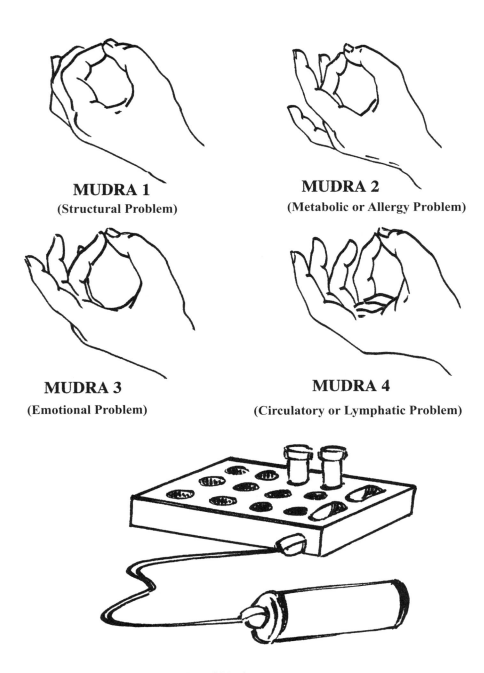

FIGURE 11.4 Mudras and Hand Electrode and Block.

doctor with the meridian or organ ampoule in circuit to understand the pathological association or causal relationship of that meridian or organ and the medication necessary to balance it. The hand modes filter out background energy and focus in on a more specific resonance. The hand modes are minicircuits and join specific meridians. For example, the emotional hand mode joins up the Triple Heater–endocrine points; the metabolic mode, the Large Intestine and Allergy meridians.

There are 5 hand modes that the doctor will hold for a second before testing the O-ring with the meridian ampoule in circuit:

1. *Structural* (thumb to index finger) — physical damage or mal-alignment, teeth problems. Use neural therapy vitamins, minerals, herbs, or organ-specific regenerational remedies.
2. *Metabolic* (thumb to middle finger) — problems due to allergies, endogenous or metabolic toxins. Use enzymes, allergy desensitization, or detox and drainage remedies.
3. *Emotional* (thumb to ring finger) — emotional stress, neurotoxins, or possible hormonal or endocrine imbalance. To evaluate further use CRA (see below) to determine if it represents mental, emotional, or hormonal problem. Mental = glabella; hormonal = cartilage of nose; emotional = epigastrium. Utilize herbs, flower essences, homeopathic remedies.
4. *Circulation/lymphatics* (thumb to little finger) — toxins in circulation, lymphatics and mesenchyme congested, and stagnant. Use detox and drainage formulas.
5. *Constitutional block/inherited miasm* (thumb to all bunched fingers) — deep cellular information, usually inherited. Use organ degeneration formula.

At this point you have all the weak meridians and their pathologic problems. For example: LR = Mudras 2 and 4 — a lot of stagnation and congestion in the organ meridian; GB = Mudra 3 — emotional issue blocking meridian; HT = Mudra 5 — predisposition to heart imbalance.

If the Mudra involved is other than emotional (Mudra 3), you need to go to Contact Reflex Analysis (CRA) to assess:

1. Gross physical organ involvement at this time. The problem is not just energetic, but physical.
2. The head organ of the causal chain.

The technique of *Contact Reflex Analysis* is the measurement of the sympathetic activity of the skin that is a direct segmental reflection of the health of the underlying organs or tissue. Instead of using an electrical probe, we use our hands. The palms of our hands are particularly good tools since they measure up to 10 to 25 millivolts more negative than the rest of our skin. Therefore, the lowered skin resistance from our palms or finger tips induces even more increased sympathetic action potentials over a cutaneous area of disturbance that is being therapy localized. This reflexes back to the spine and sympathetic pathways in the periphery (golgi tendon organs) and the CNS (reticular activating system and cortex) to cause the O-ring to go weak.

In this technique the organ area in question (Figure 11.5) is touched with the tips of the finger and within 3 seconds the O-ring is tested. If the O-ring weakens, the organ is affected. Now correlate the CRA findings with the meridian findings. You are more interested in treating the gross pathology (CRA) with herbs, remedies, and supplements and the energetic problem (the meridians) with acupuncture.

In order to simplify the process and not have a host of organs and meridians to treat, we need to establish the *Head of the Causal Organ Chain*. One needs to find the organ that is responsible for causing the primary disturbance affecting all the other organs. This is similar to finding the patient's axis in 5 element theory. The technique, called *Head of the Causal Chain* (HCC), is borrowed from Vega testing. In this technique, two organ areas are touched in succession. If the O-ring weakens, then the first organ is affecting the second organ and is primary in the pathological sequence. If the O-ring is strong, there is no relationship from organ 1 to organ 2 in that direction. Continue to try relationships between organs until you have narrowed it down to one, or at maximum two, organ pathogenic chains of influence.

In order to use the traditional Chinese medicine diagnosis of the HCC, place the organ ampoule of the HCC in the testing block. Test the O-ring — it should be weak. Now place the color filters

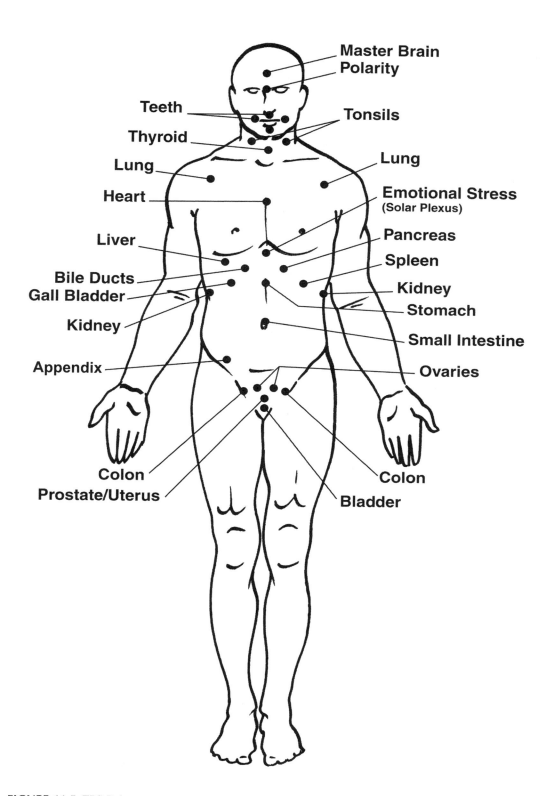

**FIGURE 11.5** EPS Points.

or the individual Chinese Modular Solutions (CMS) corresponding to the TCM syndromes or patterns one at a time in the testing block and test the O-ring. If it goes weak, there is a relationship between the organ and the TCM pathology. For example: Liver organ ampoule is weak with color filter red, lemon, and purple. This corresponds with Liver Qi and Blood Stagnation with Heat.

Now with the HCC organ ampoule (with or without the color filter) in the test block, add selected detox, drainage, degeneration, or regeneration test ampoules, Chinese herbal combinations, or supplements one at a time to see if they will strengthen the weak O-ring. These medicines will be the *oral therapies* given to the patient. Each therapeutic substance needs to be tested for efficacy and tolerance by using the PC-6 point rubbed in both directions. The O-ring should be strong in both directions. If it is not, additional therapy is needed by the patient. Keep testing until, with the organ ampoule, meridian ampoule, color filters, and therapeutics in the testing block, the PC-6 point is strong in both directions. This is the *still point*, the state of chaotic homeodynamic balance and maximum energy flow that the treatment will bring to the patient. This state can be cemented into the CNS and ANS at this time by an acupuncture treatment, while the patient is holding the electrode with all the ampoules, filters, and therapies in the test block. Select acupuncture points and technique according to your own preference or by using acupuncture indicator resonance (AIR), muscle testing which acupuncture points to use. If you have the therapeutic substances in liquid form, give the patient a small dose during the acupuncture treatment, further cementing the remedy into the CNS/ANS. If you do not have time to acupuncture, treat the ear organ points with a cold laser for 10 seconds each while the patient holds the electrode. This will suffice to cement the treatment even before the patient takes the herbs or remedies.

We have already discussed, under the section on acupuncture how to choose a particular acupuncture subsystem and then to choose the points on that subsystem. If, however, you just want to make an energy adjustment and move the Qi to help your homeopathic, herbal, or nutritional treatment, *Acupuncture Indicator Resonance (AIR)* is an easy technique to construct a quick acupuncture input.

The Bi-Digital O-ring is used as an indicator to assess the body's response to the following questions:

1. How many subsystems have to be used?
2. Which ones are they?

If the answers to the questions include one of the more esoteric subsystems such as the TMMs, Distinct meridians, or cerebral circulation, then peform those inputs. But if the body answers the Principal meridians, Curious meridians, or Five Element System, this is how you proceed:

1. **Principal Meridians** — Muscle test the ventral, lateral, and dorsal aspects of the body using CRA (touching the broad area with your palm) and the patient's O-ring. One side will test weak. Ask a yes or no question as to the possibility of another side turning weak as soon as the first side is strengthened. If the answer is yes, retest to find the second consecutive weak side. Ask if the second side needs to be treated concurrently or at a later date and note the body's answer.
   Turn your attention back to the initial weak side:
   • *Lateral* = GB and TH meridians
   • *Ventral* = LR, SP, KI, LU, and HT meridians
   • *Dorsal* = BL and SI meridians.

   Ask which meridian it is by touching the meridian line and testing — it will go weak. Also test the opposite of the Yin–Yang pair, if none of the above test weak. Next muscle touch test the Five Classical Shu or command points and ask how many points have to be used. When the number is given, point to each point and test; the weak point needs treatment. Tap on the point once; if it goes weak, acupuncture in dispersion; tap twice — if it goes weak, use tonification. Now proceed to any of the other weak indicated meridians and do likewise.

2. **Curious Meridians** — If a curious meridian is to be treated, take the patient's arm and touch TH-5, PC-6, LU-7, and SI-3 and muscle test each time — one will go weak. Now ask if it is upper body or lower body. The answer will tell which Curious meridian to use:

   1. TH-5 weak— upper body = Yang Wei Mo
      — lower body = Dai Mo (GB-41)
   2. PC-6 weak— upper body =Yin Wei Mo
      — lower body = Chong Mo (SP-4)
   3. LU-7 weak — upper body = Ren Mo
      — lower body = Yin Qiao Mo (KI-6′)
   4. SI-3 weak— upper body = Du Mo
      — lower body = Yang Qiao Mo (BL-62′)

3. **Five Element System** — If you want to treat utilizing the Five Element paradigm, have the patient lie on his or her back and imagine the Sheng and Ko diagram encircling the umbilicus. Now touch each pole of the diagram where it would be in the circle and muscle test it. One pole will be weak. Ask if there is another to be treated — there usually is. Muscle test the others for the second weak pole. Once you have the weak pole, go to the meridian of the operator (usually the Yin meridian) and muscle test for how many points are needed for treatment (is it bilateral or unilateral), and then follow the meridian testing for the first, second, and third points required. Tap once (dispersion) or twice (tonification) to see how to needle each point. Ask the body if moxa, the heat lamp, or electricity is required and on what points. At the completion of the needling, ask how long the needles need to be left in, and when the next appointment should be.

This seems like a very complicated way of deciding how and where to acupuncture or what treatment a patient needs, but I assure you after a bit of practice, it takes only 15 to 20 minutes to do an entire workup including homeopathy, herbs, nutritionals, and acupuncture treatment. It may seem like a lot of time to spend on each appointment, but until the electronics are automated, this is the only rational way of treatment, because when the patient's physiology and intelligence are directing the treatment, you get a good result every time.

## ENERGETIC PATTERN MODIFICATION

One may change, or attempt to change, any manifest habitual and reactional pattern in the body (symptoms and disease) by many different modalities including regular drugs, surgery, herbs, homeopathy, acupuncture, body work, and hypnosis. However, because every symptom and pattern in the body has a purpose and is goal oriented (even if we cannot understand it), it is far more logical to go to the source or root of the manifestation and look at it (the implicate order) as a site of repatterning rather than the manifest or peripheral explicate order. These deep reactional patterns, set up as a protective mechanism in childhood or during times of unanswered stress, have a peculiar illogical affinity for concurrent happenings at the time of the stress that are incorporated into the pattern as if they belonged there.

Let me give you an example. I had a patient come to me with a complaint of an acute allergy to turkey. She had had this allergy as long as she could remember and, once having ingested turkey, she proceeded to immediately throw up, felt very restless, and would break into tears. Washing her face in cold water almost always relieved the attack, which could go on for 20 to 40 minutes. This was a very interesting case because it had some unusual components that, on the surface, did not make much sense. If we analyse the case, we have the following facts: a violent reaction to turkey from a young age, feelings of restlessness, emotional outpouring with tears, symptoms relieved by washing her face in cold water. This actually makes a nice homeopathic case for repertorization, but I chose to treat her with Allergy Desensitization by Autonomic Nervous System Repatterning (ALR-G-ANSR). In this technique, which I will descibe below, it was found that she did indeed have an allergy to turkey, that this allergy was associated with fear, and that the allergy desensitization would be successful only if she was also desensitized to cold at the same time. We will get back to this case in a moment and what it means for the treatment of the root of disease. I have chosen allergy as a typical symptom that has no apparent purpose other than to make us miserable and keep the allergists busy.

## ALLERGY DESENSITIZATION BY AUTONOMIC NERVOUS SYSTEM REPATTERNING (ALR-G-ANSR)

*Allergy* is defined in medicine as a condition of unusual or exaggerated sensitivity of one individual to one or more substances that may be harmless to a majority of other individuals. As many as 90% of all Americans suffer from some kind of "allergic" symptom from what they ingest, inhale, or otherwise contact in their environment every day. Many of these symptoms are minor or just "lived with" and not recognized as such by either the patient or doctor.

Allergy has been around since the history of man. In 400 B.C., Hippocrates, the Greek physician, noted that cheese caused severe reactions in some people, while others could eat and enjoy it without unpleasant effects. The Roman philosopher Lucretius said 300 years later, "What is food for some may be fierce poison for others." So, "One man's meat is another man's poison."

The allergic diathesis is an inherited condition. It may not manifest, however, until later in the patient's life. When both parents are allergic, 75% to 100% of their offspring are allergic to everything to which the parents are allergic. When neither parent is allergic the number drops to 10%. Sometimes allergy can skip generations and reappear in grandchildren and great-grandchildren. Allergy, then, is an inherited reactional pattern with moderate to severe penetrance under the right circumstances.

In clinical reality, allergy is mostly unrecognized by doctors unless it corresponds with our narrow symptomatic definition of hay fever, itchy eyes, runny nose, hives, or similar acute reactions. These allergic responses relate to mucosa or skin, with IgE, basophil, or eosinophil interaction with histamine release and an exudative mucosal response. But what about brain fogginess, irritable bowel or bladder, muscle pain, or blurred vision? These reactions, which can, with careful questioning, be related to specific allergens, seem to mediate their effects via the autonomic nervous system. Allergy really represents a "protective" hyperactive or exaggerated response by the organism to any perceived "stressor" in the environment, internal or external. Our definition of allergy is a special case of this general phenomenon as outlined by Selye.[60] The internal and external nature of these stressors is very similar to the Chinese concepts of Internal and External pathogenic factors such as Wind and Cold. It could then be said that when the body is in balance, it will not be susceptible to pathogenic, exogenous, or endogenous factors. In other words in a balanced state, no diseases or allergies are possible and we are not susceptible to them.

Then what makes allergic patients so susceptible to common or minimal stressors? The secret lies in the neutral impressionability of the central nervous system. At a time of perceived danger of whatever sort, all perceived stressors in the immediate environment are lumped together as dangerous without any interpretation or discrimination and imprinted in the CNS as a whole picture. The response that is triggered by the perceived danger is then encoded as the response for all stressors perceived at that time, including common allergens that are more likely to produce a biological reaction if presented at any time to a primed host. So, anger at a parent during dinner produces wheat allergy when the bread is eaten in a huff after storming off to your room. Whenever bread is eaten in the future, the patient feels irritable with pain in the pit of the stomach. If the CNS is so neutral to impressions, then it can be reprogrammed with a different input to bread. The autonomic ganglia can be neutralized, the nerve roots and body segments innervating the affected organ put at rest, and the acupuncture meridians balanced in the presence of bread. Then, no anger or irritable response ensues with the presenting of bread, but a quiet and calm interior and exterior. This is the essence of acupuncture desensitization, the reprogramming of the autonomic nervous system and balancing of the meridians in the presence of the offending allergen. So, how do we do that?

**Step 1 — Determine if the patient is allergic.** The diagnosis of allergy can be made by many traditional and nontraditional means. One can employ a patient history, physical exam, scratch testing, intradermal skin testing, RAST testing, electrodermal screening, or biokinesiology. While single allergens can be desensitized, it has been found that adherence to a protocol that addresses the foods, vitamins, and minerals of the body first, irrespective of symptoms, has the best long-term results for permanent removal of environmental allergens at a later date.

The technique of choice in the doctor's office after assessing a regular allergy test (scratch/RAST) is to do biokinesiology (muscle testing). This testing is quick and reliable and enables you to assess the patient immediately for allergic status with respect to any allergen. It enables you to check if he or she is holding the allergen on recheck and also enables you to assess times between desensitization and times of abstinence from the offending allergen.

The techniques described are a mix of mainly NAET (Nambudripad's Allergy Elimination Technique) with some OMEGA (Dr. Roy Martina) and ART (Autonomic Response Testing of Klinghardt) and biokinesiology. The common method of doing muscle testing in the acupuncture room is to have the patient, legs uncrossed, lying supine on the acupuncture table with the doctor at the right side of the patient at shoulder level. The doctor is facing the patient, hips parallel to the table and should be alone with the patient. The patient's eyes should be gazing down toward his or her toes with his or her right hand, palm open and facing upward, next to the body, and the left hand at 90 degrees to the body, palm facing outward, thumb facing the big toe on the same side. The doctor stands on the side opposite the raised arm of the patient. The doctor leans across and into the patient and with his left hand applies downward pressure to the patient's raised arm to bring the arm down toward the big toe as the patient offers resistance to the pressure. If the arm holds, the reaction is strong (not allergic or cleared of allergen or negative response); if the arm is pushed down toward the table, the result is weak (allergic to allergen, not cleared, or affirmative result).

The patient must first be assessed as to whether their CNS and ANS are connected and functional and open to biokinesiology. The position of the hand during testing will usually obviate any problems with laterality (only one side of the body responding) or switching (going weak and strong). You have to assess the polarity of the patient who should be in the Yang or sympathetic state for testing. Testing for polarity is done by placing the index fingernail or back of your hand on the patient's glabella (Yin Tang). The patient's arm should test weak. If it tests strong, then test with the pad of your finger. It should now test weak. If it does not, then the patient is blocked (tests weak, weak or strong, strong) and the cause of the blockage has to be assessed. The common causes of blocks of autonomic regulation, excluding allergy, include:

1. Heavy metal toxicity,
2. Toxic petroleum solvents,
3. Dominant foci/toxic ganglion,
4. TMJ/malocclusion,
5. Acute psychological stress,
6. Geopathic stress.

All the above can be diagnosed with homeopathic test kits by placing the ampoule on the patient's solar plexus or testing block and retesting. If the patient is open, the ampoule can be left in place while testing. If you do not have these testing ampoules, then the patient can be temporarily unblocked as follows:

**Tests: strong–strong** — have surrogate or yourself touch patient's hand to ground and drain energy, or rub CV-6 counterclockwise and then CV-17 counterclockwise to weaken the system and brain (too Yang).

**Tests: weak–weak** — rub CV-6 clockwise and the CV-17 clockwise to increase the energy in the system (too Yin).

**Switching:** If the patient should suddenly give erratic strong/weak results, rub CV-6 and KI-27 (both points) with both your hands simultaneously.

Note: In my office I use the bidigital O-ring to assess the allergenic activity of the test ampules or substances, as using the deltoid muscle for an extended period of time on many samples causes weakness of the muscle and erroneous results. One may also test allergens in batches using an EAV or MSA machine and protocol. The point that is used is Voll's Allergy point (Ting point on the ulnar side of the middle finger), or the palm point, which is in the hollow of the palm abutting against the thenar muscle mass. An easy entry into the allergy of the body is to treat the patient's blood, urine, and saliva first. This knocks out obscure allergens and sometimes gives enough balance to eliminate all manifest allergy after one treatment.

You are now ready to treat for the sensitivity to the allergen. The sample of the allergen is placed in the aluminum block with the patient holding the attached brass electrode while you test the raised left arm for strength (not allergic) or weakness (allergic). It is rare that a patient is found who is not allergic to some food or vitamins. The energy economy of the body must first be addressed before environmentals, chemicals, or such. So, the following 15 allergens (part of Dr. Nambudripad's Allergy Test Kit) are tested for and treated first:

1. **Protein** — Egg white and yolk and chicken (enzymes and structural proteins).
2. **Calcium** — Carbonate, gluconate, ascorbate, citrate, cow's milk, goat's milk, milk casein, milk albumin.
3. **Vitamin C Mix** — Ascorbic acid, oxalic acid, citrus mix, berry mix, fruit mix, vinegar mix, chlorophyll, hesparidin, rutin, bioflavenoids.
4. **B-Complex** — B-1, 2, 3, 4, 5, 6, 12, 13, 15, 17, paba, inositol, choline, biotin, folic acid.
5. **Sugar Mix** — Cane sugar, beet sugar, brown sugar, corn sugar, rice sugar, maple sugar, molasses, honey, fruit sugar, sucrose, glucose, dextrose, maltose, lactose, date sugar, grape sugar.
6. **Iron Mix** — Ferrous sulfate, ferrous gluconate, pork, beef, lamb, gelatin.
7. **Vitamin A Mix, Fish, Shellfish Mix** — β-carotene.
8. **Mineral Mix** — All the minerals.
9. **Salt Mix, Chlorides** — Sea salt, table salt, rock salt, sodium and chloride.
10. **Corn Mix** — Blue corn, yellow corn, white corn, cornstarch, corn silk, corn oat, corn syrup.
11. **Grain Mix** — Whole wheat, rice, oats, rye, millet, barley,
12. **Artificial Sweeteners** — Equal™, NutraSweet™, Aspartame, Sorbitol, Sweet'N Low™, Saccharine, Twin.
13. **Brewer's and Baker's Yeast**
14. **Coffee Mix, Chocolate Mix, Caffeine Mix** — Coffee, tea, tannic acid, cocoa, cocoa butter, chocolate, carob, caffeine.
15. **Animal and Vegetable Fats** — Butter, lard, chicken fat, beef fat, lamb fat, fish oil, corn oil, canola oil, peanut oil, linseed oil, safflower oil, palm oil, coconut oil, olive oil.

After years of trial and error it became apparent that the desensitization repatterning would not hold in some patients. The cause of the problem is a noncompliance of either the left or right side of the brain. The brain, either the conscious left (in righthanders) or the unconscious right, has decided, for some adaptive reason, that it does not want to give up the reaction to the allergen. The patient will then sabotage you by giving incorrect information or by not accepting the repatterning. In order to facilitate the technique and not waste time, you should ask:

1. Which side of the brain am I talking to?
2. Will you tell me the truth?
3. Are the right and left halves of the brain Ready, Able, and Willing (RAW) to accept and hold this treatment?

If any of the answers is negative, you need to stop and find out by Neuro Emotional Technique (NET) or hypnosis why this antagonistic situation exists.

**Step 2 — Balance the patient's organs without allergen.** Having ascertained that the patient is allergic to the selected antigen, remove the allergen from the aluminum block and perform contact reflex analysis (CRA) of the patient's organs utilizing the testing arm. For every organ that is weak, strengthen it by rubbing vigorously over the contact area and retest. It should now be strong.

The technique of CRA is the measurement of the sympathetic activity of the skin that is a direct segmental reflection of the health of the underlying organs or tissue. Instead of a machine, we use our hands. The palms of our hands are particularly good tools since they measure up to 10 to 25 millivolts more negative than the rest of our skin. Therefore, the lowered skin resistance from our palms induces even more increased sympathetic action potentials over a cutaneous area of disturbance that is being therapy localized. This reflexes back to the spine and sympathetic pathways in the periphery (golgi tendon organs) and the central nervous system (reticular activating system and the cortex) to cause a strong indicator muscle to weaken. This technique will be used to assess the affected organ involved with each allergen.

**Step 3 — Find the Mudra (hand mode) associated with the allergen.** Place the allergen in the aluminum block, with the patient holding the brass electrode, and have the patient touch his or her thumb and index finger pad to pad. This represents Mudra 1 and relates to a structural problem (skeletal, muscular, etc.). If the patient goes weak with this hand mode, he or she may need manipulation and/or acupuncture before using allergy desensitization. The allergen is usually a contactant or chemical. Now have the patient touch the thumb pad to the middle finger and test. This represents Mudra 2 and relates to nutritional and metabolic problems with the allergen. The allergen is usually a food or a chemical that has entered the body by ingestion, injection, or inhalation. Next have the patient touch the thumb and ring finger and test. This represents Mudra 3 and relates to an emotional issue with the allergen. These allergens can vary and relate to the environment at the time of the emotional stress. Most often the allergens are foods such as milk products, sugar, or chocolate. Almost 80% of all allergies have an emotional component. Mudra 4, thumb to little finger, relates to vascular problems and is only used in desensitizing patients to cholesterol.

**Step 4 — Do CRA with the weak Mudra and assess the involved organs.** Usually only one Mudra is weak with the allergen. Have the patient hold that Mudra and test for the associated organs that are affected by the allergen. This is done by touching the reflex contact points of the organs on the patient and assessing weakness of the testing arm with each point. Note which organs are involved.

**Step 5 — Reset the autonomic nervous system in the presence of the allergen and the weakened organs.** Have the patient lie on the abdomen (prone) while holding the Mudra in the left hand and the electrode in the right hand. Place homeopathic ampules of the organs involved in the test block, which will open those organs up for energy transfer and repatterning. Now stimulate the Hua Tuo Jia Ji points (1/2 cun lateral to spinous processes) on both sides of the spine from T-1 to L-5. The spinal ligaments and facet joints have the highest autonomic innervation of any skeletal or segmental structure. One could stimulate only the segmental level associated with the weak organ or organs, but it is easier and safer to stimulate all levels because there is neurological overlap between segments and you may miss one. The stimulation can be done by purposeful clockwise rubbing with the thumbs or by using an activator device to percuss the area and shock the associated segmental ganglia into resetting.

Now stimulate the spinal nerve root segments as they emerge from the spinal canal at 1 cun lateral to the spinous processes (not quite the Shu points) from T-1 to S-3. Sixty percent of nerve fibers come from the organ while the other 40% interact with the rest of the body. Multiple levels above and below the segment in question will be involved, so just do all segments as with the Hua Tuo Jia Ji points.

If the Mudra involved is Mudra 3, the hand holding the electrode is placed in contact with the forehead during the spinal treatment. If the organ involved is the brain, the brass electrode is held in the hand and, instead of the spinal treatment, a special brain resetting technique is used. With the patient lying on his/her back:

1. Have the patient take a deep breath in (cerebro spinal fluid [CSF] out). As the patient exhales, (CSF in) massage the face from the glabella to CV-20. Repeat this procedure 3 times.
2. Repeat breathing procedure, this time massaging the side of the face from ST-5/6 across the TM joint to CV-20. Repeat 3 times.
3. Go to the head of the table and with the same breathing, cradle the patient's occiput in your hands with your finger tips on GB-20 and exert gentle traction toward yourself. Repeat 3 times.

Practically speaking, if you have the liver as an affected organ in the aluminum block, this is sufficient treatment for the brain (the sea of marrow).

**Step 6 — Retest patient to see if treatment is holding.** Turn patient onto the back and retest the CRA weak organs with the appropriate Mudra. All the organs should now be strong. If not, repeat the back treatment. Retest the other mudras to make sure that no other mudra is involved. If it is, test for involved organs, place them in the block, and redo the back treatment.

**Step 7 — Acupuncture 8 Gates to consolidate the state of balance.** After being tested against the allergen and showing no weakness, the patient continues to lie on the back with the electrode in the right hand, and the left hand holding the Mudra. Insert acupuncture needles into the right hand LI-4, right wrist HT-7 (if Mudra 3 is weak), right arm LI-11; left arm LI-11, left wrist HT-7 (if Mudra 3 is weak), left hand LI-4; left leg SP-6, left foot LR-3; right foot LR-3, right leg SP-6. The patient then lies quietly for 15 minutes. At the end of that time the needles are removed and all the involved mudras and associated organs are retested for strength. If any is weak, the back points with held mudra are repeated once. The patient is then instructed to wash the hands with water only to remove energy from the fingertips. The patient should be desensitized as soon as he or she gets up from the table and may eat or be in contact with the allergen.

**Step 8 — Allergen Retesting.** The patient should be retested within a week to ascertain the state of sensitivity to the allergen. All mudras, organs, and combinations should be checked.

Many allergens are layered with other environmental issues such as hot, cold, RNA, DNA, acid, base or other allergens that were sensitized simultaneously. They may have to be done together with the original allergen desensitized to be cleared. If the patient is clear and holding strong on the allergen, all mudras, and combinations, then a new allergen can be done. If the patient has symptoms from the previous desensitization, wait until the patient feels better before continuing with a new allergen. If the patient is very weak, you may have to break down and individualize some of the more complex allergens, such as B-Complex. Very weak patients may not be able to hold the allergen during the 8 Gates treatment. Have the normal patient eat a small amount of the allergen after a successful completion of treatment to reinforce the new memory in the brain. The minimum time between desensitization is 5 hours (there are ways of circumventing this problem). If the patient becomes emotional after treatment, immediately retreat with Mudra 3, if it was not used during the treatment. After treating for vitamins, supplement the patient with the vitamin.

The patient's dog and cat are far better allergen samples than you can get from an allergy supply house. Always use the actual substance if possible. Have patients bring in their vacuum cleaner bags and use that as a sample (contains everything in the house). You can also set out a jar of water inside or outside a house and collect whatever is floating about as a sample. I do this weekly in our area and also go on field trips and collect the predominant flowering and pollinating weeds, grasses, trees, and flowers.

Most patients are permanently free of allergy to that allergen after treatment. Occasionally allergen will resensitize, usually because you have not treated the emotional component. Of all the allergens, mold, fungus, and yeast are the most difficult to treat.

**Step 9 — Treatment of the emotional component of allergy.** It is clear from many patient encounters that when allergy is based on a Mudra 3 or emotional connection, the emotional connection must first be treated before the allergen can be cleared. You can use any number of emotional repatterning or release techniques. I use either hypnosis or Scott Walker's Neuro Emotional Technique (NET). Once the connection between the allergen and the emotion is broken, the allergen may be treated successfully. Kind of makes regular allergy shots seem somewhat superficial.

And now, back to the lady and her turkey allergy. On testing it was found that the turkey allergy was a Mudra 3 and connected to the Kidney (fear) and Stomach (cause of her vomiting — Rebellious Stomach Qi). On careful questioning it turns out that as a child, she would go to her aunt's farm during the school holidays. Her aunt required everybody to work while they were at the farm. Her job was to slaughter the turkeys. She hated it, as she was a very sensitive girl, and would be nauseous and sick to her stomach as she cut off their heads. She remembered the blood squirting onto her face and how she would run crying from the barn to the water pump and wash the blood and tears from her face. Need I say more?

Every patient is an individual and needs to be tested before being treated by asking if it is appropriate to do so. Doctors with little experience in allergy should proceed cautiously and err on the conservative side when treating weak or chronically ill patients.

# 12 Ayurvedic Medicine

## HISTORY AND CONCEPTS

*Ayurveda*, derived from *ayur* meaning life and *veda* meaning knowledge, is the Indian systematized medical art of the "science of life." The philosphy has developed over 5000 years and embodies concepts integrating the nature and origin of man and the cosmos.

The *Divine Mother* or *Prakruti* creates the universe, observed by the passive male energy, *Purusha*. The combination of the two primordial energies gives rise to *Mahad*, the *Universal Intelligence*, which creates the individual's intellect or *Buddhi*. Within the center Buddhi is a central core called *Ahamkar* or the ego. The ego then divides into the components of all of creation:

1. **Sattva** — the principle of light and correct spiritual purpose, the concept of space in the universe, clarity of *perception*;
2. **Rajas** — the principle of movement, atmosphere of the planet, movement of perception, which becomes *attention*;
3. **Tamas** — the principle of inertia and darkness, body of the planet and all of nature, precipitation of perception, which becomes *experience*.

## THE FIVE FUNDAMENTAL ELEMENTS

These three universal qualities influence our minds and bodies. Rajas is the actual life force and it vivifies the organic (Tamas) and inorganic (Sattva) nature of man. All organic and inorganic substances are made of the Five Fundamental Elements — space, air, fire, water, and earth. These all have functions and qualities much as we have already seen in the Five Elements paradigm of Chinese medicine.

1. **Space** — a difficult concept to grasp other than it defines what is not matter. It is the first expression of consciousness and necessary for the existence of matter, and in the bodily context, the cells.
2. **Air** — the vital life force or *Prana*, the Qi of TCM, and the Vital Force of the homeopaths. Prana represents the flow of consciousness and all movement within the body.
3. **Fire** — the metabolic process in the body related to the absorption and transformation of food into energy. All transformative activities are governed by the Fire element, including the transformation of perception into knowledge.
4. **Water** — the container and transporter of the energy and nutrients for life.
5. **Earth** — represents the solid material nature of all things on earth, including our bodies, soil, rocks, etc.

## THE THREE ENERGY TYPES

Ayurveda defines three basic types of energy or functional principles that are present in everyone. These are the *three Doshas* — *vata, pitta,* and *khapa*. The dosha concept is another fractal system which every vata, pitta, and kapha has within itself in elements of the other two doshas. Each dosha is made up of a predominant contribution of two of the basic Five Fundamental Elements. All people have a combination of all three doshas. According to Ayurveda, there are 7 possible combinations, body types, or constitutions, also known as *prakuti*. This constitution was established at conception as a combination of the prakuti of your mother and father. The seven types are:

- single dosha predominant (3 types).
- two doshas, equally predominant (3 types).
- three doshas, equally predominant (1 type).

The cause of disease in Ayurveda is viewed as the lack of proper cellular function because of an excess or deficiency of *vata*, *pitta*, or *kapha*, and/or the presence of toxins, *ama*, that interfere with dosha balance. If you know your dosha constitution, you will also know your biological weaknesses and strengths, and this will enable you to take steps to strengthen your weaknesses and avoid activities or habits that will weaken you further and disturb your homeodynamic balance.

**Vata** is composed of *space* and *air* in the body and is about movement in the body.
**Associated with:** the lung and all its pathology.
**Governs:** breathing, blinking, muscle and tissue movement, heartbeat, and all intracellular activity.
**In balance:** promotes flexibility and creativity.
**Out of balance:** promotes fear and anxiety.
**Predominant period:** increases with age.

**Pitta** is composed of *fire* and *water* and represents the body's metabolism.
**Associated with:** inflammation, fevers, jaundice, skin rashes, and ulcers.
**Governs:** digestion, absorption, assimilation, nutrition, metabolism, and body temperature.
**In balance:** promotes understanding and intelligence.
**Out of balance:** arouses anger, hatred, and jealousy.
**Predominant period:** in adulthood.

**Kapha** is composed of *earth* and *water* and represents the body's structure.
**Associated with:** water issues or phlegm and mucus, sinus congestion, sluggishness, excess weight, diabetes, water retention, and headaches.
**Governs:** the bones, muscles and tendons, lubricates the joints, moisturizes the skin, and maintains immunity.
**In balance:** promotes love, calmness, and forgiveness.
**Out of balance:** promotes dependency, attachment, greed, and possessiveness.
**Predominant Period:** in infancy and through late childhood.

## ETIOLOGY AND DIAGNOSIS OF DISEASE

The Ayurvedic physician uses the same seven examinations as outlined in the Chinese medical exam. The pulse diagnosis is very important in Ayurvedic medicine.

The *etiology of disease* is quite definite in Ayurvedic medicine. All Vata disease has its origin in the colon; all Pitta disorders have their origin in the small intestine and all Kapha disease has its foundation in the stomach and gastric mucosal secretions. If the doshas are in balance, then the patient is not susceptible to disease.

## PATHOPHYSIOLOGY OF DISEASE

According to Ayurveda, all disease goes through six progressive stages, which are very reminiscent of the stages of disease in homotoxicology. These stages are *accumulation, provocation, spread, deposition, manifestation,* and *differentiation.*

1. **Accumulation** — The aggravated dosha begins to accumulate in its GI organ of predilection. This may happen at the change of seasons, and so ritual cleansing or purification is advised as a preventive measure at the turn of the seasons.
2. **Provocation** — The dosha accumulation tends to extend into neighboring organs and affects their function and vitality. Treatment is by purification and herbal tonification of the affected organs.
3. **Spread** — The aggravated and accumulated dosha now metastasizes throughout the body. The dosha may move in any direction. For example, if Vata moves upward (like Rebellious Stomach Qi) it causes nausea and vomiting or light-headedness; or if it moves downward (like deficient Spleen Qi) it causes diarrhea. The doshas will travel along three pathways of disease propagation:
   a. the internal pathway — gastrointestinal tract;
   b. the intermediate pathway — vascular system;
   c. the deep or vital pathway — musculoskeletal system, nerves and brain, endocrine and productive system, and all major organs.
4. **Deposition** — The aggravated dosha now settles in a weakened organ or area and begins to accumulate. Prodromal clinical symptoms begin to appear.
5. **Manifestation** — The cardinal signs and symptoms are now apparent as the body tries to balance out the doshas.
6. **Differentiation or Destruction** — Structural and degenerative changes have occurred. The disease is very difficult to treat at this stage.

## TREATMENT OPTIONS

Treatment is aimed at creating balance among the components of the constitution, the *doshas, dhatu* (tissues), and *mala* (urine, feces, and sweat) again. There are many modalities including surgery, herbs, nutrition, gemstones, crystals, metals, mantras, and sound.

Ayurveda recognizes the important root of illness in unexpressed and suppressed childhood negative emotions. Each of the doshas has its negative emotional tendencies, and these are watched for, observed, and released in treatment.

The hallmark of Ayurvedic treatment is the detoxification or ritual purification of the body called *Panchakarma*. To remove aggravated doshas and toxins (ama), Ayurveda suggests the use of Panchakarma (Pancha = five; and karma = actions), or the *five therapeutic actions*. These five actions are therapeutic vomiting, therapeutic purgation and laxative use, medicated enemas, nasal administration of medication, and purification of the blood. Before these ritual treatments can be initiated, the body is prepared for detoxification by *oil massage (snehana)* to encourage lymphatic drainage and toxin movement from soft tissue and by *therapeutic sweating (swedana)* to excrete toxins through the skin.

Different doshas respond better to individualized therapy. For instance, kapha (mucus) responds to therapeutic vomiting, pitta responds to purgatives and laxatives, and vata repents best to medicated enemas. Nasal insufflation clears and energizes the prana of the body and the mind. Purification of the blood actually refers to venisection and bloodletting, which can be accomplished, if need be, by donating at your nearest blood bank.

The Ayurvedic material medica is vast with more than 1000 cataloged herbs available for use. The administration of herbs is very similar to the Chinese system, with cold herbs being administered for a hot disease, etc. In the West, the out-of-context use of a specific Ayurvedic herb, such as Commiphora mukul (Guggul Gum Resin Extract) for the treatment of hypercholesterolemia, is the only general evidence of the use of this holistic, complex, and interesting medical philosophy.

## CLINICAL USE

Apart from the out-of-context use of a single Ayurvedic herb for a single Western diagnosis or symptom, the constitutional assignment, or *prakuti*, of a patient has some valuable clinical and prognostic value. For instance, both penicillin and aspirin have pitta-provoking attributes, so it would be clinically disadvantageous to prescribe these substances to a predominantly pitta person. Steroids, similarly, have a kapha-type action.

Ayurveda is similar to homeopathy and Chinese medicine, as it looks for the root and degree of penetration of the disease, rather than merely the name of the disease or treating its manifest symptoms. This description of Ayurvedic medicine is similar to the concepts described in Traditional Chinese Medicine and bespeaks of a common source or root. When people are given enough time and intellect to contemplate the nature of man and the cosmos, their perception usually ends in a final commonality of thought.

For the sake of space only, Traditional Tibetan Medicine is not discussed, as it represents a true marriage between Ayurvedic and Chinese medicine, and apart from the Buddhist philosophical base, and a partially different material medica, it is not appreciably different than either medical system.

# 13 Western Herbology or Phytotherapy

## HISTORY AND BACKGROUND

Just like Chinese medicine and homeopathy, Western herbology could be a book in itself, so I have contained my discussion to a little background, terms used in Western herbology, and a description of a number of the more popular herbs, their uses, side effects, and interactions with regular medications.

Although herbal use and prescribing is as old as civilization itself and has been used by the Native Americans for hundreds of years, the use of herbals in the United States has only become popular in the last five years. Because of the complexity of Chinese herbal prescribing, the general population has opted for single use Western herbs for single indications. This has led to a quasi drug usage, where a single herb is used instead of a pharmaceutical drug for a common indication.

In the United States, herbal preparations fall under the jurisdiction of the Food and Drug Administration (FDA), which regards them as food supplements. Under pressure from the pharmaceutical industry, the Dietary Supplement Health and Education Act was passed in 1994, in which the FDA allowed manufacturers to list use and safety information on herbal product labels, but they could not make any claims as to medicinal, curative, or preventive actions.

The European model is far more intelligent and pragmatic. The herbs are referred to as phytomedicine and are regulated as drugs. The German Commission E, an expert panel, was organized in 1978 to determine the use and safety of herbal medicines. In order for an herbal product to be registered, it has to pass the stringent testing, quality control, and literature search of the Commission E scientists. In 1995, 7% of prescription drugs covered by the German health insurance providers were herbal preparations. The German Commission E has assessed 360 herbs and produced 462 monographs. Each monograph addresses a single herb or a fixed herbal combination. Issues of use, potential toxicity, and interactions are addressed. The European Scientific Cooperative of Phytotherapy (ESCPO) has also published monographs in an attempt to bring consistent standards to botanical drug use throughout the European Union.

In the United States most herbal preparations are sold through multilevel marketing, direct marketing, the Internet, health food stores, or over the counter in pharmacies. Almost no phytotherapy is used by doctors. Patients are medicating themselves all the time, and have no clue as to the dosage, interactions of different herbs, interactions of herbs with regular medications, or the quality of the herbs they are using.

## TERMS USED IN PHYTOTHERAPY

### PHARMACOLOGY OF WESTERN HERBS

The pharmacology of an herb can be studied at three different levels:

1. Actions (traditional)
2. Individual chemical components (orthodox)
3. Pharmacological effects of the whole crude drug (phytotherapeutic)

Herbs, however, differ from drugs in:

1. **Chemical complexity** — This induces synergistic actions of the many different chemicals in the plant. Many of the different chemicals exhibit different actions such that an herb will manifest multifaceted actions in a single prescription. The combinations of additive and diverse actions, rather than a single focused action, usually results in less toxicity and fewer side effects.
2. **Subtleness and gentle activity** — Patient susceptibility will be more likely to be present in response to a multifaceted chemical herb than to a single chemical. Herbs, when prescribed for some time, exhibit cumulative effects as the organism slowly starts to respond to the herbal nudging. Herbs are often not forcing the biology in any one direction, but allowing better regulation of the body itself in response to the herbs' mild stimulation.
3. **Application with a different therapeutic strategy** — Often the drug is being used for gentle physiological support rather than trying to suppress a physiological response. Herbs seem to have multiple levels of effect, on the CNS, organs, and at the molecular level, all in one single herb. Many herbs are used to tonify or to allow adaptogenic responses to take place.

The main active constituents of herbs are:

1. **Volatile Oils** — All contained in the highly scented plants and usually used in aroma therapy. These oils are obtained by steam distillation and all the other components of the herb are left behind. Volatile oils are usually not a single compound, but a mixture of compounds such as azulene, cineol, borneal, camphor, menthol, and pinones.
   **Action:** Antiseptic and antibacterial, and quite often anti-inflammatory. Most of them are stimulants.
   **Example:** Oil of Oregano, which is a good antiviral.
2. **Tannins** — are widely distributed throughout the plant kingdom. Tannins can precipitate proteins and are used for tanning leather. Tannins are astringing and their action on cells in the body is to make them "astringed" or tight. For example, in diarrhea we astringe the mucus membranes to stop the mucus and fluid flow.
   **Action:** Astringent.
   **Example:** *Camellia sinensis* (Black tea).
3. **Saponins** — Lower the surface tension and produce a lather. They can emulsify the fat in the intestines and can facilitate the absorption of other fat-soluble herbal constituents in mixtures. Saponins are also slightly irritative to mucous membranes and produce a reflexive cough reaction. Saponins can hemolyze red blood corpuscles. They should not be used on open wounds.
   **Action:** Emulsification, irritant to mucous membranes, expectorant, hemolytic.
   **Example:** *Saponaria officinalis* (Soapwort).
4. **Alkaloids** — are widely distributed in the plant kingdom. All of them contain a cyclic nitrogen. They have many actions.
   **Actions:** Soporific, among many.
   **Example:** Opium, morphine, and codeine.
5. **Glycosides** — are complex organic molecules that contain some kind of sugar. The molecules can be split from their sugar (the glycone) to form an aglycone. The glycone enables the molecule to be absorbed and pass through membranes into cells, while the aglycone is the active principle. These molecules can spontaneously split with poor storage and lose a lot of their activity because they can no longer be absorbed.

**Action:** Whatever action the aglycone exhibits. '

**Example:** *Digitalis purpura* (Foxglove).

6. **Bitter Principles** — all stimulate the digestive system. They increase the production of digestive enzymes, hydrochloric acid, stomach peristalsis, and the absorption of food from the small intestine. They also increase the production of bile and stimulate the liver. They are the basis of the well-known aperitifs or drinks that are used as appetizers.

    **Action:** Stomachic, cholagogue, choleretic.

    **Example:** *Cinchona officinalis* (Quinine).

7. **Mucilage and Gums** — are the sticky and slimy constituents of herbs. They are complex carbohydrates that can be broken down into simpler sugars. They form gels with water and produce slimy protective layers on the internal and external surfaces of the body. They can absorb large quantities of water and swell, and are used as bulking agents for constipation.

    **Action:** Demulcants, bulking agents.

    **Example:** *Tussilago farfara* (Colt's Foot).

8. **Anthroquinones** — are very complex compounds. Known for their laxative action. Also have many flavones and flavonols.

    **Action:** Laxative, antioxidant.

    **Example:** *Cassia angustifolia* (Cascara sagrada).

9. **Enzymes** — are high in many plants, usually within the flesh of the fruit.

    **Action:** Depends on the activity of the enzyme, but most are proteolytic.

    **Example:** Pineapple (bromelain) and Papaya (papain).

## HERBAL PREPARATIONS

Herbal preparations can be used internally or externally. The most common pharmaceutical forms used in Western herbal traditions are infusions, decoctions, tinctures, and liquid extracts. Pills and capsules have appeared only recently.

Preparations for internal use include:

1. **Infusions** — not to be confused with herbal teas since they are much stronger. A typical infusion is 1 oz of herb to 1 pint of fluid, about 30 gm of herb to 600 ml fluid, or 10 gm of herb to about 200 ml of fluid (1 glass). Water is boiled and poured on the divided herb, covered, and left to stand for 5 to 10 minutes. The liquid is then strained and may be taken hot or cold.

2. **Decoction** — usually used for roots, bark, or seeds that do not extract well under conditions of infusion. Similar herb/water ratios are used but that the herb is simmered for 5 to 10 minutes in a covered pot. Some decoctions are done in an open vessel and are based on reducing the fluid from 600 ml to 300 ml.

3. **Tinctures (Tr)** — is defined by the strength or the ratio and the alcohol strength used in extraction. For example, Tr Taraxacum radix 1:5, 25% alcohol. Ratios are always expressed as the amount of dried herb in grams to the amount of corresponding liquid in mL. Alcohol strengths are given as a percentage of pure ethanol in a given volume of final extracting liquid. For example, 250 mL of pure ethanol made up to 1 litre final volume gives an alcohol strength of 25%. Tinctures are made by a process of maceration, in which the "marc" or macerated herb, is left to soak for 2 to 3 weeks with the "menstruum" or alcohol–water mixture. The mixture is covered and mixed daily. After 2 to 3 weeks the liquid is decanted, the marc pressed, and the resultant liquids combined.

4. **Liquid (L.E) or Fluid Extracts (F.E)** — usually a 1:1 or 2:1 ratio. These very concentrated liquids are made by percolation or reserved percolation of concentration of a maceration.

Preparations for external use include:

1. **Ointments** — These are thick and greasy and are used where a protective barrier is required.
2. **Creams** — These are more watery, penetrate better than ointments, and are used where the herb needs to be absorbed.
3. **Lotions** — These are water-based mixtures for adding moisture to the area where they are used.
4. **Poultice** — Raw warmed herbs are placed on the affected area and covered with a cloth.
5. **Douches** — An herbal infusion or liquid is diluted with warm water and used as a douche, usually for vaginal placement.
6. **Pessaries and Suppositories** — The liquid herb is mixed with wax or some other solid substance that will melt in body heat and placed vaginally or rectally.

Most prescriptions that are liquid are based on 5 mL three times a day. Powdered and solid forms of dosing depend on the concentration of active ingredients and the herb in question. Herbs may be administered for months, weeks, or days depending on the therapeutic intent. Acute problems will have a shorter duration of treatment, while chronic problems and tonification require extended periods of treatment.

## THERAPEUTIC ACTIONS OF HERBS

1. **Abortifactant** — herbs that will induce abortion. Blue and Black Cohosh, Rue, Rosemary, all laxatives (downward action).
2. **Adaptogen** — herbs that act to strengthen the body and increase resistance to stress. Panax and Siberian ginseng, Tang Kuei, Withania, Gotu Kola, Shizandra.
3. **Alterative** — herbs that favorably alter the course of an ailment and restore health; improves the excretion of wastes from the circulatory system. Echinacea, Blue Flag, Red Clover, Clivers.
4. **Analgesic or Anodyne** — herbs that relieve pain. Opium Poppy, California Poppy, Jamaica Dogwood, Wild Lettuce, Corydalis.
5. **Antasthmatic** — herbs that help resolve asthma. Grindelia, sundew, lobelia, ephedra.
6. **Antemetic** — herbs that prevent nausea and vomiting. Ginger, Black Horehound, Chamomile.
7. **Anthelmintic or Vermifuge** — herbs that destroy worms. Garlic, Wormwood, Tansy, Butternut.
8. **Anticatarrhal** — herbs that stop catarrh. Golden Seal, Fenugreek, Eyebright, Golden Rod, Garlic.
9. **Antilithic** — herbs that stop stone formation. Gravel Root, Stone Root, Pellitory of the Wall, Wild Carrot.
10. **Antimicrobial** — herbs that stop bacterial infection. Echinacea, Uva Ursi, Bone Set, Yarrow, Inula, Sage, Thyme, Garlic, Baptisia.
11. **Antiphlogistic** — herbs that counteracts inflammation and fever. Willow bark, Wintergreen, Licorice, Wild yam, Sarsaparilla, Comfrey, Peppermint, Elder Flowers, Bone Set, Ephedra.
12. **Antirheumatic** — herbs that help arthritis. Celery Seed, Black Cohosh, Bog Bean, Devil's Claw, Guiacum.
13. **Antitussive** — herbs that stop coughing. Wild Cherry, Colt's Foot.
14. **Antispasmodic** — herbs that break spasms. Chamomile, Lemon Balm, Betony, Valerian, Scullcap, Mistletoe, Cramp Bark.
15. **Antisialogue** — herb that stops salivation.

16. **Aperient** — herbs that are laxatives. Psyllium seed, Linseed, Rhubarb Root, Yellow Dock, Cascara Sagrada.
17. **Aphrodisiac** — herbs that increase sexual appetite. Damiana, Saw Palmetto, Cola, Panax Ginseng, Withania.
18. **Astringent** — herbs that tighten mucosa or other structures. Oak Bark, Rhatany Root, Tormental, Witch Hazel, Cranesbill.
19. **Bronchodilators** — herbs that bronchodilate. Ephedra.
20. **Cardioactive** — herbs that have cardiac activity. Hawthorne, Mistletoe, Motherwort, Panax Notoginseng.
21. **Carminative** — herbs that relieve gas or colic from the alimentary canal. Cinnamon, Dill, Fennel, Aniseed, Ginger, Parsley, Peppermint.
22. **Cathartic** — herbs that cause diarrhea. Senna, Cascara Sagrada.
23. **Cholagogue** — herbs that stimulate the flow of bile from the gallbladder to the duodenum. Greater Celandine, Peppermint, Dandelion, Boldo.
24. **Choleretic** — herbs that stimulate production of bile from the liver. Globe Artichoke, St. Mary's Thistle.
25. **Circulatory Stimulants** — herbs that cause increased circulation. Cayenne, Ginger, Prickly Ash, Rosemary, Gingko Biloba, Panax Ginseng.
26. **Demulcent or Emollient** — herbs that protect, lubricate, and sooth gastrointestinal linings. Comfrey Root, Marshmallow Root, Slippery Elm, Fenugreek.
27. **Diaphoretic or Sudorific** — herbs that cause sweating or excessive perspiration. Ephedra, Yarrow, Elder Flowers, Peppermint, Boneset.
28. **Digestive Tonic** — herbs that help appetite and digestion. Gentian, Meadowsweet, Fringe Tree, Ginger, Parsley, Golden Seal.
29. **Diuretic** — herbs that increase urinary output. Dandelion Leaves, Celery, Birch, Clivers.
30. **Emetic** — herbs that cause vomiting. Lobelia, Ipecacuanha.
31. **Emmenagogue** — herbs that stimulate menstrual flow. Blue Cohosh, Life Root, Pennyroyal, Yarrow.
32. **Expectorant** — herbs that encourage coughing up mucus. Inula, White Horehound, Thyme. For dry coughs and asthma, to soothe the mucous membranes and loosen the phlegm, use Colt's Foot, Licorice, Aniseed, Ephedra, Sundew. Some herbs have a broader range of action and can be used in both clinical situations such as Lobelia, Garlic, Ginger, Mullein, Red Clover, Elder Flowers.
33. **Galactogogue** — herbs that increase breast milk. Fennel, Fenugreek, Nettle, Vervain, Clivers, Celery Seed, Vitex.
34. **Hypoglycemic** — herbs that decrease blood sugar. Gymnema, Goats Rue, Garlic, The Bitters, Fenugreek, Jambolan Seed, Nettle.
35. **Hypertensive** — herbs that increase blood pressure. Licorice, Broom.
36. **Hypotensive** — herbs that treat high blood pressure. Hawthorne, Lime Flowers, Garlic, yarrow, Coleus.
37. **Hypnotic** — herbs that calm and induce sleep. Hops, Passion Flower, California Poppy, Valerian, Corydalis.
38. **Lymphatic** — herbs that increase lymphatic flow and drainage. Poke Root, Wild Indigo, Blue Flag, Clivers, Fenugreek, Calendula.
39. **Muscarinic** — herbs that contract smooth muscle, causes salivation and perspiration, abdominal colic, and excessive bronchial secretions.
40. **Nervine** — herbs that relax and sooth the nerves. Oats, Damaina, Scullcap, Cola, Panax Ginseng, Rosemary.
41. **Oxytocic** — herbs that will stimulate labor. Blue Cohosh, Golden Seal.
42. **Parturifacient** — herbs that induce abortion. Raspberry leaf, Beth Root, Squaw Vine.
43. **Purgative** — herbs that are stimulant laxatives. Jalap, Bitter Apple, Scammony.

44. **Rubifacient** — herbs that cause local vasodilitation and redness. Cayenne, Ginger, Wintergreen.
45. **Sedative** — herbs that relax and are anxiolytic. Jamaican Dogwood, Henbane, Valerian.
46. **Sialogogue** — herbs that cause salivation. Gentian, Calumba, Snake Root.
47. **Stomachic** — herbs that promote digestion and improve appetite. Parsley, Meadosweet, Dandelion, Daminana, Valerian.
48. **Stimulant** — herbs that stimulate circulation such as Cayenne, Ginger, Prickly Ash; stimulate digestion such as Bitters, Gentian; or stimulates smooth muscle such as Bayberry.
49. **Styptic** — herbs that stop bleeding. Panax Notoginseng, Calendual, Horsetail, Cranesbill, Tormentilla.
50. **Tonic** — herbs that increase energy. Dandelion Root, Kelp, Alfalfa, Oats, Damiana, Helonias, Chamomile, Panax Ginseng, Withania.
51. **Uterine Remedies** — herbs that regulate the uterus and hormones. Vitex, Helonias, Blue Cohosh, Chamomile, Motherwort, Squaw Vine.
52. **Vasoconstrictor** — herbs that constrict vessels. Bugleweed, Ephedra, Broom.
53. **Vasodilatory** — herbs that dilate vessels. Feverfew, Buckwheat, Garlic, Lime Flowers.
54. **Vesicants** — herbs that produce skin vesicles. Croton Oil, Turpentine, Formic Acid.
55. **Vulnery** — preparation applied externally.

## POPULAR HERBS, THEIR USES, INTERACTIONS, AND TOXICITY

As there are over 400 commonly used Western herbs in the materia medica, I have chosen the top 20 most popular herbs. They will be named according to their common names, with the Latin names following. The main indication for each herb in common clinical practice will be in italics.

AHPA safety rating provides four categories of herb safety:

Class 1 — Herbs that are safe with appropriate use.
Class 2 — Herbs that have restrictions:
   2a. For external use only unless otherwise directed by a professional with expertise in using the particular substance.
   2b. Not for use during pregnancy unless otherwise directed by a professional with expertise in using that particular substance during pregnancy.
   2c. Not for use while breast-feeding unless otherwise directed by a professional with expertise in use of the particular substance while nursing.
   2d. Other restrictions according to professional guidance.
Class 3 — Herbs that can be used only with the guidance of a qualified professional (prescription only).
Class 4 — Herbs with insufficient data for classification.

The biggest problem with Western herbs is the lack of herbal product standardization, and the paucity of clinical and toxicological data and documented experience with the herbs.

The top 20 most popular herbs are:

1. **BILBERRY** (*Vaccinium myrtillus*, Family Ericaceae)
   Description: Dried ripe fruit contains tannins, anthocyanins (15 different), and flavenoid glycosides.
   Clinical Uses — Oral  - nonspecific acute diarrhea
                        - venous insufficiency of the lower limbs including varicose veins; reduces platelet aggregation; can be used for hemorrhoids in pregnancy.

                - retinopathies and visual disturbances related to microcirculatory disorders especially night blindness, diabetic retinopathy, and macular degeneration

                - hyperglycemic states

    Topical    - oral and pharyngeal inflammation

This herb is most often used in a combination with vitamins and minerals in products designed to treat or prevent the ocular complications of diabetes, night blindness, and macular degeneration. Interest in the herb started in the Second World War when British pilots noted increased night vision when eating the berries. It is used more in Europe for varicose veins, hemorrhoids, and peripheral vascular disease.

Actions and Mechanisms: Antioxidant, astringent, hypoglycemic, antiedemic, antidiarrheal. The astringent tannin components are responsible for the observed benefit in diarrhea and irritation of the mouth and throat mucosa. The anthocyanoside constituents decrease vascular permeability, and aid in the redistribution of microvascular blood flow and the formation of interstitial fluid.

Dosage — Preventive: In eye disorders, 80 mg 2x/day of a fruit liquid extract standardized to contain 25% anthocyanidins.

Therapeutic:          In eye disorders, 240 to 640 mg/day, results in 6 to 8 weeks.

Topical use:         10% decoction for gargling and swishing.

Contraindications and Side Effects: Some digestive disturbance in higher dosages, which disappears on taking the herb with food. Safe in pregnancy and lactation.

Herb–Drug Interactions: Should be used with caution in patients on Warfarin or antiplatelet medications, or those who have hemorrhagic disorders.

AHPA Safety Rating — Class 1.

2. **BLACK COHOSH, SQUAW ROOT** (*Cimicifuga racemosa*, Family Ranunculaceae)
Description: Root contains actein, cimicifugoside triterpine glycosides, and formomonetin. Also contains salicylic acid.

Clinical Uses — Oral: - perimenapausal and menapausal symptoms, both physiological and emotional, instead of, or as an adjunct to, hormone replacement therapy

                - hormonal replacement therapy in women under 40 years of age, in situations of oophorectomy/hysterectomy.

Most of the data comes from a German product called Remifemin®, which has been on the market for some time. There have been multiple clinical trials of the product, which seems to have good efficacy for menapausal symptoms.

Actions and Mechanisms: Estrogen mimetic, LH suppressant, estrogen receptor binding, emmenagogue, and uterine stimulant. The rhizome and root contain the therapeutic principals. The action of Black Cohosh is related to the binding of estrogen receptors and the suppression of leutinizing hormone by the triterpine glycoside 27-deoxyactein. Black Cohosh has an estriol-like activity.

Dosage — Equivalent of 40 mg of root extract, standardized to contain 2.5% triterpine glycosides, 2x/day. Therapy needs to be for 8 weeks to assess effect. Black Cohosh should not be taken without a break for longer than 6 months.

Contraindications and Side Effects: Not to be taken if pregnant as it may induce uterine contractions. A history of breast cancer does not seem to be a contraindication because of its estriol effect. Physician should review use after 6 months of therapy. Side effects include occasional allergic reactions, gastric irritation, and nausea and dizziness on overdose. Patients with extreme sensitivity to aspirin and who are asthmatic may have a problem with this herb.

Herb–Drug Interactions: Black Cohosh appears to potentiate the actions of some hypertensive and hypoglycemic medications. The herb may be given concurrently with estrogenic preparations without any siginificant problems. Theoretically, concomitant use with other salicylate-containing herbs could potentiate the aspirin effect. These include Aspen Bark, Poplar, Sweet Birch, White Willow, and Wintergreen.

AHPA Safety Rating — Class 2b and 2c.

3.  **CHAMOMILE** (*Matricaria or Chamomilla recutita,* Family Asteraceae or Compositae)
Description: The dried flower heads contain 0.4% essential oil with the constituents alpha-bisabolol or bisabolol oxides A and B, chamazulene, flavenoids, coumarins, and mucilages.

Clinical Uses — Oral  - as a digestive aid and carminative
                           - as a mild sedative
                           - some anti-ulcer activity
                           - infantile insomnia
           Inhalant  - upper respiratory and sinus inflammation
           Topical  - inflammed, cracked, and sore skin
                           - minor infections, insect bites, etc
                           - hemorrhoids, anogential inflammation
                           - oral infections of the mucosa

Chamomile is most often used as a tea to soothe the nerves. In cardiac catheterization patients it was found to be an effective anxi0olytic and sedative with minimal effect on cardiac functions. Studies have shown efficacy as a topical astringent and mild analgesic. It speeds up healing of minor wounds.

Actions and Mechanisms: Anti-inflammatory, diuretic, vulnerary, antimicrobial, mildly sedative, antiplogistic, musculotropic, and deodorant. The flower head or flos of German Chamomile possesses many actions, including antiallergic, antiflatulent, antis-pasmodic, mild sedative, antiinflammatory and antiseptic actions. It also soothes mucus membranes. Chamomile's antiallergic and anti-inflammatory actions result from the azulene constituents, which inhibit histamine release. The sesquiterpene bisabolol con-stituents also possess anti-inflammatory and anti-ulcer properties.

Dosage — Tincture of 1:5 extract in 45% alcohol (standardized to 1.2% apigenin), 1 to 4 ml 3x/day.

Decoction: 3 to 4 gm boiled for 10 minutes in 150 ml, 3 to 4x/day as a tea or gargle.

Topical: 3 to 10% infusions, or ointments and gels.

Contraindications and Side Effects: Relative contraindications in people with cross-reactive allergy to other members of the Asteraceae and Compositae families (ragweed, chrysanthemums, marigolds, daisies). The usual problem is contact dermatitis in the use of topical preparations. Side effects are minimal.

Herb–Drug Interactions: May potentiate both herbs and drugs that have sedative and anticoagulant or antiplatelet properties.

AHPA Safety Rating — Class 1

4.  **ECHINACEA** (*Echinacea purpura*, Family Asteraceae or Compositae)
Description: Flower head, leaf, and root contain caffeic acid derivatives, flavonoids, alkylamides, and polysaccharides.

Clinical Uses — Oral  - resistance to infection, colds, and flus
                                 - general immune stimulant, recurrent infections
                                 - upper respiratory infections
                                 - as antiinflammatory in arthritis

A commonly used herb by patients as either a prophylactic immune stimulant or an acute therapy for colds and upper-respiratory tract infection. It should not be used for an extensive period of time to increase the Wei Qi energy of the body. I have just seen a case of extensive fixed drug reaction due to long-term use of Echinacea.

Actions and Mechanism: Antiviral, immune stimulant, antispasmodic, antibacterial, anti-inflammatory, hyaluronidase inhibitor, adrenal cortex activity stimulant, lipoxygenase inhibitor. The macerated juice of the whole plant has multiple effects on wound healing. It inhibits tissue and bacterial hyaluronidase, and induces the formation of phagocytes and fibrocytes from fibroblasts. It stimulates the adrenal cortex and, therefore, has anti-inflammatory activity. Echinacea purpura has potent antiviral activity to many common viruses including influenza and the herpes group viruses. Lymphocytes are stimulated to release tumor necrosis factor.

Dosage — Tincture: 225 mg (2 to 4 ml) 2x/day of a 6:1 echinacea purpura root extract standardized for content of alkenoic acid amide, cichoric acid, and mutivariant polysaccharides.

Encapsulated Freeze Dried Plant: 325-650 mg 3x/day Use at first sign of cold or flu symptoms. Do not use for long-term prophylaxis.

Contraindications and Side Effects: Contraindicated in any patient with an autoimmune disease because of the possibility of worsening of the process. Also should not be used in patients on immunosuppressive or antirejection drugs. Relative contraindication in allergic individuals with cross reactivity to other herbs of the Compositae family. May exacerbate asthma in allergic patients. Some evidence suggests that Echinacea may inhibit oocyte fertilization and alter sperm DNA and should be avoided by couples trying to conceive. Side effects include mild nausea, vomiting, and diarrhea. Tinctures have a vile taste. Avoid long-term prophylactic use.

AHPA Safety Rating — Class 1.

5. **FEVERFEW** (*Tanacetum parthenium*, Family Asteraceae)

Description: Dried flower and leaf containing 0.1-1% the sesquiterpene lactone, parthenolide.

Clinical Uses — Oral  - migraine prophylaxis
- prevention or treatment of other inflammatory and spasmodic disorders including asthma, rheumatoid arthritis, and dysmenorrhea
- reduces tinnitus

Feverfew use is pretty much restricted to those relatively few patients who respond to it for migraine prophylaxis. Side effects are not uncommon.

Actions and Mechanisms: Antispasmodic, anti-inflammatory, inhibits platelet serotonin secretion and synovial cell and mitogen-induced proliferation of polymorpholencocytes. Feverfew leaf can cause uterine contractions in humans and cattle. It inhibits platelet aggregation and serotonin secretion.

Dosage — Prophylaxis of migraine: 25 to 250 mg/day for 4 to 6 weeks of a standardized extract containing at least 0.2% parthenolide. Treatment of migraine: up to 2 grams a day.

Contraindications and Side Effects: Contraindicated in pregnancy. Cross-allergenic reactions with other members of the Asteraceae and Compositae families including ragweed. Side effects are important and include sore and swollen lips and tongue and loss of taste from chewing the leaf. Also seen are indigestion, diarrhea, flatulence, nausea and vomiting, and hypersensitivity reactions.

Herb–Drug Interactions: Care must be taken with patients on anticoagulants and antiplatelet drugs, as well as other anticoagulant active herbs, as it may potentiate their action.

AHPA Safety Rating — Class 2b.

6. **GARLIC** (*Allium sativum*, Family Liliaceae)

Description: Fresh or dried clove contains alliin, its degradation product, allicin, essential oil ajoene, and sulphur compounds such as allyl sulphide.

Clinical Uses — Oral  - lowering LDL, VLDL; increasing HDL lipids.
- hypertension
- arteriosclerosis
- reducing reinfarction and post MI mortality
- immune stimulant, antiviral, antibacterial, and antifungal
- liver protectant
- lowering blood sugars in diabetes
- heavy metal detoxification

Garlic has been used for centuries for the above indications, and will continue to be used as such. Easy to use in food. Very useful as an alternative medication in mucocutaneous candidiasis. Difficulties include the odor (even in "odorless" preparations), the poor standardization of products, and the deactivation of the active compounds by gastric acids.

Actions and Mechanisms: Antibacterial, antimycotic, fibrinolysis inhibitor, lipid reducer, blood-coagulation time enhancer, atherosclerosis preventer, hypoglycemic, gastric secretion and motility stimulant, anti-inflammatory. Possible cancer preventive. The intact bulb and the clove contain the odorless amino acid alliin. When the cells are broken, alliin comes into contact with the enzyme allinase and turns into allicin, an unstable, odiferous compound with all the antibacterial activity. Further conversion yields the essential oils E-ajoene and Z-ajoene, which are antithrombotic and inhibit the fibrinogen receptors on platelets. Allylpropyl disulfide has been shown to decrease blood sugar and increase insulin levels.

Dosage — 1 clove or 2 gms of fresh garlic or equivalent. About 650 mg of garlic powder containing 6 mg allicin. Enteric-coated products are prefered as they control after-odor and prevent breakdown of the active principals in the stomach.

Contraindications and Side Effects: Unsafe in large amounts in children and in pregnant and lactating mothers. Regarded as safe in amounts used in foods. Side effects, usually due to overuse, include nausea, diarrhea, flatulence, and burning of the mouth. Contact dermatitis has been documented in an industrial exposure setting.

Herb–Drug Interactions: Use with caution in patients on anticoagulants, antiplatelet drugs, insulin, and hypoglycemics. Will increase the bleeding potential of nonsteroidal anti-inflammatory drugs and works synergistically with EPA oils (eicosapentaenoic acid).

AHPA Safety Rating — 2c.

7. **GINGER** (*Zingiber officinale*, Family Zingiberaceae)

Description: The fresh or dried rhizome contains essential oil with sesquiterpene hydrocarbons (zingiberine and bisabolene) and also pungent compounds (gingerols and shogaols).

Clinical Uses — Oral  - antinauseant in cases of motion sickness, morning sickness, chemotherapy, and indigestion
- anti-inflammatory in arthritic conditions
- carminative
- cardiotonic

Ginger is an extremely good settler of the stomach, and can be prepared at home by grating some fresh ginger into boiling water and steeping for 5 minutes. In spite of the German E monographs, it is safe in these doses in pregnancy for morning sickness. It is quite a hot herb and this should be in mind when prescribing it.

Actions and Mechanisms: Antispasmodic, anti-inflammatory, peripheral circulatory stimulant, antinauseant, and carminative. Ginger has many different actions depending on its different constituents, but is often used to balance a Cold pattern or to restore a Yang deficient pattern. It stimulates stomach acid secretion, inhibits prostaglandins, and is a cardio-tonic and antitussive.

Dosage — In nausea: use 1 gm of dried or powdered root, or the equivalent in extract, standardized for more than 5% gingerols and shogaols. Dosing can start 1 to 2 days before a trip and may be taken every day.

Contraindications and Side Effects: Is not contraindicated in pregnancy. It is contraindicated in gallstones. Side effects include heartburn (too hot) and CNS depression and cardiac arrhythmias when used in large amounts.

Herb–Drug Interactions: Ginger will antagonize the activity of H-2 and proton pump inhibitors. Ginger might affect oral hypoglycemics (potentiate), barbiturates (potentiate), and anticoagulant and antiplatelet drugs (potentiate).

AHPA Safety Rating — Class 1 (fresh root); Class 2b (dried root).

8. **GINKGO** (*Ginkgo biloba*, Family Ginkgoaceae)
Description: The dried leaf extract contains 22 to 27% flavoneglycosides (quercitin, kaempferol, isorhamnetin), 5 to 7% terpene lactones (ginkgolides A,B, C, and bilobalide), and no more than 5 ppm ginkgolic acids.
Clinical Uses — Oral   - dementia, including Alzheimer's and vascular dementia.
                    - cerebral vascular deficiency in the elderly
                    - tinnitus and vertigo
                    - peripheral vascular disease, intermittent claudication
                    - macular degeneration
                    - asthma and bronchoconstriction

Ginkgo has had good long-term results in mild to moderate dementia, memory deficits, and tinnitus caused by vascular deficiency. It also shows a good response in some patients with intermittent claudication with improvement of pain-free walking distance.

Actions and Mechanisms: Antioxidant and PAF (platelet aggregating factor) inhibitor. The leaf constituents, Ginkgolides A, B, C, and M, contain the PAF inhibitory activity. PAF causes many different physiological changes that are antagonized by ginkgo. These include platelet aggregation, bronchoconstriction, chemotaxis, inflammatory compound release, decreased cardiac contractility, and hypersensitivity reactions.

Dosage — About 120 to 240 mg per day in divided doses of a 50:1 standardized leaf extract containing 22 to 27% ginkgo flavone glycosides and 5 to 7% terpene lactones. Should be taken for 4 to 8 weeks.

Contraindications and Side Effects: Contraindicated in patients exhibiting allergy to the herb, and in pregnant and lactating females. Side effects include the severe allergic reactions which can occur on the skin, mouth, GI tract, and anus. Cross reacts with allergy to poison oak, poison ivy, poison sumac, mango rind, and cashew nut shell oil. It may reduce fertility.

Herb–Drug Interactions: Ginkgo may potentiate the activity of MAO inhibitors and antiplatelet drugs.

AHPA Safety Rating — Class 2d.

9. **GINSENG** (*Panax ginseng* — Family Araliaceae)

Desciption — The root and root hairs of white and red ginseng contain 1.5% ginsenosides, peptides, and polysaccharides.

Clinical Uses — Oral  - adaptogen, a substance that enhances nonspecific resistance to stress and increases stress tolerance
- mental and physical fatigue
- enhance mental performance
- adrenal exhaustion and steroid use

Ginseng is used as a general "pick me up." Chinese, red, Korean, or Siberian ginseng are all warming and can damage patients if they already have deficient or false heat with their exhaustion. It is better to use American ginseng, which is cooling, in these patients. I use a mixture of three ginsengs that is neutral in temperature.

Actions and Mechanisms: Hypoglycemic, adaptogenic, antioxidant, antidepressant, antidiabetic, antiedemic, antihypertensive, immune stimulant, anti-inflammatory, anti-ulcer, and cholesterol reducing. Improves mental functioning and increases resistence to stress. It is the different ginsenosides that contain all the regulating and stimulating activity that ginseng exhibits.

Dosage — Taken before a meal, 100 mg 2x/day of a 5:1 standardized root extract. Use for 3 weeks without interruption followed by a one-week rest period before resuming the next cycle. Otherwise, as a powder or tea taking about 200 to 600 mg a day.

Contraindications and Side Effects: Contraindicated in infants and children, who are already "Hot." Also contraindicated in pregnancy (a "hot" state) and in lactating females. Should probably be avoided by cardiac patients. Side effects in sensitive patients include skin eruptions, mastalgia in older women, estrogenic effects in postmenopausal females, diarrhea, headaches, and hyperpyrexia. In excess use susceptible patients will experience hypertension, nervousness, imsomnia, and increased libido.

Herb–Drug Interactions: May potentiate MAOs (especially Nardil®), hypoglycemics, and anticoagulants. Exercise caution when using with other stimulants such as caffeine, ephedra, and guarana — may precipitate hypertension.

AHPA Safety Rating — Class 2d (hypertension).

10. **GOLDENSEAL** (*Hydrastis canadensis*, Family Ranunculaceae)

Description: The dried rhizome and roots contain the potent isoquinoline alkaloids hydrastine and berberine.

Clinical Uses — Oral  - broad spectrum antibiotic with activity against bacteria, yeast, and parasites
- antisecretory in diarrhea
- cardiotonic and cardioprotective

Goldenseal is usually found in combination with echinacea and used as an antibiotic combination. This combination is to be deplored, because of the relative inequalities in toxicity between the two herbs, goldenseal being far more toxic. Patients end up taking this combination for months with consequent side effects.

Actions and Mechanisms: Antibacterial, antifungal, antiparasitic, cholegogue, and cardiotonic. The alkaloid berberine has a very broad spectrum antibiotic activity that includes the following organisms: staphylococcus, C. diphtheriae, salmonella, streptoccus pneumonia, pseudomonas spp, shigella, trichomonas, N. gonorrhea and meningitidis, T. pallidum, giardia, fungi, and amoeba.

Dosage — 250 to 500 mg per day of a 4:1 standardized root extract containing 5% total alkaloids, calculated as hydrastine. Can be used for "traveler's diarrhea" by taking a dose daily for one week before and one week after travel. Needs alkaline pH for best antibiotic activity.

Contraindications and Side Effects: Contraindicated in pregnant and lactating females. Also should not be used if patients are on antihypertensives or have inflammatory bowel disease. Side effects include nausea and dizziness, irritated mucous membranes, constipation, depression, dyspnea, bradycardia, cardiac damage, hypotension, spasms, and death. Large doses of hydrastine can lead to hyper-reflexia, convulsions, paralysis, and death from respiratory failure.

Herb–Drug Interactions: Goldenseal increases stomach acid, potentiates barbiturates, causes hypertension, inhibits heparin, and potentiates sedatives.

AHPA Safety Rating — Class 2d.

11. **GRAPE SEED** (*Vitis vinifera* — Family Vitaceae)

Description: The grape seed is a potent source of bitter tannins called procyanidin oligomers (PCOs), as well as essential fatty acids and vitamin E.

Clinical Uses — Oral
- microcirculatory disorders
- varicose veins
- diabetic retinopathy
- macular degeneration, night blindness
- capillary fragility
- antioxidant activity

Grape seed extract is found in many antioxidant products as a cheaper alternative to Pycnogenol, the similar pinebark extract. It is a very active antioxidant and also potentiates the activity of Vitamin C.

Actions and Mechanisms: Antioxidant, anti-inflammatory and radioprotective. Grape seed PCOs are potent antioxidants, free radical scavengers, and have antilipoperoxidant activity. The extract also noncompetitively inhibits various proteolytic enzymes including collagenase, elastase, and hyaluronidase.

Dosage — Treatment dose is 75 to 300 mg per day for 3 weeks. For maintenance: 40 to 100 mg daily.

Contraindications and Side Effects: None known at this time.

Herb–Drug Interactions: May increase action of Warfarin due to the tocopherol content of grape seed.

AHPA safety Rating — Class 1.

12. **GREEN TEA** (*Camellia sinensis* — Family Theaceae)

Description: Steamed, dried fresh leaf contains polyphenols (epigallocatechin gallate, or EGCG), flavenoids, and methylxanthines.

Clinical Uses — Oral
- antioxidant for protection of cells, tissues, and organs
- cancer chemopreventative
- cardiotonic and anti-atherosclerotic
- prevention of gingivitis and dental caries
- improved resistance to infections

Green tea has been used in the Orient for centuries to good health effect. It is found as a powder as a constituent of antioxidant mixtures, but is more commonly consumed as a refreshing tea as a healthy lifestyle choice.

Actions and Mechanisms: Lowers cholesterol, reduces platelet aggregation, lowers blood pressure, antimutagenic, anticarcinogenic, radioprotective, anticariogenic, antibacterial, diuretic, stimulant, and astringent. The leaf bud, leaf, and stem have the following properties: caffeine (60 to 70 mg per 6 oz of tea) is responsible for the diuretic and CNS effects; the catechins are responsible for the antioxidant activities; tannins are responsible for the antidiarrheal activity. Ingestion of 9 cups a day will decrease total cholesterol only. Tea leaves contain potent antioxidants that will prevent the oxidation of LDL-cholesterol and reduce platelet aggregation.

Dosage — 1 teaspoon of tea leaves in 8 oz of boiling water. Up to 10 cups a day have been recorded. The average is about 3 cups, an equivalent of 240 to 320 mg of polyphenols. One should limit ingestion to a maximum of 5 cups per day. Powdered, decaffeinated green tea capsules are available and are equivalent to 4 cups of tea.

Contraindications and Side Effects: Contraindicated in infants as it leads to binding of iron and microcytic anemia. Contraindicated in lactating mothers because it can cause insomnia in breast-feeding infants. Side effects are those of excessive caffeine. Green tea by itself can cause gastrointestinal upset and constipation.

Herb–Drug Interactions: Ephedra will potentuate the stimulant activity of the caffeine in green tea. More than 40 drugs are affected or have an interaction with green tea. [(A) is antagonistic to drug; (P) potentiates the drug]. These include: antacids (A), aspirin/acetominophen (P 40%), antipsychotic drugs (A), barbiturates (increases caffeine), beta-adrenergic agonists (P), benzodiazepines (A), beta blockers (A), Thorazine® (A), Cimetidine® (decreases caffeine clearance), Clozapine® (P and also causes psychosis), CNS depressants (increases caffeine), hypoglycemics (A), Disulfiram® (increases caffeine), Ergotamine® (P), Diflucan® (increases caffeine), lithium (P with withdrawal), MAO inhibitors (hypertensive crisis), oral birth control pills (increases caffeine), Phenytoin® (decreases caffeine), Phenylpropanolamine (increase BP and mania), quinolones (increases caffeine clearance), Theophylline® (P), Verapamil® (increases caffeine), and Warfarin® (A).

AHPA Safety Rating — Class 2d.

13. **HAWTHORN** (*Crataegus oxycantha*, Family Rosaceae)
Description: Dried fruit contains oligomeric procyanidins, vitexin, quercetin, and hyperoside.

Clinical Uses — Oral - cardiotonic and cardioprotective
- prevents atherosclerosis and reduces hypertension
- helps CCF, senile heart, cor pulmonale, and mild arrythmias
- improves digestion

Hawthorn is an exceedingly safe and effective cardiotonic and should be used with CoQ10 and magnesium as a treatment for all your CHFs.

Actions and Mechanisms: Increases coronary blood flow due to dilatory effects resulting in an improvement of myocardial blood flow. The herb is positively inotropic and negatively chronotropic. It also reduces peripheral vascular resistance and is antilipemic. The flavenoids and proanthocyanidins are the active substances in the herb. Its cardiotrophic properties are due to increased membrane permeability for calcium and phosphodiesterase inhibition that increases intracellular cAMP. Hawthorn also decreases uterine tone and motility and is antilipid.

Dosage — The average dose is 5 gm of berry per day, 80 to 300 mg of extract in capsules or tablets of a standardized 2.2% bioflavenoid, or 18.75% oligomeric procyanidin content in tincture of 4 to 5 ml per day. Effect is felt at 4 to 8 weeks and should be continued indefinitely.

Contraindications and Side Effects: Contraindicated in pregnant and breast-feeding females. Used with caution in cardiac patients on multiple drug therapy (needs careful supervision). Not to be self-prescribed (happens all the time). Side effects include nausea, fatigue, perspiration, and skin rash on the hands.

Herb–Drug Interactions: Be careful of additive effects in coronary vasodilators, cardiovascular drugs in general (will potentiate digoxin, watch for toxicity), and CNS depressants (additive).

AHPA Safety Rating — Class 1.

14. **HORSE CHESTNUT** (*Aesculus hippocastanum*, Family Hippocastanaceae)
Description: The seed extract, leaves, and pealed nuts contain esculin and aescin.
Clinical Uses — Oral  - veinous insufficiency
                       - veinotonic, for varicose veins and hemorrhoids
                       - anti-edemic
                       - anti-inflammatory
                       - used for leg cramps and poor circulation

A very effective herb for patients with bad familial varicose veins that cause the legs to feel stiff, heavy, and achy.

Actions and Mechanisms: Anti-inflammatory, analgesic, reduces swelling in chronic venous insufficiency, inhibits varicose vein producing enzymes, reduces capillary permeability and has antigranulation effects. The Horse Chestnut leaf contains the potent toxic glycoside aesculin, which is a hydroxycoumarin with potential antithrombin activity. The Horse Chestnut seed contains triterpene saponins referred to as aescin and aesculin. Escin decreases the permeability of venous capillaries caused by histamine and serotonin, and constricts veins. It has a weak diuretic actvity.

Dosage: 200 to 500 mg of the extract per day, standardized to contain 16 to 21% aescin (150 mg aescin per day). Capsules of the herb contain 250 mg and are taken 1 to 3 x/day. Topical applications may be done 4 x/day.

Contraindications and Side Effects: Contraindicated in pregnancy, breast feeding, children, anticoagulant therapy, and kidney or liver impairment. Side effects with excessive ingestion include gastrointesinal irritation, toxic nephropathy, liver damage, shock, spasm, mild nausea, vomiting, hives, and a pseudolupus syndrome.

Herb–Drug Interactions: Take care with anticoagulant drugs and hypoglycemics.

AHPA Safety rating — Not yet rated.

15. **KAVA** (*Piper methysticum*, Family Piperaceae)
Description: The dried rhizome contains kavalactones.
Clinical Uses— Oral   - anxiolytic and sedative
                       - muscle relaxant
                       - stress relief

Kava is used in many proprietary compounds for the relief of stress, anxiety, and insomnia. It has relatively good short-term efficacy, exhibits minimal tachyphylaxis, but no dependence, if used for prolonged periods.

Actions and Mechanisms: Sedative, analgesic, soporific, anticonvulsant, muscle relaxant, and local anesthetic. The rhizome and root contain the active kava pyrone constituents. All of these pyrones show evidence of CNS activity. The pyrones have analgesic activity that is not via the opiate pathway. Their muscle-relaxing properties are equivalent to the benzodiazepines.

Dosage — For anxiety and muscle tension, standardized 11:1 root extract equivalent to 70 mg of kavalactones 1 to 3 x/day. For sedation, an equivalent of 210 to 500 mg of kavalactones one hour before bedtime.

Contraindications and Side Effects: Contraindicated in pregnancy, breast feeding, and endogenous depression. Use for 3 months or less. Side effects include an allergic reversable dermatopathy with excess use (yellowing of the skin), skin rashes, gastrointestinal irritation, and drowsiness. A rare case of Parkinsonian-type effect has been reported, probably due to Kava's dopamine antagonism. Care must be taken driving or operating machinery, or engaging in hazardous occupations while taking kava.

Herb–Drug Interactions: Kava will potentiate all other anxiolytic and sedative drugs. Concomitant use with alcohol, barbiturates, and benzodiazepines is unwise. Kava will anatgonize the effects of Levodopa.®

AHPA Safety Rating — Class 2d (may interfere with driving or operating heavy machinery).

16. **MILK THISTLE** (*Carduus marianum*, Family Asteraceae)
Description: Seed from the pappus contains silibinin, silydianin, and silychristin, collectively called silymarin.
Clinical Use — Oral   - protection of the liver from damage due to toxins, ethanol, hepatitis, cirrhosis, pharmaceutical drugs, and other toxic and pathological problems
   - recovery of liver function following any pathological insult
   - as an antidote to *Amanita phylloides* mushroom poisoning
   - bile duct inflammation

Although Milk Thistle is an excellent hepato-protectant, it should be used together with substances that ensure Phase I and II detoxification of the liver, and with Chinese herbs that have Blood- and Qi-moving characterisitics, for a complete treatment.

Actions and Mechanisms: Antihepatotoxic, antioxidant (inhibits leukotriene formation, stimulates protein synthesis, and regulates glutathione), changes hepatocyte membranes, and activates nucleolar polymerase A. The liver protectant effect of Milk Thistle is based on two mechanisms of action. The first involves stabilizing the outer hepatocyte membrane and preventing toxin penetration; the second is its activation of nucleolar polymerase A, which increases ribosomal protein synthesis, which in turn stimulates hepatocytic regeneration and healing. Silymarin undergoes enterohepatic recirculation, and is, thus, concentrated in the hepatocytes.

Dosage — 400 mg daily dose of a standardized 70% silymarin extract for 8 to 12 weeks, at which time the dose is reduced to 200 to 250 mg a day.

Contraindications and Side Effects: No data on pregnancy and lactation, but avoid using. Side effects include a mild laxative effect, which is probably desirable anyway.

Herb–Drug Interactions: Will protect the liver from pharmaceutical hepatotoxic drugs when they are used for prolonged therapy.

AHPA Safety Rating — Class 1.

17. **SAW PALMETTO** (*Serenoa repens*, Family Aracaceae or Palmaceae)
Description: The dried ripe fruit contains fatty acids, phytosterols, and polysaccharides.
Clinical Uses — Oral   - symptomatic relief of benign prostatic hypertrophy (BPH) stages 1 and 2
   - all urinary difficulties

All male patients over the age of 45 years should have Saw Palmetto, or one of the BPH products, as part of their supplement program. The herb can be given indefinitely without any long-term problems.

Actions and Mechanisms: Antiexudative, diuretic, urinary antiseptic, hormonal and endocrine effects, decreases 5-dihydrotestosterone (5-DHT) and testosterone. BPH results from increased 5-DHT in the prostate. The fatty acid fractions of Saw Palmetto reduce levels of 5-DHT by inhibiting the action of 5-alpha reductase on testosterone, and by inhibiting 5-DHT binding to androgen receptors. The anti-iflammatory effects of Saw Palmetto may also play a part. Saw Palmetto does not necessarily affect prostate enlargement or prostatic specific antigen (PSA) levels. On present evidence, it just helps with BPH symptoms.

Dosage — For BPH: 320 mg of the lipophilic extract (80 to 90% fatty acids) daily.

Contraindications and Side Effects: Contraindicated in pregnant females (some have used it for its antiandrogenic action) and breast feeding. Side effects include infrequent cramping and nausea.

Herb–Drug Interactions: Saw Palmetto can interfere with oral contraception and hormonal therapy.

AHPA Safety Rating — Class 1.

18. **ST. JOHN'S WORT** (*Hypericum perforatum*, Family Hypericaceae)

Description: The dried, aboveground parts contain hypericin and pseudohypericin.

Clinical Uses — Oral  - mild to moderate depression
- mood stabilizer, and to improve stress tolerance and sleep
- seasonal affective disorder

Topical  - wound healing and antiviral

Hypericum does have good efficacy in the majority of mild to moderately depressed patients. It does not help all depressed patients and some of the side effects preclude its use. It does exhibit tachyphylaxis in some patients.

Actions and Mechanisms: Mild antidepressant, sedative, anxiolytic. Topical preparations are anti-inflammatory, antibacterial, and vulnerary. The mechanism of action is not quite clear, as the serotonin uptake inhibition of hypericin cannot be duplicated at a reasonable drug blood level in animals. Other mechanisms that may participate in its activity include the modulation of cytokines, the inhibition of catechol-o-methyl transferase, the inhibition of receptors for adenosine, benzodiazepine, gamma amino benjoic acid (GABA), and inositol triphosphate. Hypericin is a broad spectrum antiviral.

Dosage — Oral: for depression, 900 mg/day of a 5:1 extract of a standardized 0.3% hypericin. Improvement requires several weeks. Topical: 1:10 tincture in diluted down 45% alcohol.

Contraindications and Side Effects: Contraindicated in pregnancy, breast feeding, and in patients on MAO inhibitors. Contraindicated for HIV patients on protease inhibitors and or non-nucleoside reverse trans-scriptase inhibitors, as hypericin induces the liver cytochrome P450 metabolic pathway and will result in lowered levels of HIV drugs. Use with caution in patients on serum serotonin reuptake inhibitors (SSRIs). Side effects includes photodermatitis, photosensitivity, premature cataract formation, infertility, and neuropathy.

Herb–Drug Interactions: Avoid concomitant use with antidepressants, other than for changing from drug to the herb or vice versa. Hypericin reduces digoxin levels in healthy people.

AHPA Safety Rating — Class 2d.

19. **VALERIAN** (*Valeriana officinalis* — Family Valerianaceae)

Description: The fresh or dried root contains essential oils with monoterpenes and sesquiterpenes, including valerenic acid.

Clinical Uses — Oral  - insomnia and nervousness
- intestinal cramps and dysmenorrhea

Valerian is an excellent soporific, is well tolerated, and is without the dependency issues related to the benzodiazepines. It can also improve the sleep of normal individuals and does not have any hangover effects the next morning. It does not have immediate action, but takes some weeks before its full effect can be felt. If the patient has been on the herb for some time, some tapering is necessary to prevent withdrawal symptoms.

Actions and Mechanisms: Sedative, hypnotic, antispasmodic, anodyne, anticonvulsant, hypotensive (mild depressant effects on the CNS, GABA enzyme inhibitor). Valerenic acid inhibits the catabolism of GABA, thereby increasing its levels and decreasing CNS activity.

Dosage — For insomnia: 300 to 500 mg Valerian root extract, standardized to 0.8% valerenic acid, or 5 ml of 1:5 tincture, one hour before bedtime.

Contraindications and Side Effects: Contraindicated in patients taking antidepressants and other sedatives. Side effects with chronic use include headache, excitability, insomnia, uneasiness, arrythmias, and some emotional dependence in susceptible people.

Herb–Drug Interactions: Valerian will potentiate other sedative–hypnotic drugs.

AHPA Safety Rating — Class 1.

20. **VITEX — CHASTEBERRY** (*Vitex agnus-castus* — Family Verbenaceae)

Description — The dried, ripe fruit and leaves contain iridoid glycosides, flavenoids, and volatile oils.

Clinical Uses — Oral
- menstrual irregularites and premenstrual complaints
- hormonally related acne and mastodynia
- corpus luteum insufficiency (infertility)
- hyperprolactinemia

Vitex seems to work for PMS and related menstrual and fertility abnormalities in females with a deficient luteal phase and low progesterone levels.

Actions and Mechanisms: Anti-androgenic and antiprolactin. Vitex has an active ingredient that binds to dopamine (D1 and D2) receptors and inhibits prolactin release. It decreases follicle stimulating hormone release from the anterior pituitary, but increases leatinising hormone release, thereby favoring progesterone over estrogen. The net effect is to normalize the luteal phase by increasing progesterone levels.

Dosage — Aqueous alcohol extract (50 to 70%v/v) corresponding to 30 to 40 mg of dried fruit per day; or 175 mg per day of a 20:1 standardized fruit extract containing 0.5% agnusides. Patient needs to continue treatment for 3 to 6 weeks for efficacy and can stay on the treatment for 3 to 6 months at a time.

Contraindications and Side Effects: Contraindicated in all patients on dopamine receptor antagonists such as haloperidol, as well as dopamine antagonists and dopamine-receptor blocking agents, such as metoclopromide. Not enough data to know the extent that Vitex interfers with oral contraception or hormone replacement therapy. Women who become pregnant while taking Vitex should stay on the herb until the fourth month. Vitex induces premature lactation if taken in late pregnancy and may suppress milk production during lactation. Side effects include nausea, headache, diarrhea, weight gain, itching, and urticarial rash.

Herb–Drug Interactions: see Contraindications and Side Effects.

AHPA Safety Rating — Class 2b

# 14 Therapeutic Nutrition

## INTRODUCTION

The subject of nutrition, diets, supplements, and the like is filled with controversy and opinions. I will offer my somewhat truncated outlook as befits a physician in a busy clinical environment. My opinions are definite and relate more to the role of food and supplements in the individual, rather than the role of food and supplements in any particular disease. There will not be hundreds of references to my statements of fact. If you doubt anything I say, please prove me wrong by your own research. I don't think that you will come to a different conclusion.

I will trace the history of food, because therein lie the problems that have developed in modern man. We have not adapted our eating to our changes in environment, but have opted for time-saving and convenient nutrition, over what our bodies really need. It is not possible to look at nutrition as an isolated issue in health, because it reflects our whole attitude toward ourselves and the world around us. Chinese and Ayurvedic medicine use food therapeutically, both as a preventive and as a therapeutic means of keeping man in balance with his internal and greater external environment.

### HISTORICAL ASPECTS OF FOOD

Back when we were omnivorous hunters and gatherers of food, our biochemistry was set up such that, when we found sufficient food, we could have more than our fill and store as much of the bounty as possible. Our biochemistry has changed little since that time. We would wander through the forests, plains, and mountains eating whatever food was in season or ripening, and then there would be long periods of starvation, during which we would draw on our fat to supply us with the calories for daily living. If we were lucky, we would have had a successful hunt and our fill of protein. As time went on, we eventually developed ways of preserving this meat and other foodstuffs, so that the cold winter months would not be so nutritionally harsh. Most of our food was fresh, raw, and unprocessed and grew in a fertile and unpolluted soil. The water we drank was free of chemicals and adulterants. We walked, ran, and worked for most of the day to satisfy our basic needs and slept for the ten to twelve hours that constituted the night. It is interesting to compare this existence with some modern "cavemen," the nomadic Bushman or Koi People of the Kalahari Desert in South Africa. Their lifestyle has not changed for at least a thousand years. They exist on what they can dig out of the earth and what they can hunt. From discussions with elders of one of the larger groups, I have found that they have a sense of importance, for the different activities of life, according to their time allotments for each activity. They spend, on average, four hours a day looking for food or hunting; they tell stories and contemplate the world for four hours; and they dance or play for two to four hours every day. What an idealic existence. They are free of all chronic disease and seem not to age in the same way we do. Another interesting fact is that the average Bushman female has only about 100 menstrual periods in her whole life. She is either pregnant (5 to 10 children) or breast feeding (usually five or more years for each child), and then menopause is upon her. No osteoporosis, breast cancer or heart attacks to bother her. The average Western female has about 400 menses in her lifetime until menopause, and the use of hormone replacement therapy will extend those numbers still further. How much do the poor women have to take?

## CHANGES IN FOOD PRODUCTION

What historical changes in how we choose, grow, store, process, and eat our food have changed the balance in our bodies toward disease?

1. **Quality of Food** — The quality of food depends on the soil and water used to grow it. The soil has become demineralized and sterile, and the water is polluted with chemicals, pesticides, and herbicides over much of the country. Food that grows in this lifeless terrain is itself lifeless and devoid of essential minerals.

2. **Storage and Transport of Food** — Gone are the days when your local farmer offered his wares on the town square. Your apples come from Washington or New Zealand, your potatoes from Idaho, and your citrus from Florida or Brazil. This fruit and produce have to travel long distances to arrive at your supermarket, and they are either picked green or in some way preserved in order to get to you "fresh." In Nevada, all the produce is shipped from California to Utah (900 miles) and then shipped back to Reno (500 miles back again). No wonder I pay extra for organic and vine-ripened produce and fruit.

   The advent of international trade has made 50% of the food you eat come from another country where the criteria for the use of pesticides and human waste as fertilizer are far less stringent. Food from across the equator makes grapes available in spring and apples in summer; there is no longer a rotation of food, everything is available all the time, and addiction and binging is easy.

3. **Processing of Food** — Of all the changes that have occured in the last century in food, the differential processing and refinement of foodstuffs has been the single most harmful change to reflect on the health of our nation. It was the advent of extracting oils from seeds and nuts, refining whole wheat to white flour, and adding sugar and high fructose corn syrup to beverages, that proved to be our dietary undoing.

4. **Choice of Foods** — Because of the above points regarding the quality, storage, transport, and processing of foods, we are left with prepared foods that are high in calories, refined sugars, rancid and saturated fats, and highly allergenic proteins, foods that are low in fiber, minerals, vitamins, and nutritional value. Consequently, your patients are always hungry, fatigued, constipated, toxic, dissatisfied, putting on weight, and downright miserable.

## PATIENT-CENTERED NUTRITION

As the patient is the center of the biology that needs to be nourished, let us look at the issues that surround the patient and his or her eating. Each patient is an entirely unique individual when it comes to nutrition. Apart from a bias toward a modified vegetarian, fish and lean meat diet, I do not manadate any regimen for the patient. The diet that a patient has chosen must be looked at as part of the personality; it had a hereditary predisposition, developed over time, and has been goal-oriented and successful up until now. Most of what we are talking about is learned behavior, tempered by some of the body's cravings and individual metabolic and nutritional requirements, and influenced by interpersonal relationships, cultural and geographical issues, and significant happenings in our lives. Let us consider these issues one by one.

### HEREDITARY PREDISPOSTION

The biochemist Roger Williams, working at the University of Texas at Austin, conducted intensive studies on biochemical individuality and its genetic causes.[9] In a paper from *Lancet* in 1950, "The Concept of Genotrophic Disease," Williams defined genotrophic disease as: "one in which the genetic pattern of the individual calls for an augmented supply of a particular nutrient (or nutrients), for which there develops, as a result, a nutritional deficiency. Partial genetic blocks somewhere in the metabolic machinery are probably commonplace in the inheritance of individuals and explain to a considerable degree why each person possesses a characteristic and distinctive metabolic pattern...."

So, each of us has a unique metabolic pattern and nutritional requirements that balance the pattern and keep it in a homeodynamic equilibrium. Lifestyle eating choices, disease, and external factors can influence these patterns and cause a functional or metabolic deficit to manifest as a subclinical or frank clinical disease. What this really means is that it is not the genes themselves (genotype) that produce disease, but the influence on the gene expression by our conscious choices of food and lifestyle. These poor choices alter the expressions of the genes in such a way that the weakness or uniqueness of heredity results in the phenotypic expression of disease. Good nutritional choices can phenotypically produce positive changes of health and well being (balance). For example, since the end of the Second World War, the height of the average Japanese has increased by 6 inches. The genes are the same, but the food–gene interaction has changed. This concept of food altering the genetic expression of individuals and reprogramming the genes has been clearly outlined by Dr. Jeffrey Bland, in his recent book entitled *Genetic Nutritioneering*.[47] This is a totally new way of looking at the direction of phenotypic change, not from the chromosome to the body, but from what the body takes in, to the chromosome. Genes can be changed by influencing the rate of transcription of the message, and they can be modified in the post-translational phase by nutrients. This very integrated way of looking at food and the body is the basis of nutritional modification of gene expression.

To summarize, every patient's overall dietary pattern and ingestion of vitamins, minerals, phytonutrients, and other substances will modify his or her gene expression and hence his or her phenotype, balanced or diseased.

We have dealt with the metabolic issues of inheritance. Now let us turn our attention to the less easily identified and quantified behavioral issues. The hereditary contribution to behavior invovles two seemingly unconnected clinical observations, *addiction* and *allergy*. These two clinical concepts, which affect food intake and hence nutrition, are but two faces of the same coin. If you are addicted to something, you are also overtly allergic or have some sensitivity to the same item. When allergy testing patients by any means, whether scratch testing or biokinesiology, the allergic items are always their favorite foods. They will binge on these foods and also experience withdrawal symptoms when these foods are avoided. I learned this during a period when I used the "Four Day Allergy Rotation Diet" on my allergic patients. In my protocol, patients would go on a 4- to 5-day semifast of diluted grape juice and then rotate every single major food group every day, such that they never ingested the same carbohydrate, protein, fruit, vegetable, sugar, or fat two, or even three, days in a row. This technique would get rid of their cyclic allergies (only allergic if continually ingesting the substance) and prevent them from returning, because it seemed that they needed continual allergen exposure to mount an allergic response and to experience the associated symptoms that each food allergen caused (another example of foods producing phenotypic expression). During the fast and afterward, the patients would express with delight that they had lost the craving for sugar or wheat or for the item to which they were addicted and allergic. This loss of craving corresponded to a loss of allergy to the substance, and if it returned because of noncompliance with the program, both the allergy and craving returned simultaneously. What we are looking at is a hereditary predilection (addiction and allergy), modifiable and induced by diet, that runs in families and will affect the nutrition of those patients in a very significant way. We will discuss this issue in the next section dealing with childhood patterning. Of course, the addictive component could be manifest in other ways such as drugs, drinking, smoking, sex, or work but at some level of homeostasis, these two traits are either genetically linked or balance the body in some way that confers stability to the chaotic pattern.

Another genetic contribution to nutrition has been championed by Peter D'Amato, N.D., in his book entitled "Eat Right 4 Your Blood Type."[48] He ascertains that individuals with specific blood types react to specific foods because of the nature of the blood antigens and their expression in the mucosal cells of the gastrointestinal tract. One class of dietary substances that creates this reaction, with blood group antigens that coat the digestive tract, are the lectins. Specific plant lectins can cross-react with the lectins that form part of the blood group A or B antigens that line the gastrointestinal tract. The result can be specific, genetically linked food sensitivites and allergies, that sensitize the bowel to bacterial and parasitic pathogens, which attach the mucosa and cause an immune inflammatory reaction that can be spread via inflammatory mediators throughout the body. He advocates the avoidance of those foods with the specific cross-reacting lectins contained in your particular blood type. Blood type O individuals are specifically at risk because their ancestry developed at a time before the use of grains, and their serum contains anti-A and anti-B antibodies, which together contain the majority of anti-lectin antibodies to react with foods in the gut lumen. He advocates a high protein, low vegetable diet for those individuals. From my clinical experience, the value of a higher protein type diet in group O individuals is related to their increased insulin sensitivity, and not to any allergic anti-lectin phenomenon.

It has been only a little over a century since modern man has become transitory in nature and been able to change continents with ease. Before this time our ancestors were born, lived, and died, generation after generation, in the same geographical location and had adjusted and naturally adapted to the local environment and food supply. Their individual metabolisms matched their surroundings and local conditions. When we travel to another continent and another culture and cuisine, our ancestral adaptions do not change for at least another five to six generations. The new foods put selective environmental pressure on our biochemistry, and if we don't have the appropriate metabolism we start to slide into nutritional ill health. Certain well-documented groups have shown an absolute requirement for particular nutrients in their diet. For instance, the Scottish, Welsh, Irish, Danish, Scandinavian, and Celtic peoples have an increased requirement for essential fatty acids. This correlates with their historic increased intake of a diet high in fatty fish. The Pima Indians of Arizona have shown an exponential increase in adult-onset diabetes due to their adoption of Western food and straying from their native fare. Their traditional diet of beans, chia seeds, psyllium seeds, nopalitos, cholla buds, mesquite pods, and cactus are all extremely high in crude and soluble fiber and helped to naturally regulate their blood sugar.

Another inherited trait that bears contemplating is the issue of "slow and fast burners," or "fast and slow oxidizers." People tend to fall into one or the other category, as there are few balanced oxidizers. The slow oxidizers (Yin type) burn food too slowly, can feel lethargic and sluggish, and gain weight easily. They love carbohydrates, which they eat to excess, and they shun heavy meats, because fat slows them down. They suffer from dyglycemia and need to jump start their metabolism by balancing out their carbohydrates and meat intake. They do best with light forms of protein such as white meat poultry and white fish. The fast oxidizers (Yang type) are the opposite. They tend to burn their food too quickly, feel hyped, nervous, and easily stressed. They do better on heavy rich red meats, such as organ meats, lamb, beef, pork, cold water fish, and full-fat dairy products, which seem to offer more steadily burning fuel. They also do poorly on a high carbohydrate diet, because it is like pouring gasoline on a fire.

## CHILDHOOD PATTERNING

The first experience of food, as such, is suckling from our mothers' breasts. This pattern of nurturing, love, and safety holds a very strong imprint for our personal relationship with food, and what it represents. These emotional issues are translated into more tangible responses as we age, and food becomes the emotional tapestry upon which many a battle is fought. Food will assume an identity all its own throughout our lives, the personality depending on the role it played in childhood:

1. **Food as love** — In suckling from our mothers, we equate food with love, but as we get 'older, food may become a substitute for love. When we were suckling we were warm,

comfortable, and secure. We felt close to and attached to our mothers. We may then confuse this eating with the need to feel loved or may eat foods that remind us of that wonderful time — ice cream, mashed potatoes, or pudding. Food now masquerades as love. We will turn to eating whenever we feel unloved or whenever we want to express our love to someone else.

2. **Food as attention and approval** — Did your mother ever give you a special treat, by buying something you really loved to eat for dinner or for snack time? When my own mother wanted to please me and be loved in return, I got Romany Creams after dinner. We feel loved for who and what we are, and if we have a dim view of our value, we start to substitute how we feel about ourselves for how others feel about us, especially when we make them happy. So we reinforce this external attention and approval around food or the production of food.

3. **Food as camouflage** — Ever been nagged to death by your mate to "have something to eat"— "just a little bit." The litany of what you need to eat can encompass a whole supermarket of items, each one of which is qualified differently. One way of drawing attention away from our own food problems is to focus on feeding others, so the guilt may be shared, which it eventually is, with everyone feeling bad about not eating with us, and all of us getting into a pattern of over or specialty eating.

4. **Food replaces feelings** — Preparation of a special meal for birthdays, anniversaries, etc. may often be the only manifestation of affection between some couples or in a family. So eating becomes a form of emotional communication, even with ourselves, where instead of facing up to issues and discussing them, we resort to stuffing our faces to feel better.

5. **Food as reward or punishment** — Sounds like training a dog, but that is exactly what it's about. When food is used as a reward, for our loved ones and children — "if you stay quiet in church you can have an ice cream on the way home," — then food becomes the avenue of reward, consolation, and justification throughout our entire lives. "I had a bad day so I can have a piece of chocolate."

6. **Food as power struggle** — "Eat everything on your plate or you can't leave the table!" These words are often heard at the family dinner when asparagus or spinach is in plentiful supply. "Think of all the poor starving children in India or Kosovo." So the spinach just sits there meal after meal until you gag it down — you have lost the battle, they have won. You feel powerless and forever more will have problems with authority and lose your appetite in your boss's office.

For more detailed information, I refer you to: *My Mother Made Me Do It*, by Dr. Nan Kathryn Fuchs.[49]

These concepts may be amusing, but are nonetheless issues that mold and form relationships between people, behavior, and food. Let's get back to food sensitivities for a second. What about a child who is slapped on the side of the head as a matter of course at the breakfast table, by his father, just as he is eating his toast. The body puts the external stress of the assault together with bread, and as an adult this patient presents with wheat sensitivity due to the association of bread being a "dangerous" substance that needs to be expelled or avoided.

## CULTURAL ISSUES

Cultural issues need to be kept in mind when dealing with a diverse ethnic and religious population. One man's poison is another man's food. Do not enforce your eating concepts on anyone of another ethnic persuasion or culture. Try to find the best fit of good nutrition within their reality. This can lead to some interesting menus such as tofu chimichangas or braized chitlins with citrus sauce.

## GEOGRAPHICAL ISSUES

"Good eating" in Maine and Texas represent two very different cuisines. I deal with casino crap dealers on the one hand, and cattle farmers on the other. I try to relate to their regional and lifestyle eating preferences in order to get a workable and sustainable result.

## FOOD ALLERGY

Food allergy is perhaps the least recognized and most often ignored source of ill health in the average doctor's office. In medical school we are taught about the dramatic, acute allergic reactions that take place after susceptible individuals ingest peanuts, strawberries, or seafood. That is about the end of our medical understanding and interest. These unfortunate individuals should just avoid these items, and if not, carry some injectable adrenaline around with them. The use of skin scratch and intradermal testing only goes further to perpetuate that kind of thinking. "I went to the allergist and I am only allergic to environmentals and molds. Why do I feel so bad when I eat soy products, Doc?" Well, skin testing tests for IgE reactions in the skin, and most food-related immune responses are IgG. Whether you use a RAST test, rotational diet, or biokinesiology to assess food allergies, it is clinically clear, if you listen to the symptomatology given by the patients, that food allergy is rampant and the clinical manifestations stretch from brain fog to hemorrhoids. The clinical clues that tell you that your patient has a food allergy problem are: the patient says he or she has one; the patient has symptoms throughout the year (also seen with mold allergy), without obvious worsening in spring, summer or fall; and the patient can relate disappearance of symptoms when changing a diet or other food choice.

Food allergy is seen most commonly in susceptible individuals and certainly follows a genetic predisposition. The patients who are destined to experience food allergy are those children who have allergic parents, had problems with infant feeding, had reactions to milk or soy baby formulas, and experienced colic at an early age.

There are two clinically distinct types of food "allergy." The first group includes those dramatic "fixed" food allergies that produce severe reactions with occasional death (peanuts, etc.). They are difficult to treat and seem to have a genetic basis. Then, there are the rest of the food "allergies," best described as food sensitivities or cyclical allergies. These food allergies are only present as long as there is exposure to the offending allergen. When that allergen is avoided, the sensitivity fades away, only to return when the food is again eaten repetively. One of the most interesting clinical observations you will see is the appearance of new sensitivities in those patients who are avoiding their current food allergen. It almost seems as if the body really needs to express this sensitivity in some way, and is just waiting for the next most likely food to do that. This is one of the reasons I stopped using food avoidance, because patients would get into an ever narrower circle of available foods, as they avoided one food and gained yet another sensitivity. This tells us that food "allergy," the hyper-reaction to completely harmless food sources, is not what it seems on the surface. This reaction represents a fundamental reaction choice, to balance a deeper, usually emotionally or situationally connected issue in a very acceptable and nonthreatening way.

The foods that cause the most allergic sensitivities include, in order of severity: dairy products, wheat, sugar, B-complex vitamins, calcium, corn, animal oils, soy, and food colorings and additives. There are many subdivisions and nuances in all of these food reactions (runny, congested nose [wheat, soy or dairy], headache, abdominal discomfort, and diarrhea), but the clinical presentations that are most missed are brain allergy (brain fog, poor memory and concentration — usually wheat or carbohydrates) and urinary tract symptomatology (usually coffee). Avoiding these foods one at a time will tell us if they are affecting the patient. This may be easier said than done due to the inclusion of almost every allergenic food in most over-the-counter boxed foods. We have to read every label, and even then some ingredients are not listed or are disguised within another name.

The best way to document food allergies is to use biokinesiology. It is quick, cheap, and the patient can personally feel the weak reaction when you place an allergenic food in their hand. RAST testing has its limitations. Many foods come up that the patient has no reaction to, and other allergens, to which the patient quite clearly experiences a reaction, are absent from the result. The use of eliminatory diets, rotation diets, and the like are impractical and have poor patient compliance over the long term. The only way to get rid of these pesky food allergies is to use the ALR-G-ANSR (modification of Dr. Devi Nambudripad's NAET). The elimination of even one major food allergen produces a striking improvement in symptoms, health, and well being. It also improves immunity in most patients because the body is not wasting its time reacting to the foods.

One of the interesting clinical tidbits I have observed is the issue regarding lactose intolerance. We are taught that if you don't have the enzyme, you don't have the enzyme. Well that's not true in all cases. When you test patients with lactose intolerance, and they are positive (and not allergic to milk protein or whey), if you use the ALR-G-ANSR to desensitize them, their lactose intolerance disappears. In some way you have induced the enzyme to reappear. This effect can last for some time, usually 6 to 8 months in children and less time in adults. You can repeat the process with similar results over and over in the same patients.

Another interesting clinical experience I had was with a young man who had had a lifelong acute allergic anaphylactic reaction to shrimp. I had gotten rid of his other food allergies and he pressed me to do the shrimp. I was not enthusiastic at all. Fixed allergens are dangerous and refractory to treatment. However, I proceeded to desensitize him to shrimp, and the effort seemed successful. He was going to go out and have a shrimp dinner the next day, but I suggested an in-office trial before he did so. I had him, with blood pressure cuff on and adrenaline at hand, take the fresh shrimp and hold it in his hand while I tested him — he was not weak at all. Then I instructed him to put the shrimp in his mouth, but not to chew or swallow. In an instant his blood pressure dropped to 70/40 mm Hg and his pulse rate went up to 210 beats per minute; he went ashen pale and keeled forward. I caught him, placed him in the supine position, raised his legs, and immediately desensitized him again. In five minutes his color and blood pressure came back, and we did not have to resort to resuscitative measures. These fixed allergies can be impacted if you desensitize the patients 10 to 20 times, but I find that unacceptable, and do it once, just to give them the potential edge if they are exposed to the allergen and have no immediate therapy available.

The other clinical gem that comes from careful observation is that you have to desensitize all the food problems before you go onto the environmentals, petroleum products, chemicals, and molds. If you do not do this first, you will keep losing the desensitization of the nonfood allergens. This occurrence is because the food allergens activate gut-associated lymphoid tissue (GALT) and the mucosa-associated lymphoid tissue (MALT), which floods the body with cytokines and other allergic inflammatory mediators, thus lowering the allergenic threshold and allowing the easy and chronic manifestation of other external allergies.

What about regular allergy shots? I think, based on my experience (and I could be wrong), that shots do not work very well for foods or for chemicals and petrochemicals. I think that regular desensitization works well in a small percentage of people, especially to animal dander and some environmentals. However, a large proportion of my patients, who originally had shots for years, were still allergic to their allergens, had had some bad reactions to the shots, and, worst of all, in spite of having no clinical response to the shots for years, had never been told to stop. Most patients who do not have success with allergy shots stop of their own accord. I have not looked for a decent outcomes paper on allergy shots, but if there is one, please let me know. Patients are usually sent to allergists when the general practitioner has exhausted his repertoire of antihistamines and nasal sprays and does not want to bother with the problem any more. So, by default, the patients are shunted into an endless array of expensive testing and repetitive, useless, and often suppressively harmful shots to feed the allergic gravy train.

# FOOD GROUPS

The editions of the "Food Pyramid" espoused by the American Dietary Association, are nothing short of propaganda for the food group lobby whose foods appear in the pyramid. For years our children have been told that "milk does a body good." Well, it's bad grammar, and worse advice. The only organism that should be drinking cow's milk is a calf. Milk ingestion is certainly the predominant cause of the epidemic of allergy, asthma, otitis media, and sinusitis in young children. Calcium should be obtained from green leafy vegetables together with the magnesium used to facilitate the absorption of calcium. The emphasis on carbohydrates, without specifying the state or complexity of the carbohydrate is yet another small detail left out for obvious reasons. This focus on grains, pasta, and potatoes has led to fatigue, uncontrollable sugar cravings, reactive hypoglycemia, and chronic yeast infections. I will not even get into the adoration heaped on beef and other meats in the first edition of the pyramid. In addition to the pyramid, the ADA has fostered much potentially harmful misinformation, such as eggs are bad for you and the less fat in your diet the better, again without clarifying which fats are involved. In fact, adherence to the ADA recommendations has resulted in a higher prevalence of obesity in the population, and the ADA needs to be held legally and ethically responsible for the epidemic of morbidity and mortality that their spurious recommendations have caused. The USDA is no better with their recommended daily allowances (RDAs) for vitamins that are based solely on preventing vitamin deficiencies and have no relationship whatsoever to the lifestyles and nutritional requirements of an urbanized population.

What follows is more a preventative medicine discussion of the three food groups rather than prescriptive dietetics, nutritional pharmacology, or nutritional support, all of which have therapeutic aims.

## CARBOHYDRATES

Historically, grains and sugar are a very late addition to our food sources. Certainly the act of grinding grains and concentrating sugars is even newer. Our digestive, absorptive, and metabolic physiology has not really changed in the last 10,000 years and most of us have had some difficulty in handling these new foods in large quantities, which is what the ADA wants you to do. Carbohydrates, as glucose, are certainly the preferred source of immediate fuel from the liver and muscles (as broken down glycogen), and its availability prevents muscle mass breakdown for calories. However, the amount of caloric carbohydrate you can use is dependent on your physical activity. If you are an athlete or a carpenter, then, a higher carbohydrate mix would seem appropriate. If, however, you are a sedentary office worker, then an increased energy supply from carbohydrates would be overkill and result in storage of those excess calories as fat. The secret is that carbohydrate calories have to be immediately used, because the liver and muscles have only a small storage capacity for glucose as glycogen, and any excess carbohydrate is immediately turned into fat for storage, as it was designed to do, when regular food was not available. The single hormone that utilizes and stores glucose is insulin. So, insulin is at the core of the excess carbohydrate problem.

## INSULIN AND THE GLYCEMIC INDEX

The interaction of insulin on the rest of metabolism is a web-like interaction not only affecting glucose and the control of blood sugar, but also interacting with insulin-like growth factor, human growth hormone, cortisol, somatostatin, serotonin, noradrenalin, and leptin. Thomas Wolever, M.D., Ph.D., at the University of Toronto has constructed a table of foods that scores their insulin demands and, therefore, their influence on blood glucose control and the conversion of glucose into fat. In this glycemic index, he has rated foods based on their blood glucose and insulin-raising potential.[50] The higher the glycemic index of a food, the faster it is assimilated into the blood stream, produces an acute rise in blood sugar, increases insulin secretion and its rate of rise in the blood stream, and causes the excess glucose to be converted into fat. This increase in insulin down regulates the secretion of glucagon, which is the fat burner, and fat storage accelerates. Foods such as sugar, fruit juices, high fructose corn syrup, white potatoes, and white flour (all refined) have high glycemic indices, while legumes, whole wheat flour, whole fruits, and soy (complex carbohydrates) all have low glycemic indices and, hence, are able to control escalating blood glucose levels and their insulin response. Patients who are particularly prone to putting on weight with these high glycemic index foods have been classified as being dysglycemic and if even more sensitive, classified as having the Syndrome X. Over 75% of obese individuals suffer from carbohydrate sensitivity. Polycystic ovarian disease is only one of a number of metabolic problems having an increased carbohydrate sensitivity or insulin resistance. In many patients this switch to carbohydrate sensitivity and insulin resistance occurs only in middle age, or when the hormones start changing at menopause. The ways to control this problem includes:

1. decreasing refined carbohydrates in the diet;
2. increasing fiber and complex carbohydrates in the diet;
3. increasing daily exercise, which switches the metabolism;
4. eating small and regular meals, rather than binging at one time;
5. not eating late at night when the body is shutting down.

The problem with this metabolic fact is that the more carbohydrates you eat, the more your insulin surges and your glucose drops. You feel hungry again, and you crave more carbohydrate — it is a vicious cycle.

As manufacturers decrease the fat content in their products due to the ADA's proclamations, so the carbohydrate content goes up, and the problem is compounded. The next time you go to the supermarket, see what percentage of articles in your own or your neighbor's shopping cart is composed entirely of some form of refined carbohydrate.

Many different approaches to help this problem have been put forward in terms of the mixtures and percentages of carbohydrates, protein, and fats, and also the types and qualities of each food group. These will be discussed under diets.

Other problems with carbohydrates include the allergenicity and multiple health problems brought on by gluten sensitivity to wheat, rye, and barley and the mistaken notion that fruit sugar, fructose, is somehow not as bad as sucrose. Remember that fructose shortcuts the first part of the fat cycle through the pentose–phosphate shunt and is responsible for accelerated hypertriglyceridemia.

## PROTEIN

Protein is an essential part of the human structure and function. The protein component of the body consists of structural proteins, enzymes, hormones, neuropeptides, glycopeptides, hemoglobin, muscle, and many composite and complex protein molecules including antibodies. The activities of these molecules make protein the chief regulator and organizer of the whole body.

In terms of the effect of dietary protein on the body, we see the induction of glucagon secretion (in opposition to insulin), the breakdown of fats and gluconeogenesis, the specific dynamic action of protein in increasing the metabolic rate, and the maintenance of the osmotic and oncotic pressure of the intravascular fluid compartments, so that fluid balance is maintained.

The high carbohydrate, low fat, and low to no animal protein diets and vegetarian diets lead to alopecia, brittle hair and nails, menstrual irregularities, irritability, confusion, lack of sex drive, and constant food cravings. Other problems of the vegetarian diet lead to vitamin B-12 and zinc deficiency, which is further antagonized by the increase in copper that a high fiber and phytic acid diet promotes. Vegetarians are also at risk of not getting enough of the amino acids found in animal protein and not in vegetable protein, namely lysine, methionine, tryptophan, carnitine, and taurine.

I am not saying that vegetarian diets are all bad, I am saying that they are not for everyone and that they lack some vital elements.

The choice of protein is up to each individual, but suffice it to say that the white meat of free range chicken, lean pork and beef (preferably beef that is not corn fed and is hormone free), and cold-water fish are preferred.

## LIPIDS AND FATS

Fats are not bad for us. Bad fats are bad for us and good fats are good for us. The bad fats, which have been in our diet for the last 50 years, are the *saturated trans fats*, which include the vegetable fats of processed vegetable oils, margarine, vegetable shortening, and the baked and fried foods that are prepared and made from them. The animal fats that the ADA is so concerned about have decreased in our diet from 83% to 53% of total fat intake, while the vegetable fats have increased from 17% in 1910 to 47% in 1990. The worst of the vegetable fats are the unnatural trans fats from hydrogenated and partially hydrogenated oils such as margarine and vegetable shortening. It is the long shelf life that spurred the use of these fats in baked goods and the like. These trans fats cannot be used by the body as they are foreign to our biochemistry, and they cause lipid peroxidation, free radical formation, and inflammation *in vivo*. Trans fats raise the total cholesterol level, as well as lowering the level of HDL cholesterol and raising the level of LDL cholesterol, thus increasing the formation of arterial lipid plaques and the atherosclerotic process. We can prevent the damage from trans fats by eliminating them from our diets or by offsetting their oxidative tendencies with an adequate intake of antioxidants. We can purchase oil spreads that are mixtures of mono- and polyunsaturated fats such as Olivio™ and Take Control™, which are cholesterol lowering and more acceptable to the body.

*Saturated fats*, while not as healthy as unsaturated fats, are not the villains they are made out to be. After all, the stored fat in our adipose tissues is saturated fat and we need it for multiple functions such as caloric storage, cushioning the organs, and insulation against cold. Overindulging in saturated fats, however, can lead to the blockage of beneficial prostaglandin formation and the physiological consequences to cardiovascular, immune, and reproductive regulation.

*Unsaturated fats* contain the essential fatty acids (EFAs). Unsaturated fats are divided into two groups: the *monounsaturated fats* (canola oil, olives, olive oil, avocados, peanuts, almonds, and cashews), and the *polyunsaturated fats* (fish — salmon, mackerel, and halibut; vegetable oils — corn, safflower, sunflower, and sesame; and botanicals — borage, black current, and evening primrose). The EFAs contained in polyunsaturated fats include:

1. *Omega-3 Fatty Acids* — from flax seed, walnut, canola, pumpkin seed oils, and cold-water fatty fish such as salmon, mackerel, sardine, tuna, and anchovy.
2. *Omega-6 Fatty Acids* — found in the vegetable oils, safflower, sunflower, corn, and sesame; and in borage, black current, and evening primrose oils. These oils contain GLA-gamma linolenic acid, which is important for both the nervous and immune systems in individuals with poor sugar control.

## THE GASTROINTESTINAL TRACT

The GI tract is perhaps the most important Zang Fu system in the body. It is the only organ that stretches all 32 segments of the embryo, and is exposed to more allergens, has more associated lymphoid tissue, and produces more hormones than the rest of the body combined. If your patient has bowel symptomatology or pathology, you will never get him or her better until you get the bowel right. Included in this system are the two important organ embryological outgrowths of the gut, the liver and the pancreas. This triad is responsible for most of the nutrition, excretion, and immunity in the body.

The greater *gut–liver–pancreas system* (GLPS) is affected by a number of external and internal stressors that influence the digestion and absorption of food, the bowel ecology, general toxin handling, the excretion of wastes, and the general immunity of the organism. The most important issues that you will see in clinical practice include:

1. **Poor digestion** — due to poor diet, stress, poor food combining, food allergies and hypersensitivities, and digestive enzyme or hydrochloric acid deficiency. Treatment includes dietary counseling, a meditation and exercise program, allergy desensitization, and betaine HCL and digestive enzyme supplementation.

2. **Dysbiosis and parasitic infestation** — dysbiosis is an imbalance in the normal intestinal microorganisms, with a decrease in normal bacteria and commensals (Lactobacillus and E. coli, due to causes of decreased colonization resistance), and an increase in the pathogenic organisms including Klebsiella, Proteus, Pseudomonas, Salmonella, Campylobacter, Clostridium species, Shigella, Staph. aureus, enteropathic and toxigenic strains of E. coli, and Candida albicans and other Candida species. Common and invariably missed parasites include the ameobas, Giardia, Cryptosporidium, and Blastocystis hominis. Treatment includes removal of the pathogenic and out-of-balance microorganisms with preferably natural substances, as antibiotics will further disturb the ecology of the gut. Substances used include Gentiana lutea, Berberine, Hydrastis, Artemesia annua, Juglans nigra, Garlic, Citrus Seed extract, undecylenic acid, and caprylic acid derivatives. Chinese herbal combinations such as Artestatin, Phellostatin, and Aquillaria 22 from Health Concerns are effective and have high patient tolerance. If yeast is the main source of dysbiosis, and it often is, then you need to rotate your antifungal treatment, as the yeast will accommodate to the drug in about 2 to 3 months and start proliferating again. The addition of fructo-oligosaccharides (FOS) to the diet will aid the return of normal flora to the gut (do not use if Klebsiella is identified). Some patients will benefit with the addition of a colostrum-containing oral supplement. If systemic antibiotics need to be used for the refractory Candida case, Sporanox® is preferable to Diflucan®, and oral Nystatin® is preferable to Nizoral®.

   Reinoculate the good bacteria using probiotic mixtures of Lactobacillus acidophilus, Bifidobacteria species, and Saccharomyces boulardii (a competitive yeast).

3. **Leaky gut syndrome** — is a result of intestinal hyperpermeability due to reduced integrity of the intestinal–mucosal barrier. This increased permeability to the gut contents allows undigested and abnormal macromolecules to penetrate the integrity of the mucosal epithelial barrier, and allows access for these biologically foreign molecules to the lamina propria, into the gut-associated lymphoid tissue (GALT), into the portal circulation, and on to the liver. This abnormal presentation of foreign, and often toxic substances to the GALT, produces allergic immune-mediated responses in the mucosa, with associated mucosal inflammation in the crypts further compromise of the mucosal integrity. Treatment includes halting the process by treating the originating cause (dysbiosis, food allergy, lack of digestive enzymes, and infection). The gut mucosa is then healed utilizing simple juice fasting, hypoallergenic protein support such as Ultra-Clear or Ultra-Clear Sustain from HealthComm, or a comparable product, and anti-inflammatory and demulcant gut support such as Oxyperm and Permeability Factors from Tyler Encapsulations.

4. **Hepatic toxicity** — can be caused internally by the toxins and products of fermentation and putrefaction from the entire gut, or externally as xenobiotics or chemicals and intoxicants in the food, water, and air. Fat soluble toxins are easily absorbed but poorly excreted, and tend to accumulate in the body. To facilitate excretion, fat soluble (lipophilic) chemicals are converted in the liver to water soluble (hydrophilic) chemicals so that they can be excreted in the bile and out of the body. The enzymatic pathways that

the liver uses for this excretion are termed Phase I and Phase II detoxification reactions (there is possibly a Phase III reaction).

## Detoxification Reactions

*The Phase I detoxification reaction* is primarily a functionalization reaction, that is, it adds a functional group to the fat soluble substance by means of oxidation, reduction, or hydrolysis. These enzymes are membrane associated. There are two enzyme systems that are responsible for these reactions. The *cytochrome P-450 monoxygense system* is the first enzymatic line of defense against all foreign compounds, the predominant detoxification system, and responsible for most drug biotransformation. This system is composed of at least ten isoenzymes, each having a slightly different reactive profile and having affinity for a different drug or xenobiotic. This system is also important in the detoxification of endogenous active biological molecules such as steroids. The *mixed-function amine oxidase system* is used only for those compounds that fit the enzyme profile.

*The Phase II detoxification reactions* are all conjugation or synthetic reactions. Conjugation confers increased water solubility and the ability to undergo significant ionization at physiological pH via covalent bonding of the foreign compound or intermediate to an endogenous excretory molecule. This enables the molecule to be excreted through the urine or the bile. The major conjugation reactions include glucuronidation, amino acid conjugation, sulfation, glutathione conjugation, acetylation, and methylation. These enzymes are cytosol associated. These reactions require dietary cofactors or they will not be able to proceed.

*Phase III detoxification reaction.* Recent studies have shown the activity of another detoxification reaction called "antiporter" activity. This antiporter activity is important in the first pass metabolism of pharmaceuticals and other xenobiotics. The antiporter is an energy-dependent efflux pump that pumps xenobiotics out of a cell, thereby decreasing the intracellular concentration of the drug or xenobiotic. Two genes encoding antiporter activity in regard to multiple drug resistance in cancer cell lines (MDR1) and in the liver (MDR2) have been defined.

## Regulation of Detoxification

The two detoxification pathways may proceed independently and separately leading to the excretion of the modified xenobiotic, or Phase I may produce an intermediate by adding or exposing a functional group, which will then undergo Phase II conjugation. It is important to note that the Phase I intermediate may be highly reactive after its modification and even more toxic than the parent compound. This is termed *bioactivation.*

Chemicals with preexisting functional groups may be directly conjugated and then excreted. Due to the complexity of Phase I and Phase II interactions and the bioactivation of toxic intermediates, imbalances between these two pathways can cause chemically induced tissue injury, the basis for many chronic diseases including chronic fatigue and multiple chemical sensitivity. The body has developed several mechanisms to regulate these detoxification pathways. Parts of the detoxification sequences are up- or down-modulated depending on the presence of the xenobiotic or the mass action availability of the detoxification conjugating substances. The multifunction inducers include many of the flavenoid molecules found in fruits and vegetables. Garlic oil, rosemary, soy, cabbage, and brussel sprouts all contain compounds that induce several Phase II enzyme activities. Inhibition of the pathways depends on competition between two compounds vying for the same detoxification pathway or the rate-limiting and inductive availability of certain conjugating agents such as sulfur or glucuronic acid.

Treatment includes dietary modification to increase inductive cofactors such as fruits and vegetables, especially cruciferous vegetables; avoidance of toxic xenobiotics; dietary supplementation to ensure availability of all the Phase I and Phase II cofactors; and inducing up-modulating agents. Use a good multiphasic mixture, such as Detoxification Factors™ from Tyler Encapsulations.

# DIETING

It seems appropriate to have a small discussion on the different in- and out-of-vogue diets and fads that we have seen in the last decade. In fact a meeting was recently held involving all the different diet doctors — Atkins, Sears, Bethea, Ornish, etc., — and an ADA representative and, true to form, no one could really agree on anything. The diets can be classified according the percentage constituents of each of the major food groups:

## HIGH FIBER, HIGH CARBOHYDRATE, LOW FAT DIETS

**Macrobiotic Diet** — This is a dietary philosophy from Japan, developed by Sagen Itshitsuka, M.D., in which each person's dietary needs vary according to the level of activity, gender, age, climate, season, and individual factors. The diet is composed of 50 to 60% whole grains, 20 to 25% vegetables, 5 to 10% beans and sea vegetables, and 5% vegetable soups. Meat, dairy, sugar, and raw fruits are avoided. This a good detox diet, but type O blood patients will eventually become anemic due to insufficient heme iron in the diet. It is very bland and unappetizing.

    **Pritikin Diet** — This diet, founded by Nathan Pritikin, is a low-fat, low-cholesterol, low-sodium, and high-complex-carbohydrate diet, that is combined with regular aerobic exercise. The diet is composed of 80% carbohydrates, 10 to 15% protein, and 5 to 10% fat. This diet is far too high in carbohydrates and low in fat for the average person, unless an obsessive–compulsive athlete or exerciser.

    **Gerson Diet** — Founded by the Austrian physician Max Gerson in the early 1900s, this is a very strict detoxification diet consisting of fasting, raw vegetables and fruit juices (high potassium, low sodium), and coffee enemas to stimulate liver detoxification and bile production. This is a therapeutic diet used for cancer and has been found therapeutic to prevent recurrence of treated melanoma.

    **Dean Ornish Diet** — Developed by Dean Ornish, M.D., this diet is designed to halt the development of, or even reverse atherosclerosis and coronary heart disease. The diet is very low fat and low cholesterol and also employs exercise, yoga, and meditation as an adjiunct to the program. The diet consists of 70 to 75% carbohydrates, 15 to 20% protein, and 10 to 12% fats. The program does reduce coronary artery lesions, but has not had a reduction in all mortality in these patients.

    All of the diets outlined above are centered around a plant-based, high-fiber, high-carbohydrate, low-fat way of eating. The positive effects are a reduction in weight, blood pressure, blood sugar, and cardiovascular disease. The negatives include the development of essential fatty acid deficiencies (especially gamma linolenic acid and eicosapentaenoic acid), gluten sensitivity, and B-12, zinc, and iron deficiencies.

## HIGH-PROTEIN, LOW CARBOHYDRATE DIETS

**Atkins Diet** — Developed by Robert Atkins, M.D., this diet emphasizes protein and fats to the extreme in its initial two weeks, at all times staying away from any carbohydrates that produce the dysglycemia and reduced insulin sensitivity already discussed. He does have a step-down program that includes nutrient-dense whole grains. The effects of this diet are certainly impressive, with definite weight loss and a surprising decrease in cholesterol. Patients have more energy and are less hungry all the time, and hypoglycemics are able to sustain their blood sugars.

    **The Zone Diet** — Developed by Barry Sears, Ph.D., this diet emphasizes a high-protein, moderate-fat, and low-carbohydrate intake, a mixture that keeps you in the metabolic "Zone." Only high-fiber fruits and vegetables are allowed.

    **Sugar Busters Diet** — Developed by Morrison Bethea, M.D., this diet, like the Atkins and the Zone diet, emphasizes protein and does not allow any simple or refined carbohydrates. It is the most balanced of the diets, and the one that can be adhered to all the time, even if eating out. In fact, in New Orleans, most of the major restuarants have a "Sugar Buster" section on the menu.

The Atkins and Zone diets, in my opinion, are far too high in protein and fats for any long-term use, and are especially hard on the kidneys and liver. They may be used in the short term for quick weight loss, but are not advised in the ill, old, young, or otherwise compromised, unless monitored by a physician. A modified Sugar Busters diet is a resonable compromise, if you decrease the animal protein and emphasize legumes and fish.

The real problems in eating are overeating for your activity and lifestyle; eating the wrong fats, sugar, and white flour; and undereating fresh fruits, vegetables, and fiber. The secret to eating is Balance. All patients should be evaluated to assess the optimum balance of carbohydrates, protein, and fat in their diets, taking into account their blood group, ethnic background, social and work circumstances, oxidation status, and concurrent health status.

## NUTRITIONAL SUPPLEMENTATION

In the earlier parts of this century and the last two, when we worked in the fields and on the farms, a caloric intake of 4000 to 6000 calories was not uncommon to offset the calorie consumption that enabled that kind of physical work. Within that caloric scope it was quite possible to take in an adequate component of vitamins and minerals in the large mass of food that made up the daily intake. However, with our caloric requirements much reduced due to our sedentary lifestyle, we rarely, on a day-to-day basis, take in enough food to even satisfy the RDA requirements of vitamins and minerals. When adding in the poor quality of the soil, the processing of the food, which almost always leeches out nutrients, and the hollow caloric content of most of our foods, it is amazing that we are all still functioning.

The mantra of the ADA is that we need to take in all these nutrients in our food and they can be absorbed only from our food. If you can show me anyone who takes in dense nutrient foods in a quantity that will satifsy even minimal vitamin, mineral, and essential fatty acids requirements, I will be very surprised. Children and the aged are at the worst risk, as they have the most undernourishing diets. Every patient should be on a good multivitamin, mineral, and essential fatty acid supplement.

The following is the average supplementation that an adult requires. Different medical problems will add or delete certain vitamins and supplements from this core formula:

| | |
|---|---|
| **Vitamin A** — as natural Betacarotene with mixed carotenoids | 12,500 to 25,000 IU/ day |
| **Vitamin C** — as ascorbic acid or Ester C | 1–4 g daily |
| **Vitamin D** — as cholecalciferol | 200 IU daily |
| **Vitamin E** — as D-alpha succinate and mixed tocopherals | 400-800 IU daily |
| **Thiamine (B-1)** — **as HCl** | 50 mg daily |
| **Riboflavin (B-2)** | 30 mg daily |
| **Niacin** — as niacin and niacinamide | 70 mg daily |
| **Pyridoxine (B-6)** — as HCl and 5-Phosphate complex | 50 mg daily |
| **Pantothenic Acid** — as D-calcium pantothenate | 200 mg daily |
| **Folic Acid** | 400–800 mcg daily |
| **Vitamin B-12** — as cyanocobalamin HCl | 200 mcg daily |
| **Biotin** | 200 mcg daily |
| **Choline** — as bicitrate or bitartrate | 75 mg daily |
| **Inositvol** | 50 mg daily |
| **Bioflvavenoid Complex** | 50 mg daily |
| **PABA** | 25 mg daily |

| | |
|---|---|
| L-Cysteine/N-Acetyl Cysteine | 100–200 mg daily |
| **Calcium** — as citrate/ascorbate complex | 250–1000 mg daily |
| **Magnesium** — as aspartate/citrate/ascorbate complex | 250–1000 mg daily |
| **Chromium** — as GTF organically bound/picolinate | 100 mcg daily |
| **Iron** — as amino acid chelate | .0–15 mg daily |

All men and post menopausal females should *not* have iron in their supplements

| | |
|---|---|
| **Zinc** — as picolinate and amino acid complex | 12.5 mg daily |
| **Manganese** — as aspartate complex | 5–7.5 mg daily |
| **Potassium** — as aspartate/citrate or ascorbate | .50 mg daily |
| **Copper** — as aspartate | 0–1 mg daily |
| Iodine | 100 mcg daily |
| **Selenium** — as aspartate/glycinate/lysinate complex | 100–200 mcg daily |
| **Molybdenum** — as aspartate/glycinate/lysinate complex | 50 mcg daily |
| **Boron** — as aspartate/citrate complex | 0.5 mg daily |
| **Essential Fatty Acids** — as Flax seed oil — as Safflower or Evening primrose....1 T daily (Omega-6). | 1 T daily (Omega-3) |

This represents an absolute minimum in today's nutrient intake. You will have to increase many of these individual values depending on the patient's age and clinical condition.

# 15 More Specialized Complementary Therapies

## FLOWER REMEDIES AND ESSENCES

Between the years 1930 and 1936, the English physician Edward Bach, who was also involved with the microbiologist Patterson in the development of the homeopathic bowel nosodes, developed a system of emotional healing, using extracts of the scented blooms of English wild flowers. He described 38 flowers and their clinical uses. He felt, as I do, that the basis of disease was to be found in dysharmony between the spiritual and emotional–mental aspects of the human being. His flower essences have been used for years to great effect, and there are now flower essences from all over the world including California, Australia, and Europe. The most used and useful essence is his *Rescue Remedy*, which can be used for any state of agitation, shock, syncope, etc. It is a mix of five of the original flowers:

- Star of Bethlehem for shock,
- Rock Rose for acute fear and panic,
- Impatiens for inner tension and stress,
- Cherry Plum for fear of breaking down in despair,
- Clematis for the feeling of being "not completely here."

All the flower remedies may be used alone or in conjunction with any other drug or herb, homeopathic, or acupuncture treatment. The essences are given in tincure, a couple of drops under the tongue; or are diluted in water and sipped.

## MYOFASCIAL AND BODY WORK

As I have discussed, the energetic imprint of the body and the autonomic disturbances of the organs and segments of the body are reflected in the myofascial system, myotomes, and sclerotomes of the body. In order to heal a patient, all the elements reflecting the whole disease pattern need to be addressed. In my female patients, who are mostly touch deprived, the element of some kind of hands-on approach is mandatory. There are many different kinds of body work, and many nuances within a single discipline. I shall discuss a selection of the techniques that my patients and I use the most.

## CRANIOSACRAL THERAPY

*Craniosacral therapy* is a therapeutic technique developed by William G. Sutherland, D.O., which uses very gentle manual pressure applied to the skull, spine, and membranes to restore proper rythmic flow to the craniosacral system. The craniosacral system consists of the brain, spinal cord, cerebrospinal fluid, surrounding meninges, skull bones, and their relationship within the parasympathetic nervous system. This is a very appropriate system for your more fragile and sensitive patients, elderly patients, and children. It is excellent at relieving certain pain syndromes, such as headache, TMJ, and vertigo and regulating an autonomic nervous system that is out of balance.

## MASSAGE THERAPY

The profession of massage probably has its roots in antiquity. In modern day massage, of which there are numerous types, the client has the soft tissue component of the body kneaded or pummeled in order to relieve the disharmonious and tense muscular posture that modern life, and our reaction to it, expresses in our body. In the office practice, massage is an important adjunct in tight (physically and emotionally) and internalized patients, who will not let go and are either obsessive–compulsive or highly controlling individuals. Massage therapy can, in my experience, relieve pain, increase blood and lymphatic flow, relax tense muscles, decrease blood pressure, and has been shown to decrease the hormonal modulators of stress and improve immune function.

*Massage therapy*, which is different from physical therapy, is usually used once a week for 4 to 6 weeks and then bimonthly or monthly as the clinical situation dictates. Massage therapy can be used therapeutically in pregnancy, in infants, and certainly in animals (my golden labs love it). You may find chair massage available in airports and in shopping malls.

Contraindications to massage include infectious skin conditions, high fever, burns or open wounds, varicose veins or phlebitis, tumors with involved lymph nodes, and possibly low platelet count.

### ACUPRESSURE AND JIN SHIN JYUTSU

Jin Shin Jyutsu is a system of massage and acupressure that utilizes the Chinese acupuncture meridians to erase blockages and reduce pain. Literally translated, Jin Shin Jyutsu means "art of the Creator through man of knowing and compassion." It is an ancient art and was resurrected by Master Jiro Murai and his student Mary Burmeister in the 1950s. It is used as an advanced type of massage with special emphasis on the blocked areas of the meridians.

### ROLFING

Rolfing refers to a system of body education and physical manipulation developed by Dr. Ida Rolf over a period of 50 years. It is a method of structural integration in which the rolfer slowly stretches, loosens, and repositions the body's fascia, which has become stuck and adherent to local muscles, tendonous, and bony structures through poor posture and muscular tension. This restores normal length and elasticity to the myofascial network and allows for better posture, movement, and blood flow to occur. The standard treatment is once a week (for about an hour) for ten sessions, which covers the entire body. This ten-session treatment is usually enough to rebalance the musculoskeletal framework of the body.

### ASTON PATTERNING

*Aston Patterning* is my favorite body work, as it combines the best of holistic massage and rolfing and is not as painful as rolfing. Aston patterning was developed by a student of Ida Rolf, Judith Aston-Linderoth. Key to Judith's paradigm is the concept that the human body is an asymmetrical structure, and that its motion and form take on three-dimensional, asymmetrical, spiral patterns, which are unique for each person. Aston Patterning identifies and reinforces each person's own natural integrity of dimension and proportion, where all parts are allowed to rest in their own best three-dimensional shape and work together in cooperation for efficient function. The proper alignment of the body is important for three-dimensional energetic facial communication.

Several factors distinguish the Aston Patterning treatment from traditional forms of therapy:

1. It considers of the person as a whole.
2. It determines of the relationship between the client's focus and the overall patterns of posture and movement. Resolution of specific dysfunction is achieved by integration of the whole, versus attention to just one part.
3. In both the movement and the body work, the sequence determines the result. The body work is carefully planned so that the release of one segment facilitates the reduction of the overall muscle tension patterns.
4. Movement education supporting the structural changes is grounded in practical application, such as sitting and standing postures, bending, reaching, lifting, and walking. This brings the work into daily life rather than being an exercise that remains separate from routine function.
5. Lastly, the body work in Aston Patterning is unique. Holding patterns based on varying combinations of intellectual, physical, and emotional habits can be felt in the facial tissues and have three-dimensional directionality. When matched in direction, speed, and amount of movement, the tissue changes readily and without discomfort. Aston body work is perceived by the client to be very subtle and yet is profoundly effective.

## OSTEOPATHIC MEDICINE

Osteopathic medicine was developed by Andrew Taylor Still, M.D. (1828–1917) during the American Civil War. He was one of the first American doctors to realize that medicine was fixated on disease and not on the natural and living anatomy and physiology of the human being. He saw his work as a reformation of the restricted and dogmatic practice of medicine at the time, and never really intended to develop a new modality. He was hounded out of Kansas, where he practiced, and ended up in Kirksville, Missouri, where in 1892, he founded the first school of osteopathy. The osteopathic curriculum soon included manipulative techniques, but after Still's death, it fell prey to drug therapy, and now there is little difference between osteopathic and allopathic training.

However, most of my DO friends still put their osteopathic manipulative skills to some very good use. There are two basic techniques:

**Direct** — The dysfunctional anatomy is placed into the position of obstruction, and a direct force is applied to remove that obstruction. The force is high velocity, with a low amplitude, just enough to go beyond the obstruction. This is a passive treatment with the osteopath supplying the force. Another technique is the *muscle energy technique*, where the patient will supply the force into the direction of obstruction.

**Indirect** — Indirect techniques involve taking the dysfunctional unit away from the restriction until a balanced tension is achieved. This is held for a time, allowing the balanced tension to alleviate the symptoms. Another indirect technique is *strain–counterstrain*. In this technique the muscle in question is relaxed by approximating its insertions, and the position held for 90 seconds. The joint and muscle are retested to show an increase in movement and less dysfunction.

In my opinion, the osteopathic technique is more gentle, more efficacious, and longer lasting than the chiropractic technique.

## CHIROPRACTIC MEDICINE

There are nearly 60,000 chiropractors in the United States. The profession has taken vast strides since its inception by Daniel David Palmer (1845–1913) and his son Bartlett Joshua Palmer (1882–1961). Chiropractic is concerned with the influence of biomechanical dysfunction on the central nervous system and, in turn, on the function of the rest of the body. There are, as in acupuncture, many different schools and techniques, and a large degree of individual preferences and services are offered by chiropractors.

My experience with the profession has been varied. I have found that chiropractors who focus on their scope of practice are excellent and really help me whith those patients who have subluxations causing nerve impingment syndromes and associated segmental autonomic dysfunction. The chiropractors who are more interested in selling you something, or practicing out of their scope of practice, tend to be less effective in helping my patients.

When I perform acupuncture, if I do not get a good clinical result in 3 to 5 treatments, acupuncture is not going to work. The same is true in chiropractic. Having two adjustments a week for three months is nonsense.

The combination of acupuncture and chiropractic or of massage therapy and chiropractic seems to make more sense to me (and I do this a lot), because, if the muscles are in spasm, the adjustment will not hold — it will be pulled back out by the spastic muscle.

Contraindications to chiropractic include fractures, osteoporosis in the elderly, vertebral artery narrowing, and surgically fused bony areas.

## HYPNOSIS

Hypnosis has been used in all the cultures of the world from ancient times. Hypnosis is a form of cognitive information processing in which a suspension of peripheral awareness and critical analytical cognition can lead to apparently involuntary changes in perception, memory, mood, and physiology. To me, it is a state in which we access our subconscious and change its perception of our conscious reality. In changing this perception, we change everything associated with that "incorrect" perception or illusion — thoughts, feelings, physiology, etc. The only problem in using hypnosis in a busy clinical practice is that it takes quite a bit of time, and only works well in the busy office situation in patients who are highly susceptible to hypnosis, and who really believe in it.

However, I use hypnosis and suggestibility all the time in my practice. Each time I muscle test a remedy, I will ask the patients to close their eyes and feel the energy of the remedy enter them. If it is strong I say, "this will fix you after you open your eyes." I also use it extensively in neuroemotional technique and during desensitizing procedures where I use conditional clauses all the time. I will only send patients to psychological counseling with professionals who uses hypnosis. This cuts down on the time of therapy and results in good clinical information for me and an easier time for the patient.

## USE OF LOW INTENSITY LASERS

Since the early 1980s, low energy lasers have been available for acupuncture point stimulation. Most of the low energy lasers have outputs between 5 and 50 mW, FDA class IIIb, and do not burn the skin. The cutting carbon dioxide lasers have 300 W of power. About 500 mW (1/2 watt) will cause pain. *Red-beam lasers* (like the ones used as pointers in presentations), have a wave length of 600 to 700 nm and exhibit shallow skin penetration of about 10 to 15 mm. *Infrared-beam lasers* (Ga-Al-As solid-state diode) have a wavelength of 700 to 1000 nm and can penetrate tissue up to 5 cm. If the wavelength were any different, then water or hemoglobin would block the beam.

Low energy lasers have the following *physiological effects*: neurotransmitter release (acetyl choline), phagocytosis, ATP synthesis, prostaglandin synthesis, and an increase in serotonin levels. It is important to be able to calculate the energy density emitted by your laser: 1 watt = 1 joule/second. I use a 30 mW, infrared 830 nm Ga-Al-As solid-state laser. In order to calculate the number of seconds I have to hold the laser at the acupuncture point to deliver 1 Joule, I do the following calculation:

$$(0.030 \text{ watts}) \times (X \text{ seconds}) = 1 \text{ joule}.$$

The answer is that I have to stimulate the point for approximately 30 seconds to deliver 1 Joule to the point.

The following dosages are a rough guideline to therapy:

| | | |
|---|---|---|
| **Analgesic Effect** — muscular pain | 2–4 $J/cm^2$ |
| — joint pain | 4–8 $J/cm^2$ |
| **Anti-Inflammatory** — acute | 1–6 $J/cm^2$ |
| — chronic | 4–8 $J/cm^2$ |
| **Eutrophic Effect** | 3–6 $J/cm^2$ |
| **Circulatory Effect** | 1–3 $J/cm^2$ |

Lasers are useful for balancing refractory acupuncture points, sprains, and strains and for use in children and patients fearful of needles. Lasers have been used in alopecia areata, stroke patients, peripheral neuropathy, and spasticity of cerebral palsy.

**Do not look at the beam.** Severe retinal damage will occur even in a pointing device. Patients may buy pointer devices and use them on painful and dysfunctional areas including painful knees and carpel tunnel.

## USE OF THERAPEUTIC MAGNETS

Magnets do, in fact, have biological activity that is focused, predictable, and useful. Permanent nickel-plated neodymium magnets are the best, but are expensive. The strength of magnets is measured in Gauss (G) or Tesla (T = 10,000 G). By contrast, the Earth's magnetic field is about 0.5 G. The dosage delivered to the target tissue is difficult to measure, but it is a function of its distance from the target tissue. A magnet with a field strength of 1000 G at the surface, has a strength of 600 G at 1 cm and 400 G at 2 cm from the surface. The optimal physiological responses occur with a magnetic field strength of 450 G delivered to the target tissue. Human tissues are essentially transparent to magnetic fields. Time of exposure varies from 15 minutes for magnets greater than 1500 G to 12 hours for magnetic mattresses to weeks for acuband magnets. The curious meridians should not be stimulated with a magnet for longer than 20 minutes at a time. The nomenclature of polarity varies.

In the *geographic method*, the side of the magnet that attracts the north-seeking needle of the compass is named the south, negative, or sedating pole.

In the *Albert Roy Davis Method*, the side of the magnet that attracts the north-seeking needle of the compass is named the north, negative, or sedating pole. In this convention, the south pole tonifies and the north pole sedates. To decide which side of an unknown magnet to place down on the patient's skin, test the muscle each way. The patient will be strong the correct way down.

The physiological effects of magnets include pain relief, antiphlogistic, decreased edema, improved sleep, increased circulation, and increased B-endorphins. Magnets can be used for children, needle-phobic patients and in home treatment programs. Some practitioners use magnets together with ion-pumping cords to great clinical effect.

Magnets are contraindicated in patients with metal prostheses and near the chest with implanted pacemakers.

# Section IV

## The Practice of Integrated Medicine

# 16 The Practice of Integrated Medicine

The following sections will cover the assessment of the patient, the selection of treatment, and the assessment of therapeutic response.

## THE INTEGRATED MEDICAL EXAM

The integrated medical exam is used to bring out the state of imbalance and chaotic level of the patient. This "diseased" state is viewed from an integrated historical, circumstantial, emotional, physiological, energetic, laboratory, pathological, and physical perspective. Parts of the exam are similar to a regular medical exam, and parts will relate to specific inquiries about the energetic or emotional nature of the imbalance.

## THE INTEGRATED PATIENT HISTORY

The history is the most important part of the patient exams. If you allow a free flow of ideas from the patients, that is, you do not interrupt them as they tell their stories (I ask them to tell me their stories, not what is the matter with them), their language, sequencing of ideas, and use of words, will give you the real strange attractor that is causing the imbalance and physical manifestations. Most patients will present with a physical complaint because it is socially acceptable. This does not mean that the presenting complaint is the real issue. Allow them to finish their laundry lists of complaints and then just wait and stare at them. I have had pauses up to 10 minutes long. Don't flinch, just wait for the next statement, which is the subconscious's take on the problem — the *real issue*. When they have finished with that soliloquy, wait a few seconds to make sure nothing else is forthcoming and then ask, "What else?" You will usually now get the qualifiers of the real issue, or they may go on to another real issue of lesser importance.

The sequencing of thoughts as they come out of the patients' mouths will often distinguish the important from the minor issues. When you ask them about their childhood, the very first sentence is critical. This statement is usually how they perceived their childhoods or the dominant issue of their childhood. Look for *repetitive themes* in the narrative and close and estranged associations between members of the family. Anything that does not seem to fit should be pursued with vigor — there is a good reason for its peculiarity. Offhand comments, usually coming at the end of a sentence or discussion on a particular topic, are key. Repetitive metaphors and changes in tone and language usage when talking about a particular subject or person are extremely important. Obviously a sudden change in demeanor or tears or laughter, should alert you to the importance of the topic.

All your questions should be, to the best of your ability, open ended or, at the very least, multiple choice. "How was your relationship with your father?" Not, "Was your father good or bad?" What you want is a spontaneous recall, not a forced choice. Always pursue whole blocks of time or obvious personalities in the family that have been left out of the narrative.

After these interactions, you can begin the systematic inquiry.

## Prenatal and Perinatal History

The first questions should document the general medical history of the parents: What diseases ran in the family, or if they are deceased, at what age they died and as a result of what condition. That will give you a basic idea of constitution and weaknesses (the initial conditions). The age of parents at conception will give you an indication of the amount of Jing essence that the patient was given — the older the parents, the less Jing. This fact is more important in these times, when parents are delaying their childbearing years for careers, etc.

The pregnancy is often the initial cause of long-term imbalance in some patients. One must know:

1. Any emotional or traumatic occurrences during the pregnancy will imprint the fetus, lead to a different initial condition upon birth, and may affect the rest of the lives. These imprints need to be removed homeopathically.
2. Any illness, such as morning sickness, high blood pressure, eclampsia, threatened abortion, spotting, premature labor, or gestational diabetes may have an effect on the fetus.
3. Any ingested therapeutic or recreational drugs, smoking, or alcohol during the pregnancy. I have had a number of cases of attention deficit disorder, inattentive type, that responded wonderfully to homeopathic Cannabis indica, where there was a maternal history of marijuana use during pregnancy.
4. Length of the pregnancy — full term, premature, or overdue. Prematures tend to be more sensitive, have weak lungs, and are more reactive to their surroundings (allergy).

The birth itself has to be examined carefully if the information is available. The issues of importance include:

1. Start of labor — induced or spontaneous, caesarean section or not. Spontaneous labors produce children who are self-starters, induced labor, the opposite. Caesarean births produce children who have little regard for boundaries. These observations are, of course, generalizations, but are helpful at times.
2. Length of labor — prolonged or obstructed labor always produces some fearful imprinting on the child. Precipitous labor produces a clingy child, afraid to be away from its mother. The child may also show signs of cranial injury at a later date.
3. Premature rupture of membranes and meconium always herald a somewhat weaker child, more prone to infection.
4. Instrument delivery — forceps or ventouse with deformation of the head or obvious trauma to the face, will cause a focal weakness in the injured area that will be the anatomical location of headaches, neuralgia, etc. If emotionally imprinted on the child, they will lead to fear of the dark, night terrors, sleepwalking, and enuresis. These symptoms may become apparent only when there is a repeat trauma to the head later in childhood.
5. Apgars and apneas — any problem with low Apgar scores, fetal apnea, or meconium aspiration at birth will predispose the child to respiratory problems from there on, the lung being the most delicate of the organs.

During the perinatal period you will first see indications of the child's weaknesses and traits, as evidenced by:

1. Neonatal jaundice — the presence of jaundice will indicate hepatic weakness for the rest of the person's life, especially if it is severe.

2. Breast feeding — the absence of breast feeding produces a child with poor bonding and immunity and, depending on its reaction to formula, allergies and gut problems for the rest of its life. Difficulties in suckling and feeding in general will spawn a finicky and picky eater. Remember that whatever the mother eats, or whatever drugs the mother ingests, will usually come out in the breast milk and affect the infant. For this reason, I rarely use herbs in breast-feeding mothers.

3. Colic and diarrhea — if the child suffers from colic or diarrhea due to formula intolerance, especially to milk, then that child will always be a gut manifester when stressed or unhappy.

4. Diaper rash — severe diaper rash may herald a skin manifester or food sensitivities.

5. Perinatal infection or puerperal sepsis — if either of these unfortunate issues occurs, the child will be prone to the specific organism involved and needs homeopathic nosode treatment to rid his or her body of this early energetic imprint.

## INFANCY AND CHILDHOOD HISTORY

The patterning of little adults starts to take place as they start to construct their external realities of objects and people, and they learn to respond appropriately to the family inner circle. Directed inquiry needs to address the following issues:

1. Developmental milestones — Walking, talking, teething, and fine and gross motor coordination are all developmental milestones. Delays in talking, with a sudden spurt of long sentences at age of two or beyond, will be the hallmark of the "internalizer," but only if he or she does not have an older brother or sister to talk for them. A friend of mine adopted a little girl from Russia who during her early years would talk to her older brother in a language, neither Russian or English, and he would translate. Delays in teething are a reflection of calcium and bone metabolism, and these children have to be watched during their growing years.

2. Diseases — The advent of eczema or ear infections from birth, or very soon after birth, is an indicator of hereditary weakness and an inherited trait, as the child has not had enough exposure to the environment to acquire these problems. These weaknesses need to be treated miasmatically with homeopathic remedies. Ear infections may be the early clue to milk or soy allergy, depending on what formula is being used. Bad strep infections or a history of chronic urinary tract infections in childhood, will predispose to throat and lower urinary tract or Lower Heater symptoms in the patient. A bad case of infectious mononucleosis will impair the liver until it is treated. All severe infectious disease occurrences in childhood have their pathogenic imprint and will, to some extent, limit the physiology or patient's response to other like stressors, which is how repetitive infections or chronic disease starts. The chronicity of certain diseases — otitis media is a classic — is encouraged by suppressive therapy such as repetitive antibiotics.

3. Relationships (Family) — The infants are starting to work out who everybody is, and where they fit into the family picture. The pecking order is soon worked out and appropriate responses as well, depending on the perceived stressors at this point. Being a first, last, or middle child will have its own problems and joys; or being a girl or boy, its own tribulations and rewards. Find out what the rules were in the family. Relationships, perceived personalities, and influences of each parent and sibling need to be understood to work out the family dynamics. This is the imprinting time of one's life. Ask the patients to describe themselves as children or to compare and contrast their concept of selves with either parent or with siblings. Who were they most like, or who do they not want to be like? This is the time in which the initial conditions of heredity, *in utero* influences,

and birth are now further stirred to come up with a semipermanent chaotic picture that will be their triggering and responsive anchoring attractors for life.

4. Relationships — school and friends — Identification of relationship patterns at school and with friends, especially if they are markedly different from those at home, will often reveal stress issues that have shaped the personality and its manifestation as disease. Children will often escape to school from a bad home life and will state their love of school. Other children will be meek at school and domineering at home, showing their need for family boundaries or exhibiting dysfunctional home behavior for attention or personal gain.

5. Physical, emotional, and sexual abuse — The discovery of abuse in a childhood is perhaps the single most significant finding that affects patients' lives and their manifestation of disease. Most of these childhood experiences are extremely painful, deep seated, and disturb the core of the developing personality. *Physical abuse*, if it does not maim or kill the child, is the least harmful. It will, however, pattern the individual to respond with physical violence when stressed.

   The more insidious stressor is the *emotional and verbal abuse* suffered by many children — "you are no good," "you never do anything right," "why are you not more like your brother?" These issues are pretty clear-cut in their effect on self-image, but what is even more surprising is the devastating effects of subtle expectations even in the best of homes. High achieving parents give a message of obligatory high achievement to their children, even if the words are never spoken. The children then take it upon themselves to be high achievers, and if they fail in their own eyes, they have no one to blame but themselves, and self-destructive behavior ensues. This is not an uncommon pattern to encounter in upper class families.

   *Sexual abuse* is the most destructive of all and happens to both girls and boys, by either sex. As procreation is our most important biological "purpose," the distortion of this function at too early an age, or in a violent, nonconsenting, noncognitive manner, produces a permanent, discordant record on every level of the organism. In girls, on the physical plane, it causes a permanent disturbance in the Lower Heater (pelvis), that predisposes to menstrual problems, pelvic and low back pain, infertility or spontaneous abortions, frequent infections, fibroids, and gynecological neoplasia. On an emotional level it plays havoc with hetero- and homosexual relationships and with trust and self-image in general, and predisposes the patient either to sexuality as a major means of expression or to frigidity and a fear of intimacy. In boys, depending on the perpetrator, they will equate sex with love or will be unable to relate to females normally and may be able to relate only to males sexually.

6. Sequencing — All happenings in one's life are in relationship to some stressor or stressors. Every incident of disease, infectious or otherwise, has some emotional background terrain to it. In childhood, the big emotional landmarks are weaning, kindergarten, changing schools, changing locations, puberty, divorce, and the loss of a loved family member.

## PUBERTY AND THE TEENAGE YEARS

By the time puberty arrives, children have more or less formed their core beliefs, their concepts of the greater world, and their place within it. Puberty brings about a shattering of some of these foundations, and the next 8 to 10 years are an emotional and physiological roller coaster, with both the children and their parents hanging on for dear life. Sex first raises its ugly head, as do drugs (we hope that exposure has not yet occurred). One must question young children about sexual and drug-related practices, which in my area are quite shocking. School gangs and other serious pressures at school to drink, to do drugs, and to have sex, all make this time a very dangerous and potentially disastrous developmental period. Even my own youngest son, when he left middle school and went into high school, said he was so happy to leave middle school because he had not been shot or stabbed, and had not had to choose between joining a white supremacy, hispanic or red neck gang. A far cry from the stresses at my high school, where being caught smoking was a high crime.

The problem I see most often in teenagers in my practice is quite surprising. Many of my teenage patients are quite exhausted and burned out from the enormous load that is thrust upon them by teacher and parental expectations, and all the options that are now open to them. Most of them have after-school jobs to keep up their car insurance or to buy the latest electronics and clothes. They are poorly nourished and do not get adequate rest or sleep. Many of them are stuck in a sport or sports that have very rigorous schedules, with coaches that would make Hitler look like a sissy. All this adds up to a serious mismatch of time and energy, resulting in a stressed biology that was ill-designed for this lifestyle and, in time, will fail and make the quantum jump into a "diseased" chaotic pattern of survival. These are supposed to be the best times of our lives, but they rarely are. Treatment includes both parents and child, with serious reduction in extraneous commitments, and a focus on those pursuits that are relaxing, enjoyable, and under the control of the child. Dietary modification and enforced rest periods and sleep make up the full complement of resuscitation required for these "old and worn out" children.

Patients who cannot remember much of their early childhood are purposely blocking it out for good reason and need to be gently coaxed, maybe at the next visit once they feel more comfortable, to talk about the issues, no matter how difficult they may be. If this is not done, you are playing with half a deck of cards and will not be able to get to the bottom of all the issues presented to you.

## ADULT HISTORY

Finally, we start to come to the near present, and see what has happened to our beat up children as they ventured away from the nest into the real world. Again, the big milestones, and their reasons for being, seem to define the course of events and the "disease" that accompanies them. These include but are not limited to:

1. Leaving Home — This is a major change from the past patterns and comfort zones. Some patients do it with glee, even doing it early to get away from a hostile home environment. Others do it reluctantly and fearfully and may end up coming back again, as their sense of self-reliance without the family is too low to survive alone. They have been ill-prepared during childhood, and do not have the tools necessary for survival. Some do not leave. This is not normal, and the reasons for this aberration need to be explained.

   Some go out and work and establish their freedom at once, while others pursue higher learning as their first taste of freedom. During the college years, all kinds of adjustments are made and new lifestyles experienced. This is often a turbulent time of trial and error, with new ideas and repressed old ideas and identity coming to the surface. In my practice, the percentage of college-going patients actually completing a degree the first time around must be in the low 20th percentile. This time supports far too radical a change for all but the most devoted to focus on more learning. Infectious diseases such as mono, herpes, and miscellaneous viral syndromes abound, sometimes for the very first time. Therapeutic abortions are not uncommon, as is the addiction to alcohol, drugs, and sex with new-found freedoms.

2. First Jobs — These are usually not too much of a problem, unless one is severely disillusioned as to the nature of day-to-day work (as opposed to the colorful picture painted by out-of-touch professors) and is left up in the air and discombobulated as to what to do next.

3. Work History — This is often an indicator of the general nature of the personality function imprinted during childhood. High work ethics and obsessive–compulsive behavior seem to go together, as does type-A personality and workaholism. Work time being out of balance with family time, rest time, or play time is a big problem in modern families. I believe from my patient observations that so-called "quality time" does not make up for no time. Total immersion in work as the only indicator of worth is another problem. One also sees the opposite, changing jobs at the drop of a hat, and even just plain not wanting to work.

Work history is also important as to industrial exposure and work injuries over the years. Certain industries, such as the casino industry in my town, have their own associated dangers of drug addiction, alcoholism, and transiency.

Being laid off is a very devastating and not uncommon occurrence. This is especially so in single parents (usually mothers) with little backup or family support and, for older or long-term employees, where retraining and loss of dignity are difficult issues to address.

Mothers who are working 40 to 60 hours a week, try to be perfect wives and look after 2 or 3 children soon end up in my office in a burned out condition similar to those teenagers I was describing. These superwomen exist only on TV and in movies. Something has to give in these situations, and it is usually the woman's health.

4. Marriage(s) — My average patient has been married 2 to 3 times, with my all-time record of a lady at age 80 on her 10th wonderful marriage. Marriages can be categorized into three types — good, bad, and "we live in the same house." The "good" and the "we live in the same house" types are not of too much importance, unless the patient is totally suppressed, doesn't know the difference, and is totally deluded about the marriage by norms, customs, and expectations. The bad marriage needs to be examined in detail, especially if there are multiple bad marriages and a common thread joining them. Often the bad marriage is the cause of the presenting disease. This scenario is seen in patients who feel trapped and have no other means of emotional or monetary support. This picture is often seen in breast cancer cases. Often women stay in the marriage for the kids — a very bad idea as kids are not stupid and will be more damaged and dysfunctionally programmed as to the nature of marriage by the charade. The most important fact to elicit in these situations is, what is staying in a bad marriage providing for the patient's biology and, even more interesting, what leaving the marriage will do to the patient. Most of the answers to these questions will be gleaned in the childhood patterning section. This dysfunctional behavior is repeating an early survivalistic action that unfortunately has few redeeming qualities in the adult situation.

Never having been married is also a red flag and needs to be further explored. The epidemic of living together, while not married, sets up a pattern of disingenuous commitment that is the pattern for the marriage that may follow it. Obviously, this is not the case in every instance, but the theory holds true in many cases.

Other stresses in the marriage besides the controlling and abuse issues include: financial issues (a big one); sexual issues, too much, too little, or just plain weird; mixed families (his children, her children, and our children); and interracial marriages, interethnic marriages, and marriages across religious barriers. All of these can have their place in the manifestation and presentation of "disease."

5. Children — The extra dynamic of a child is enough to either break or make the marriage. More than one child just adds a logarithmic complexity to the equation. Children take up all your time, money, and energy. If there is some left over, it is rarely spent on self. The kind of juggling of time and energy that the activities of today's child demands is a wonder of modern logistics. As the children age, the demands become more stringent and expansive, and a strain is put on the whole balance of the marriage. There may

always be one bad apple in the bunch, and this child will often be the precipitating factor that causes disease to manifest, especially in mothers.

Competition and inappropriate role playing may occur between mothers and daughters for father's affection, or if one parent is continually absent, a daughter will become the surrogate mother and wife or a son the surrogate father and husband. These roles will stay with them for life. Parents may also try to live spuriously through their children, and when the role fails or is not to their liking, they may manifest disease.

A conscious decision not to have children needs to be fleshed out as to cause and logic. Sometimes it is quite correct as the patient would have made a bad parent while at other times it reflects their personal perception of their experience as a child (not good, and does not want to be reminded of it in any way), or just plain selfishness.

6. Disease patterns and events — All diseases are in response to some inner imbalance (the explicate and the implicate order of nonlinear dynamics). You need to be able to correlate the temporal sequencing of the disease with an issue or an event that triggered or was the background terrain (physical or emotional) for this bodily response. Without this knowledge, you will just be skimming over the surface and will never reach true cure.

## THE LATER YEARS

After 50 and beyond, if you are not faced with midlife crises, which appear to be prevalent in the male gender in my area, the work of the physician is to keep all systems functioning at peak capacity with as little downtime and degeneration as possible. This is the time period where the sins of the youth come visiting, and the physical body and mind take the brunt. I don't get too involved in the emotional issues of childhood unless really pushed, I just look at the cards dealt in front of me and try to play a winning hand.

In females it revolves around menopause, the empty nest syndrome, and trying to live with a retired husband who is in their hair all day. Dietary and hormonal changes give the body and face a different look, which is either happily accepted or fought against like a mortal enemy. The ravages of multiple births take their toll, the bladder and uterus (if they are lucky enough to still be present) start to sag, and the varicose veins and hemorrhoids make their appearance. Amazingly enough, if properly hormonally attended to, most postmenopausal females feel better and have more energy than they have had for some time. If this is not the case, find out where the block or obstacle to cure is and remedy it. Attention to osteoporosis and cognitive decline is an important part of the interview.

In males, after they have come to their midlife crisis, the issues are with loss of worth and prestige in retirement, for those who live to work, and a feeling of fear and insecurity, in those who have not made long-term preparations for this eventuality. Both of these situations will cause Kidney Yin deficiency (which increases with age) with associated fatigue, low back pain, and insomnia. Having to live a different lifestyle is hard for some, but joyful to many. I may seem a little gloomy as I discuss old age, but only a few people come to me when they feel great, and this *is* a book about what to do for the ill and diseased.

## THE INTEGRATED REVIEW OF SYSTEMS

1. **Main Complaint** — In spite of what I have said about the origin of disease, the main complaint is important. It represents to the patient the reason, or one of the reasons, for the visit. It has been selected out because it has made an impact on the biology. It may be metaphorical, or it may just be unbearable. The complaint should be qualified, as should all complaints, under the following subheadings:
   a. Score the symptom on a scale (1 to 10, 1 being best, 10 being worst). This enables you to quantify the progress or lack thereof with treatment. You want to know about quality, sensations, and severity of the symptom.

b. How long has the patient had the symptom, and how has it changed over time? This defines the time sequences and possible prior triggers. It also tells you the progression or regression of the pathological process and may offer some clues to the pathogenesis or inner issues.

c. Did the symptom start after any particular event? This is sometimes quite enlightening. "I have never been the same since my hysterectomy," or "since the accident," or "since I started birth control pills," etc.

d. Is there a pattern to the symptom? Does the patient have it all the time? Does it start at the same time of the day? Is it only on weekends or at work? Does it disappear when leaving the house, the spouse, or when on vacation? Does it occur before menses or only after a viral infection, or after eating cheese? The list is endless, but most of the time if you just flat out ask the question, the patient will give the connecting answer.

e. What makes it better or worse? These questions are called modalities and refer to almost any situation and circumstance you can think of. Examples include the vertigo is worse lying down or moving; the abdominal cramping is better with bending over and a hot water bottle. All these individualizing reactions of the patient will lead you to the correct and specific homeopathic remedy or Chinese herbal pattern and mixture.

f. What does it stop the patient from doing, or what could the patient do if he or she did not have it? This is very revealing question as to the body's reason for having the manifestation. The answers may surprise you.

g. Who made the diagnosis and how was the diagnosis made? An important question for integrated practitioners, as many patients are self-diagnosing or being diagnosed by crystal healers or the like. This will also help you know what has not been done in terms of investigation.

h. What treatment has the patient had and what did it do? A lot of good information can come out of this question. First, it will tell you, by reason of successful treatment, what pathophysiology is being positively impacted; and if unsuccessful, you can rule out a whole line of proposed treatments. It also reveals the patient's process through the disease and the present state of mind and body.

i. What does the patient want you to do about this problem? This establishes the dual role of patient and physician in the healing process and empowers the patient as to the direction of cure. It also will catch outrageous expectations that you sometimes encounter, which can immediately be rectified before misunderstandings and mismatches occur.

2. **Other Symptoms** — Other symptoms may have equal or less significance. Many of these symptoms will have energetic connections to the main symptoms, such as the case of migraines, fatigue, and hip pain in my South American professor, a perfect example of Gall Bladder Yang excess. In my intake form I have a list of complaints that patients can tick off any they have ever had. This usually gives me a snapshot of the organ or Five Element pole around which they are clustered.

3. **Drug History** — This includes both regular Western drugs and, more importantly in my practice, any herbs, homeopathics, or nutritional supplements being taken. I also want to know who prescribed them and for what purpose. Some people have been on some drugs for years for no apparent reason, because nobody stopped them, and their ever-changing doctors did not adequately know them. Overdosing and drug interactions must also be looked at as a cause for morbidity. This is especially important in the elder population who are not properly supervised or who now live alone.

4. **Family History** — This should have already been gleaned from the previous data concerning the parents, etc. Reasons for parental demise or demise of siblings is important. It may also be useful to ask about sibling morbidity and current state. This information may give you some insight into your patient's long-term prognosis if siblings are

much older or a premorbid pattern appears. The arrival of stepparents, stepbrothers and sisters, or the disappearance of a loved parent or sibling are important.

5. **Geographical History** — Place of birth and upbringing are important in regard to lifestyle, local and extended family support, and influences such as issues of environmental pollution including farming with pesticides and herbicides, polluted water basins, local polluting industries, or being involved in working with parents in a toxic environment. Moving schools at critical emotional times and leaving friends or relatives also have their influence on the disease process.

6. **Habits and Activities** — Any recreational or other drug habits or addictions should be discussed. Smoking as a premorbid risk is extremely important. The same is true of alcoholism. Dangerous or excessive compulsive activities should be highlighted and the reason for their existence questioned. I had a young man who exhibited cerebral edema and hyponatremia after a grueling 100-mile race. He almost died, but was back training for the next one as soon as I had homeopathically successfully treated his absent short-term memory, that was a direct result of the self-induced brain injury.

7. **Energy** — If the patient does not have any energy, then you cannot change anything, and you certainly cannot get the patient to start to formulate a new lifestyle or eating habit. Low energy or fatigue can come from many different problems including emotional, constrained Liver Qi or Blood deficiency, poor aeration of the lung with hypo-oxygenation of the blood, anemia, Spleen Qi deficiency, Heart Qi and Blood deficiency, Kidney Yin and Yang deficiency, and reduced Essence or Jing. It is one of the most important symptoms to monitor in assessing the success or failure of treatment.

8. **Stress** — I ask about stresses as a matter of course to try and assess the residual total resources and reserves of the patient. Different inventories can be used to assess this issue. It is playing a bigger and bigger part in the etiology and presentation of disease. All the individual contributory components need to be assessed, and I do it like this: I ask patients to make lists of the things they do, all the people they have contact with or are responsible for, all the organizations and other activities in which are involved, and then to do an energy and stress audit of each entry, asking: Does it give me energy and is it unstressful, or does it take energy away and stress me out? They are all very surprised at the outcomes of this compilation. I then ask them to unplug from the big offending drains on their energy and resources. This always seems to focus them on the big issues, with better success at decreasing their biological burden.

9. **Sleep** — Patients are almost never asked how they are sleeping unless they bring it up to the doctor as a problem. I can tell you two facts for sure: insomnia is endemic, and until you get the patient adequately sleeping, he or she will not improve whatever it is you are treating them for. Insomnia is also a serious sign of some imbalance, usually emotional. Difficulty in getting to sleep is a Heart Shen disturbance (issues of love and nurturing), while not being able to stay asleep is a Kidney Yin deficiency (issues of prolonged stress and anxiety). Grinding of teeth at night is an important notable symptom, and relates to Tuberculinum as a remedy, and the Liver-Gall Bladder meridian as an energy treatment.

The state of heat or coldness at night is also of some interest to me. Most people are either a "hot" (kick the covers off and stick the feet out) or a "cold" sleeper (wear bed socks and are like a baby in a cocoon). Of passing interest is that in husband–wife pairs there will seldom be two "hots" or two "colds" married to each other; one is usually hot and the other cold. If the woman was cold before menopause, and then becomes hot after the menopause, the husband usually begins to cool down at that time as he loses his Yang energy, and the bedroom thermal homeostasis is maintained. Sweating at night is a bad sign of Kidney Yin deficiency, with the inability of the Wei Qi to hold in the moisture. It is also a sign of some febrile infectious diseases such as tuberculosis, another sign that the Wei Qi is weak.

Dreams are very important if they are repetitive and have a common theme running through them. We tend to work out issues at night in our dreams that we cannot deal with, for one or another reason, during the day. These narratives often lead to the cause of some physical disturbance or unexplained attitude.

10. **Digestion and Excretion** — I have already stated in the nutrition segment that a dysfunctional bowel is the bedrock of most bodily diseases. I ask about swallowing problems, heart burn, GERD, indigestion, abdominal pain, bloating, food allergies, etc. Most chronically ill patients have some gastrointestinal problem. The belly-achers, that we identified with colic in infancy, are here in droves, with non-ulcer dyspepsia, irritable bowel syndrome, or ulcerative colitis (all emotional diseases) and they are going to show any stress in their bowels. Gut dysbiosis (usually yeast overgrowth) with sugar craving is endemic. You have to treat these symptoms at every encounter to get to biological homeodynamic equilibrium. I screen all my patients energetically for *H. pylorii* and will treat them if found to be positive.

Bowel activities are as equally important as indigestion. The colon needs to be flushed out at least once a day (my artificial norm) in order not to entoxicate the liver with the fermentation and putrefaction products of the large bowel. Constipation also causes stagnation in the Lower Burner (pelvis) and will affect menses, the lower back, and the kidneys. Most patients with this problem have been that way since childhood, as a reflection of anger and suppression as a child, and the pattern is sometimes difficult to break, especially in females.

Diarrhea on the other hand is very exhausting to the body, as you are losing vital fluids. The history of the diarrhea is very important, especially relating it to ingestion of water from streams (Giardia), or the result of a visit to a foreign country. Parasites are much underdiagnosed and should be looked for in this very cosmopolitan and mobile society. The testing of well water and city water should also be undertaken in resistant and unexplained cases. Patients with alternating diarrhea and constipation usually have IBS.

Beware the changing bowel habit with no energetic findings and an indicator drop on Meridian Stress Testing — time for colonoscopy.

11. **Respiratory Tract** — I am interested in defining the patient's childhood infectious patterns: whether they are all in the nose and ears, or always straight to the lungs. The treatments and the remedies used are totally different. Chronic sore and strep throats yet again are a different animal. We need to know about past or present smoking patterns and any repetitive pneumonias or, if the patient has not been well since an influenza or other virus. Color of sputum and nasal discharge, white or pale is a Cold process, yellow or brown or green is a Hot process.

Asthmatics have a whole protocol of their own and are granted special treatment, never having to call in for an appointment, just turning up when the two big No-Nos occur together: tight chest and feeling tired.

I look for allergy as a contributing cause to all lung problems, as well as industrial exposures and family animals including parrots and other exotic birds. Tuberculosis in the patient at one time or in parents or grandparents is very important as a premorbid trait and can be treated homeopathically. The same is true of Coccidiomycosis — Valley Fever.

The lung is the delicate organ in Chinese medicine and must be treated with great respect. You can still lose a patient to asthma or pneumonia, even in the best of academic/medical institutions.

12. **Cardiac History** — The most important antecedants to cardiac disease are a cardiac family history, and a childhood history of scarlet fever or repetitive sore or diagnosed

strep throats. Chest pain and palpitations are usually caused by Kidney Yin deficiency in conjunction with Coxsackie B virus. In fact, Dr. Tang said that in his experience of 30 years he had never seen a myocardial infarction that was not positive for Coxsackie B at the same time. I routinely screen for and eradicate Coxsackie B whenever I find it. Most EKGs and holter monitors in young or middle-aged adults show very little treatable findings. I now energetically screen all my patients for Chlamydia pneumonia (possible cause of atherosclerosis) and will treat them if found to be positive.

There is a homeopathic relationship between suppressed or treated gonorrhea and heart disease, and one should ask about a history of gonorrhea in all cardiac patients. This predilection can be altered with homeopathy.

To put it all in perspective, most cardiac problems originate in a broken heart!

13. **Hepato-Biliary Tract** — The liver and gallbladder are severly impacted by emotional issues including anger, suppressed anger, and resentment — all common emotions of our time. Historic evidence of infantile jaundice, a bad infectious mononucleosis, hepatitis, or chemical exposure will alert you to problems in the liver. Some patients have never been well since their Hepatitis B immunizations, and energetically still carry the imprint in their livers. Other patients have always shown detoxification reactions with coffee, or show an absolute intolerance to fats or rich meals. Patients who suffer from ingrown toenails of the inner aspect of the big toe (Ting point of the Liver meridian), migraines, or occipital headaches, TMJ, fatigue or hip pain, all have a problem with this organ system.

It is interesting to note that almost half of my patients who have undergone cholecystectomy for abdominal pain in the right upper quadrant, still have the pain. The organ was removed, but the energetic imbalance lives on.

14. **Hormones** — The *thyroid gland* is the most undertreated and misunderstood endocrine organ. Most patients with thyroid problems will have a maternal history of some kind of thyroid problem. In females, all thyroid problems reflect a dysfunction of the fifth chakra (throat chakra) due to suppression of its energetic and actual function, communication. Look for the communication issue and correct it if possible, before you blithely prescribe Synthroid®. The other issue regarding thyroid is the fact that the TSH normal ranges are incorrect. Because of the high number (up to 20% by recent figures) of subclinical hypothyroid patients, the normal upper limit of the TSH level is much too high, and any patient with a TSH above 2.5 is actually hypothyroid and needs to be supplemented. How do I know? (1) Because I have tested these patients and asked the question regarding whether they need supplementation or not, and (2) the ultimate test, the patients felt so much better without any toxic signs or symptoms. Their energy improved, their hair stopped falling out, their menses normalized, and their skin became more moist. The other issue is many of these patients, particularly those patients with fibromyalgia, have a problem utilizing just T4. Either they cannot convert it to T3 or they have refractory T3 receptors, and have an absolute need for a mixture of T4 and T3, which I give them as Thyrolar®, or Synthroid® with Cytomel®, or as Armour® Thyroid. It is also of great interest that very large doses of oral Cytomel (100 to 200 microgms or more), in 50% of my fibromyalgics, takes away most of their pain, with absolutely no toxic hyperthyroid side effects. For some sensitive patients I have had Cytomel® and Ketoprofen® mixed in a gel for local application to muscles,with great symptomatic relief.

Female hormones are an absolute nightmare unless you have a systematic way to handle them. Chinese medicine has a very nice separation of the pre- and postovulatory phases of the female cycle — the preovulatory estrogenic phase is related to the buildup of Yin and Blood (Liver), and the postovulatory progestational phase is related to Yang and Qi. Likewise, the hot flashes in menopause are related to either Liver Yin or Kidney Yin deficiency with blazing Fire, and can be successfully treated.

15. **Kidneys and Prostate** — A history in the family of renal stones or any other kidney or bladder problem, especially any congenital structural problem with ureters or urethra, will inidicate Kidney weakness. Most bald-headed males have a propencity for Kidney deficiency, this trait being passed from mother to son and from father to daughter and so on. Children will often manifest this deficiency early on as enuresis (usually inherited from father). Females with chronic urinary tract infections should be investigated for structural defects, and then asked about sexual abuse.

    The prostate will always have some energetic problem if there is a history of gonorrhea. Otherwise the regular screening of digital exam and PSA should be routinely done.

16. **Allergy** — This symptom has so many manifestations that questioning is mandatory. Above and beyond the normal hayfever and allergic rhinitis, symptoms such as poor concentration and brain fog, headaches, urinary irritation, and gastrointestinal complaints are important. Allergy to cats is almost specific for the homeopathic remedy Tuberculinum. Investigate the effects of petroleum products such as perfumes, paints, and gasoline fumes. Common household products may also produce symptoms in the sensitive. Differential symptoms at home, in the car, or at work may provide clues. Food sensitivity is often overlooked but, with mold sensitivity, accounts for more than 70% of symptoms. Any allergic symptom that does not fluctuate through the year and get worse in spring, summer, or fall, is not an environmental, but is related to mold or foods. Appearance of symptoms in the winter usually relates to petroleum sensitivity to forced air gas or oil heating, or reaction to the smoke of wood burning. In Nevada and California the pollution from forest fires is an important allergen. Many allergens are integrally connected to old childhood memories and will be triggered by emotional events as discussed earlier in the book. The multiple chemical sensitivity syndrome, in my experience, is an emotional disease, with allergy being the surrogate symptomatology for unresolved emotional issues. I say that with some assurance due to the following clinical observation in not one, but many of these unfortunate patients. If you test these patients for allergy, they will demonstrate 20 to 30 allergens. If you desensitize them, and they show a good clinical response and have lost sensitivity to those allergens, retesting them against the original panel of 200 or so allergens, will now result in positive tests for another 20 to 30 different allergens to which they were not sensitive originally. You can go on doing the allergy round robin until you are blue in the face with these patients. This is not to say that they do not have allergic symptoms, they certainly do, but their origin is self-induced to balance the whole.

17. **Menstrual History** — Most girls will follow their mother's menstrual pattern. If puberty is early, then menopause will be late; and if puberty is late, then menopause will be early. Girls who stutter and start at puberty, with irregularity at the beginning, will maintain that pattern throughout life. Anemia and Blood deficiency severely affect the menstrual period and need to be corrected. The Liver and the hormone line (Triple Heater) are connected, and the Liver controls the menstrual blood, so that the Liver is extremely pivotal in menstrual irregularities. Any issue impacting the Liver, emotional or physiological, will impact the menses. The hormones of the body do not work in isolation, so look for other hormonal abnormalities, especially thyroid problems. Young girls with dysmenorrhea are sometimes suffering from Cold invasion of the uterus due to too scanty clothing in the pelvic region during cold winter days, sometimes seen in cheerleaders or swimmers.

18. **Food and Cravings** — Each patient will demonstrate a particular food preference or preferences. These preferences will indicate old childhood food imprinted patterns, organ deficiency connections, or focal physiological needs. The table of the Five Elements gives the relationships of the organ pole and the associated food craving: salt = Kidney, sour = Liver, bitter = Heart, spicy = Lung, and sweet = Spleen. Many women will demonstrate a craving for chocolate at menses, as an indicator of magnesium deficiency.

Some patients will chew ice, an observation connected with iron deficiency and certain homeopathic remedies. Any departure from, or significant change in normal tastes is an indicator of a major shift in the body. Abstinence from food with the craved flavor will usually decrease the craving, this being the connection between allergy and addiction. The emotional components of food and addiction were discussed previously.

19. **Affinities** — This is a mixed bag of facts that relate to things and preferences that seem to characterize or otherwise affect the patient or his or her disease manifestations. Some patients will respond positively or negatively at the change of the seasons, during the full moon, on wintery overcast days, and in the bright sunlight. Some patients hate the wind, some the damp, some love the rain, some hate the mountains and love the coast. All these affinities will characterize your patient and allow the correct remedy to be prescribed.

## THE INTEGRATED PHYSICAL EXAM

The physical exam will confirm, with physical correlates, the impressions of the integrated medical history. The essence of the exam is to assess three areas of interest that fully document the "dis-ease":

a. Surface energy and meridian blockages, usually experienced as pain, muscle spasm, and limitation of movement;
b. Status of the internal Zang Fu organs;
c. Relationships and interactions of the affected organs and associated symptoms.

Of course, a regular physical exam is included with the energetic exam, but is not documented here for reasons of brevity.

1. **General Observations** — It is useful to observe the patient in the waiting room, walking into your consulting room, or their interplay with your office staff before you get to see them formally. First, get a gestalt of their whole demeanor. Are they type-A, are they withdrawn, are they embarassed, apologetic, defiant, or compliant. Observe their complexion, coloring, state of their skin and hair; e.g., pale, ruddy, dark rings under the eyes (allergic or Kidney deficiency), dry, oily, unkempt, or well-groomed. Are the lips full, red, chapped, or pursed? Do they look refreshed and eager, or tired and depressed? Do they face you and talk into your eyes or never look directly at you? Are they seductive, spacey, or boring? Do you struggle to make them talk or are they loquatious and hard to stop? The patient's voice is important — is it pitiful, wailing, quiet, overbearing, angry — try and imagine what the patient looks like just by hearing his or her voice. The way the patient is clothed will give an indication regarding his or her background and the personality involved. I remember as a child when I would catch the public bus, I would look at the shoes of people sitting opposite me and try to guess what they did for a living based on their shoes.

    All these individualized qualities make up the personality housing the imbalance that you are about to assess, and you should get an early start in understanding and appreciating the background on which this manifestation has been superimposed.

2. **Pulses** — The Chinese pulses, taken on the radial artery at the wrist, can be used to assess the present state of the Yin and Yang organs, or they can be felt before and after treatment to monitor the effects of treatment. The Chinese, some American practitioners, and Ayurvedic practitioners are able to use the pulse to diagnose the entire imbalance of the individual. The radial pulse becomes the arbitor of the clinical state. I have adopted a much simpler use for the pulse — finding out which is the weakest Yin organ. This is

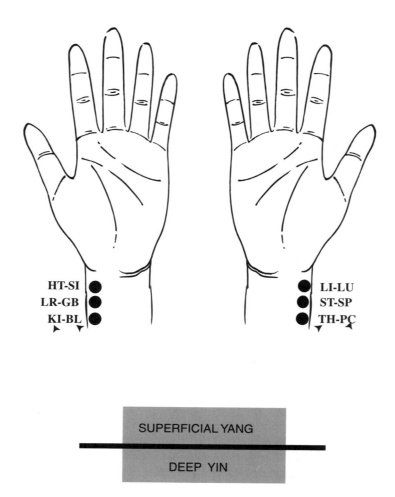

**FIGURE 16.1** Radial pulses.

a more Japanese meridian style of approach. I then do a minor superficial needle tonification of that Yin organ before proceeding to more definitive acupuncture treatment.

The radial pulse is taken with three fingers, the second, third and fourth fingers, which are placed with the third finger over the radial styloid process, the examiner's hand curling over from the dorsal aspect of the patient's arm, and the other two fingers on either side of the styloid process over the radial artery (Figure 16.1). The artery is compressed to feel its pulsatile strength, and then slowly released to appreciate its depth and fullness. The Yang organs are felt superficially, the Yin organs are felt deeply. The three positions of the pulse — proximal, middle, and distal correspond to the Lower, Middle, and Upper Heaters respectively. The Yin and Yang organs are represented on one side or the other of the left or right arms:

|  | RIGHT ARM | LEFT ARM |
|---|---|---|
| **Proximal Position** | | |
| Superficial | Triple Heater (TH) | Bladder (BL) |
| Deep | Pericardium (PC) | Kidney (KI) |

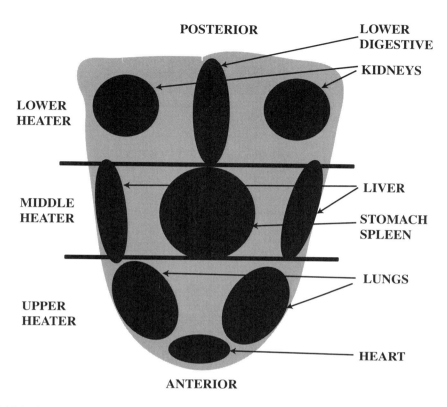

**FIGURE 16.2** Organs on the tongue.

**Middle Position**

| | | |
|---|---|---|
| Superficial | Stomach (ST) | Gall Bladder (GB) |
| Deep | Spleen (SP) | Liver (LR) |

**Distal Position**

| | | |
|---|---|---|
| Superficial | Large Intestine (LI) | Small Intestine (SI) |
| Deep | Lung (LU) | Heart (HT) |

3. **Tongue Diagnosis** — The tongue is the indicator of what the organs look like from within the body. The tongue takes some time to change, and so is more like a HbA1c as opposed to a static blood sugar, which would represent taking of the radial pulse.

   The tongue is divided into regions representing the Upper Heater (anterior 1/3), the Middle Heater (middle 1/3), and the Lower Heater (back 1/3). It is also divided into regions representing the Yin–Yang organ pairs, as yet another somatotopic microreflex system (Figure 16.2):

ANATOMICAL AREA YIN — YANG ORGAN PATTERN

| | | |
|---|---|---|
| Tip | Heart and Pericardium | Red — excess Yang |
| Lateral Sides | Liver and Gall Bladder | Orange/red — excess Yang |
| Center | Stomach and Spleen | Red or pale — Heat or deficient Yin |
| Anterior 1/3 | Lungs | Red — Heat or deficient Yin |
| Posterior 1/3 | Kidney and Bladder | White — Yin; Yellow — Yang |

The color, shape and size, coating, and moisture of the tongue are also diagnostic clues to the inner body.

a.  **Color** — The tongue color is the single most important aspect of tongue diagnosis. The normal tongue color is pale and pink and slightly moist with little or a thin translucent coating. The color of the tongue reflects the state of the Organs, Blood and Qi. Heat and Cold, Yin and Yang, and stagnation of Qi or Blood can be diagnosed from the tongue.

*   *Pale tongue* indicates a Blood deficiency (dry, mostly in females) or a Yang deficiency (wet, mostly in males) that has failed to supply the tongue with Blood.
*   *Red tongue* is always pathological. It represents Heat; from excess has a yellow coating, while Heat from deficiency (False Heat) has no coating.
*   *Red with red points or spots* indicates Heat with Blood stasis, the bigger the spots, the more stasis is present.
*   *Red with prickles* (red and raised papillae) indicates Heat in the Upper Burner, usually seen in febrile diseases.
*   *Red and peeled* indicates long standing Kidney Yin deficiency with excess chronic Heat.
*   *Purple* always indicates Blood stasis.
*   *Blue* indicates Internal Cold with Blood stasis.

b.  **Body Shape** — Here we include body shape, consistency, texture, and motility. They will reflect deficiency or excess and the state of the Blood.

*   Thin tongue suggests deficiency of Fluids and Yin.
*   Swollen tongue is usually a sign of deficient Yang and Excess Dampness.
*   Stiff tongue is due to extreme Heat from some Excess condition.
*   Flaccid tongue indicates Heart and Spleen Qi deficiency with Blood deficiency.
*   Cracked tongue indicates an exhaustion of Blood. Long horizontal cracks indicate an exhaustion of Yin; ice floes indicate Yin deficiency from old age; transverse cracks on sides indicate chronic Spleen Qi deficiency; vertical crack in the center is due to stomach Qi deficiency; a vertical crack that extends to the tip is related to Heart Qui deficiency and Heat.
*   Deviated tongue indicates wind, External or Internal.
*   Quivering tongue indicates Qi and Blood deficiency with associated Spleen Yang deficiency.
*   Tooth marked tongue indicates Spleen Qi deficiency.

c.  **Tongue coating** — This is an indicator of the digestive function of the Spleen and the Stomach. Coatings can change quickly in response to treatment and pathology.

*   *Thick coat* indicates Excess; *thin coat* or no coat Deficiency.
*   *Root or attatchment* to underlying tongue — If the coating cannot be brushed off indicates a normal situation if the coating is thin, but a pathogenic situation if the coating is thick. If the coating is rootless, that is can be brushed off with ease, it indicates Stomach, Spleen, and Kidney deficiency.
*   *Greasy coating* indicates Phlegm. It is thicker in the middle than at the periphery.
*   *White coating* indicates a Cold condition.
*   *Yellow coating* indicates a Hot condition.
*   *Black, dry, and cracked coating* indicates serious Yin depletion.

d.  **Moisture** — The moisture of the tongue reflects the balance between Heat and Cold, Dry and Wet states.

*   *Dry tongue* indicates excess heat and loss of Yin and fluids.
*   *Wet tongue*, if just moist, is normal; if wet and swollen, it indicates Dampness and decreased Yang.

4. **Ear, Nose, and Throat** — The ENT examination is important as it reflects the status of the associated Yin organs. It also is an indicator of the state of the tissue derived from the embryonic endoderm.

   - *The ears* are controlled by the Kidney, and any symptoms are related to the Kidney Yin, such as tinnitus, deafness, and vertigo. The state of the drum and mucosa is an inner view of the entire local pharyngeal area, and is most useful in diagnosing allergic mucosal responses and viral and bacterial invasion of the sinuses, pharynx, and eustachian tube. The auricle should also be examined at this time, both visually and with a blunt probe or an electronic resistance device, to assess the somatotypic information of the ear microsystem. The Principal meridians controlling the ear anatomical area are the TH and GB meridians, which wrap around the ear.

   - *The nose and sinuses* are controlled by the Lung. If pressure elicits local pain or discomfort over the maxillary sinuses (LI and ST meridians) or the frontal sinuses, ethmoids and sphenoids (BL and GB meridians), or the sinuses are congested and blocked, then the sinuses should receive a local and distal acupuncture treatment.

   - *The lips and mouth* are controlled by the Spleen. Inspection of the lips will reveal the state of the Spleen. The lips and pleen are normal if the lips are full, red, and moist. Lips that are thin, dry, and cracked indicate Stomach Heat and Yin deficiency because the paired Stomach tends to dryness; and, if the lips are pale and swollen, this indicates Spleen Qi and Yang deficiency.

   - *The eyes* are controlled by the Liver. The sclera and conjunctivae will demonstrate the state of Heat, Blood, or Yin in the Liver. If the eyes are red, or the sclera yellow, this indicates Liver Heat and deficient Liver Yin. If the conjunctiva is pale, this indicate Liver Blood deficiency.

5. **Palpation of Principal Meridians** — the large points of the Yin and Yang Principal meridians should be palpated to document the area of disturbance. First determine if the primary area of imbalance is the ventral, lateral, or dorsal suface of the body. The Yang meridian will usually be the tender one of the pair. The Yang meridians of the upper zone, the head and neck and arm, will have the most tender points. You should already have a good idea from the history:

   - *Ventral surface problems* include cardiovascular disorders, high blood pressure, chest pain, facial neuralgias and palsies, asthma, maxillary sinusitis, hiatal hernia, nausea, dyspepsia, vomiting, loss and increase in appetite, bulemia, colitis, constipation, hypo- and hyperthyroidism, testicular problems, inguinal hernias, shin splints, and weakness.

   - *Lateral surface problems* include high blood pressure, facial twitches and ticks, TMJ, ear problems, lateral neck problems, headaches and migraines, shoulder tension, tight chest, varicose veins, phlebitis, stomach ulcers, constipation, hemorrhoids, gallstones, sweating disorders, hip pain, and lateral sciatica.

   - *Dorsal surface problems* include frontal sinusitis, neck stiffness and pain, vertex headaches, high blood pressure, constipation and diarrhea, urinary and prostate problems, impotence, amenorrhea, all back pain, Cushing's syndrome, ankylosing spondylitis, epilepsy, convulsions, vertigo, insomnia, psoriasis, eczema, acne on forehead and upper back, paranoia, and dorsal sciatica.

6. **Palpation of the Dorsal Musculature** — Start with the posterior occiput at GB-20 and also feel the sternocleidomastoids. Then palpate the neck, checking each cervical segment for tenderness and assessing the range of motion of the neck. Palpate the musculature of the shoulders, especially trapezius, and note if the muscle spasm or tenderness extends down the arm. Remember that carpal tunnel syndrome begins in the cervical spine and shoulder musculature, not in the wrist. Check the scapular associated muscles (levator

scapulae, the rhomboids, supra and infra spinatus, and terres major and minor) as well as the serratus anterior.

Check every segment level of the paraspinal muscles at each Shu point for regional spasticity and tenderness. Note the level and the associated organ. Palpate the post superior iliac sping, the glutei, and then bladder meridian points BL-40 and BL-59 for tenderness.

The upper back and neck reflect SI and BL blocks; the mid-back reflects liver and stomach organ problems, the lower lumbar area reflects kidney organ problems, and the sacral area reflects large intestine and bladder organ and uterine problems.

You should now have a good idea of where most of the surface and meridian blocks are located, and which energy subcircuits are involved. Remember you can have a surface meridian block without organ dysfunction and pathology if the perverse energy has not penetrated deeper than the Wei Qi layer.

7. **Inspection and Palpation of the Abdomen** — First get a general impression of the abdomen. Is it scaphoid, bloated, and swollen? A normal abdomen should be flat, warm, and soft. Next feel the quality of the temperature coming from the upper abdomen (CV-12 to tip of sternum), middle abdomen (umbilicus to CV-12), and lower abdomen (pubic bone to umbilicus). The heat or coldness of each segment will give you an indication of the state of activity of the three Heaters. You should then palpate the abdomen for tenderness bearing in mind all the different examinations of the abdomen (Korean Hand Acupuncture, YNSA, and "Hara" palpations) that are available. If I am not going to use a specific acupuncture subsystem, then I am looking for tenderness in the epigastrium (ST), RUQ (LR and GB), LUQ (SP and ST), LLQ (LI), RLQ (LI and SI), and suprapubic area (BL and female organs). Small enlargements of the liver are significant and represent Blood stagnation and portal venous system congestion. I then slide my hands around dorsally to the renal angles and palpate firmly. You may be surprised how often that maneuver brings out a negative patient reaction.

8. **Scars and Lesions** — You should do a systematic search for all scars, both large and small, and document them. At the same time, do a skin lesion and soft tissue tumor survey. Note if any of the scars is livid, hypertrophic, or itchy, or happens to cross one of the affected meridians or organ lines. Muscle test to see if any of these scars is causing a problem. If a positive response is elicited, the scar should be infiltrated with 1% lidocaine and homeopathic Silica. The most significant scars are those of operations, after which the patient has never felt well, or horizontal scars, such as a Pfannenstiel incission (bikini cut), for hysterectomy or Caesarian section.

## THE INTEGRATED ENERGETIC EXAM

In the energetic exam, the patient's energetic past and present are revealed by the use of *meridian stress assessment*. This is a measurement of the energetic standing waveform, which disturbs and influences the patient's reactive chaotic choice and is the primary arbitrator of the eventual physical manifestation seen on the physical exam. These energetic anomalies are appreciated as a *focus of interference* or a *field of interference* that causes changes in the autonomic nervous system, hypothalamus and the connective tissue mesenchyme. Thus, energetic disturbances in one part of the body can affect any other part of the body, sometimes at a distance from the original interference field.

This focus, or localized area that has lost its homeostatic regulating capacity, acts like a hidden energetic disturbance, causing dysfunction and imbalance in organs, systems, and meridians. The presence of these occult energetic disturbances can be suspected from the history including a history of repeated streptococcal infections and then the sudden appearance later in life of nonspecific arthralgias; a history of severe mononucleosis that produces a patient that always tests weak on the liver; or a patient who has not been well since that dental work, or since being on that antibiotic, etc.

The *common energetic foci* include:

- *Bacteria* — usually inadequately treated or suppressed with antibiotics. Most important include Strep, Staph, Salmonella, S. pneumoniae, Mycoplasma pneumonia, Chlamydia, and other sexually transmitted diseases.
- *Viruses* — influenza, infectious mononulceosis, cytomegallo virus (CMV), Coxsackie B, Rabies (from pet innoculation), Herpes group, Hepatitis B immunization, and polio.
- *Teeth* — bad root canals, devitalized teeth, dry sockets, root cysts, granulomas, jaw osteitis, incompatible dental material with electro-microcurrents, and impacted teeth.
- *Anatomical sites of chronic infection* — tonsils, sinuses, mastoids, appendicitis, cholecystitis, pyelonephritis, and pelvic infection.
- *Scars* — any or all of them.
- *Antibiotics, drugs, and immunizations* — any of these suppressive treatments may leave mesenchymal residuals of their activity that causes a local energetic disturbance.

The protocol of measurement is as follows:

a. The *Control Measurement Points* (CMPs) of all the organs are measured, and the values (normal, inflamed or irritated, or degenerated) are recorded.
b. The *pattern of disturbance* is analyzed as to the probable cause. For instance if you see the lymph, lung, nerve, and endocrine points irritated, the probable cause is a virus.
c. The *disturbed meridian is provoked* with the energetic signature of the proposed cause e.g., the virus, and a resonant return to a normal or below normal reading indicates harmonic resonance or "identity" with the provoking frequency. Each abnormal meridian is addressed in the same way, until all abnormal meridians have been balanced by the provoking frequencies. If the cause of imbalance is unknown, each meridian is screened for problems with the following stressors: viruses, bacteria, fungi, parasites, dental problems, hormones, heavy metals, chemicals, allergy, electromagnetics, radiation, neurotransmitters and emotions. The resonant frequency library has over 30,000 different items to choose from for this job.

You now have an energetic picture of the patient's organs and the pathophysiology affecting those organs. Depending on the resonant frequency multiple chosen to provoke the abnormal meridian, you can determine whether the pathophysiological process is active, or recent or in the long past. So, you can build up a longitudinal picture of the historic disease and responses of an organ, up to its present state of being.

Now use biokinesiology to construct the relationships between the organs and their pathology. The protocol is as follows:

a. Determine the *head of the causal chain* — In every patient there is usually a dominant weak organ that is causing most of the trouble and influencing adjacent or energetically related organs. It is important to treat this organ first, as most of the complaints will disappear with treatment of the root cause organ, instead of treating every single symptom.
b. Determine *the number of causal chains* — The head organ may have influence in two different directions, and you may decide to support one direction and not the other, according to your clinical experience with this patient. An example of this might be a Kidney that is deficient and head of the causal chain. Its one causal chain is affecting the Lung and causing Kidney deficient asthma, while the other causal chain is not feeding into the Liver and causing deficient Liver Qi and, hence, generalized fatigue. The asthma is more important than the fatigue, and so this causal chain is addressed first (you can test which one the body wants to be treated first), and, usually, the secondary causal

chain will also get some help in the process. This is done by nudging the direction of preferred reaction utilizing the acupuncture Sheng and Ko cycle rules, specific herbal blends, nutritional therapy, or constitutional or organ-specific homeopathic remedies.

You now have all the information regarding the patient's history, the physical exam, and the energetic exam, and all that is left is an appropriate laboratory exam. I am not going to say much about the laboratory, even though I am a pathologist, apart from the fact that static testing is almost useless and that all your testing, to be of any real value, should be dynamic, that is, provoke the patient and look at a response, to get an idea of the function and individual weaknesses and strengths of the liver, kidney, or gut. The only static testing of value relates to levels of nutrients and toxic substances such as heavy metals, or the documentation of a culture or sensitivity.

It is now time to put everything together into a patient assessment and develop a therapeutic plan of attack.

## THE INTEGRATED PATIENT ASSESSMENT

The only criteria of success in the patient's eyes is the disappearance of symptoms and the appearance of wellness. You may have to go through a circuitous route to get there, not quite what the patient had in mind, but with mutual information sharing and consent, it is possible to get there together and still be intact.

The rules of treatment are a little different in the different modalities. In Chinese medicine you have to decide if you are going to treat the acute superficial symptoms first or tonify the deeper root from which these acute symptoms arise. You could also address the Yin organ pathology first, and the Yang organ pathology later. In *homeopathy*, you are trying to treat the whole picture layer by layer, last disease first, backward through time. What you end up doing is using your common sense. If the acute picture is causing marked morbidity, treat it first, the root will wait. If there are too many presenting symptoms to treat, treat the common root, and let the body weed out the symptoms by the next visit. When in doubt, detoxify the liver, improve lymph flow, get the bowel moving, and renal output adequate and smile a lot. The body is a wonderful thing — it won't let you down.

The second encounter is the difficult part. I see patients after two weeks, not before. This gives time for the body to appreciate the input and to respond and manifest again. Check all the original symptoms and what happened to them. Segregate the ones that are left (usually half of the original total) and add any new ones. Disappearance of a symptom or group of symptoms indicates the preferential causation of the body. Get rid of the superficial issues first, but the body still has to manifest the deeper problems. The symptoms that remain are more important, irrespective of what the patient's priorities were. New symptoms can indicate a second underlying layer, or may be part of the residual symptom group that was not able to manifest (or did not need to be manifest) until this time. No response or a worsening response can be interpreted in many ways, but you have to know the patient. The first interpretation is that you really missed the assessment. This is highly unlikely, due to the kinesiological testing of the therapy. It is more likely that you were too vigorous in your treatment, or that the patient was very sensitive and you caused an aggravation of the symptoms. Back off the treatment and wait to see what happens (it's really hard to wait, but it often makes the difference between an inappropriate second prescription and success). If the patient still worsens, you have a bad dense pathology going on and need to investigate further or refer the patient, or the patient has a hidden agenda, does not want to get better, and is using the disease for various personal purposes. Integrated medicine is very efficient at reconstituting functional imbalances (remember, the problems to the left of the biological wall), but less effective in degenerative and neoplastic diseases.

The patient's perception of change for the better or worse is the most important criteria of success (within reason). Often, one will cause old pathologies to reappear as the patient's biology moves backward in time (Hering's Laws of Cure), and the ride may be rocky. Reassure the patient and let the body have some time to recapitulate and then divest itself of these old patterns of disease. After you have seen the patient once or twice, you end up treating what presents, that is, whatever is in front of you at the time. This is more or less a mopping-up operation of residual chaotic subpatterns.

If you have impacted the patient at the core of his or her problems, the patient should experience a disappearance of symptoms, a marked improvement of overall health, and a feeling of well-being. One should at some point remove hereditary patterns of weakness utilizing homeopatic miasmatic therapy. This will prevent degradation of the genome from generation to generation. This can be done for potential parents before conception or during the pregnancy.

## SELECTION OF MODALITIES AND TREATMENTS

This is not as hard as it may seem, because the problem usually selects the treatment. What modality works with what problem is learned over time with experience, but suffice it to say that using a little of each modality is far superior to using a lot of one modality. Most patients will receive constitutional homeopathic care (for the pure energetic component of the patient) and organopathic homeopathy (for detoxification and regulation); a Chinese herbal combination for tonification of the root imbalances; therapeutic nutritional support and dietary modification for focused therapeutics and to replenish any nutrient deficits, respectively; acupuncture to regulate the Qi imbalance; and emotional support to understand the meaning and origin of the imbalances. Body work and hypnosis is added as necessary. Regular drugs are added and used in conjunction, or as stand-alone therapies if appropriate. The combination of regular drugs and alternative therapies is tricky for the uninitiated, but allows a more global bodily response and usually a decrease in the amount of regular drugs used. At all times, energetic and global therapies are preferred to suppressive therapies. Replacement therapy, such as insulin or thyroid hormone, is regulated within the total treatment input (it may change up or down depending on what other therapies you are using) and is dosed using biokinesiology (what does the body say it needs, not what the lab test says it needs).

In selection of the medications for each patient, the following protocol is used:

a. *Modality* — Muscle test to find out which modalities are appropriate at this visit. Which is the most important modality for the whole body? In what sequence should they be administered?

b. *Therapeutics* — Provoke each selected substance against the abnormal meridian readings and see what substance balances the reading. Select the least number of substances that balance the most readings. When complete, the entire meridian stress assessment (MSA) should be balanced. Now, test the combination of substances — homeopathics, herbs, nutritionals, and drugs together — for efficacy and tolerance using biokinesiology (should be strong in both directions when rubbing PC-6 up and down the arm) (Figure 16.3). This now represents the prescription for the first two weeks. At each interview this process is repeated until the MSA is balanced and the patient has no symptoms and is visibly better. If the MSA is in balance and the patient is still symptomatic, you are dealing with a nonorganic lesion (emotional block), or a neoplastic problem or you have missed a pure gross physical obstacle to cure. MSA cannot diagnose anything, it just shows the resonant relationship of the frequency composite standing waves to each other and to your provoking frequency stressors.

We, as all other physicians, don't cure everybody, but our percentages and patient (and doctor) satisfaction are better. Most diseases have their origin, as I have discussed, in an emotionally blocked core and are mostly functional, not organic problems. Integrated medicine, by reason of its broad therapeutic focus, is able to address the mass of functional disease without further damaging the patient or compromising the cybernetic energy flow of the organism. While most of Western

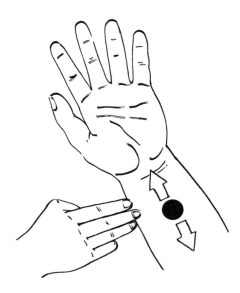

**FIGURE 16.3 PERICARDIUM 6 TEST.**

medicine focuses on suppressive therapy and smaller and smaller therapeutic targets (now single cytokines and the genome), it will miss the true interaction between patient and doctor, that is, *to heal*, not to cure.

## THE ASSESSMENT OF THE BIOLOGICAL TERRAIN

### BIOELECTRONICS OF VINCENT — BTA S-2000

Assessment of the biological terrain was first attempted by Professor L. C. Vincent, a French hydrologist and epidemiologist, in the early 1900s. He was charged with the responsibility of providing potable water to France and her colonies. He noticed in his investigations that there were marked variances in the types of diseases in different areas and postulated a relationship between the quality of water and the occurrence of disease.

He developed the *Bioelectronics of Vincent* (BEV), an objective and scientific way of looking at the biological status of the human body related to its fluid milieu, and its relationship to its state of biological age. His evaluation was able to predict the organism's vulnerability to developing a chronic degenerative condition. BEV does not diagnose a specific disease, it documents the terrain of the individual and the subsequent susceptibility to a group of diseases. BEV has been updated and improved with electrode and computer technology to a single interfaced instrument, the *BTA S-2000*. The Biological Terrain Assessment (BTA) instrument is able to produce a computerized analysis (Figure 16.4) of blood, urine, and saliva for pH (acid/alkaline balance), $rH_2$ (redox potential, oxidative stress), and $r$ (resistivity, reflecting the mineral content). These three measurements are able to assess the nature of the individual's biochemical makeup and provide information regarding the status of the patient's enzymes, amino acids, and other biological parameters. Variations on these parameters are indicative of an individual's predisposition to different pathophysiological states, relating to the associated biophysical terrains.

The pH measurement can indicate the state of alkalinity or acidity of the blood. If the blood is too alkaline or acidic, this will cause a differential function of many pH-specific enzymes and

## Balance Chart

Utilize the "Balance Charts" to assess your patients' pH, redox, and resistivity balance, and compare the results to optimal values.

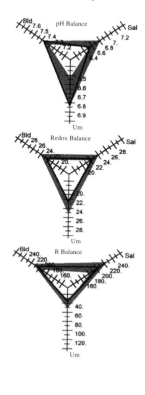

## Histories

Quickly monitor your patients' progress with our "Histories Chart", an exceptional tool for increasing patient compliance.

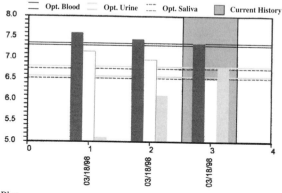

## Plot

Educate your patients with our colorful "Plot", which gives an immediate graphic representation of the biological terrain.

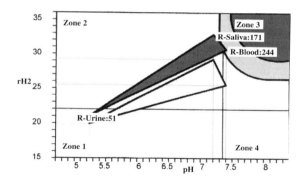

**FIGURE 16.4** Some of the valuable graphs and charts of patient data created by the BTA S-2000 software.

the conformation of certain biological proteins in the body. The digestion and absorption of vitamins, minerals, and nutrients are all dependent on an optimal pH. Environmental xenobiotics and industrial pollutants will all have their effect on the pH.

*Oxidative-stress values* indicate the electron movement and concentration in the patient's system. The effects of stress, poor air quality, and food lacking in nutritional value, along with lack of aerobic exercise, generally result in values much higher than optimal. If these values continue to remain in an elevated state for prolonged periods of time, then the body becomes more susceptible to illness, disease, degeneration, and premature aging.

*Resistivity* indicates the gross mineral concentration of the fluid. If minerals are deficient, enzymatic reactions cannot occur; conversely, if mineral content is elevated, congestion, stagnation of vital fluids, and dystrophic deposition of minerals will occur.

Plotting of the pH and redox potential along the horizontal and vertical axes, respectively, with intersection of the neutral values of each, result in four quadrants of biological terrain:

Quadrant 1  - acid reduced terrain
            - abundant protons
            - abundant electrons
            - area of active life forms
Quadrant 2  - acid-oxidized terrain
            - abundant protons
            - few electrons
            - area of fungal life forms
Quadrant 3  - alkaline-oxidized terrain
            - few protons
            - few electrons
            - area of viral/neoplastic life forms
Quadrant 4  - alkaline-reduced terrain
            - few protons
            - abundant electrons
            - area of bacterial life forms

One of the most significant uses of BTA is as an objective control of the efficacy of any therapy. Using serial measurements over days, weeks, or months, you can determine objectively the direction of clinical response at a biophysical level, and modify your therapy appropriately. The BTA is also able to provide you with a theoretical *biological age* that can be compared to the chronological age of the patient. Serial measurements of biological age can assist you in therapeutic decisions.

### THE INTEGRATED BIOENERGETIC SCORE INDEX (IBS)

The IBS Index was developed by Roy Martina, M.D. as a practical way of assessing the biological terrain of the patient using biokinesiology and index vial filters.

The patient is tested against three groups of homeopathic filters arranged on a three-dimensional graph that includes biological data pertaining to:

1. *Entoxification* — 0 to 10 on the horizontal axis;
2. *Elimination Block* — 0 to 15 vertical positive axis;
3. *Degenerative Scores* — 0 to 15 vertical negative axis.

Serial testing of the patient after therapy will indicate which of the parameters have improved and where treatment needs to be concentrated. It will also tell you if you are treating too fast for one of the parameters that cannot catch up. For example, if the tox score and the block score are high, you had best go carefully and treat the block first before you try and detox too quickly (Figure 16.5). If the tox score is high and the block score is low, you should begin detoxification slowly, or you will cause a massive dump of toxins into the system, and make the patient feel very uncomfortable.

## DOCTOR ISSUES

Not all physicians can practice Integrated Medicine, nor should they. We need the great surgeons, psychotherapists, and other specialties. Some could incorporate a more holistic approach to their practice and enhance their own satisfaction and results. Practicing in the energetic field (your own and the patient's) has some serious drawbacks. It is very exhausting. It is difficult to practice more than four days a week. Each patient requires focused attention at every level of his or her being, and energetic information is being transferred back and forth during the interview. The doctor needs to be balanced, healthy, and impartial in order to take accurate readings to treat the patient for

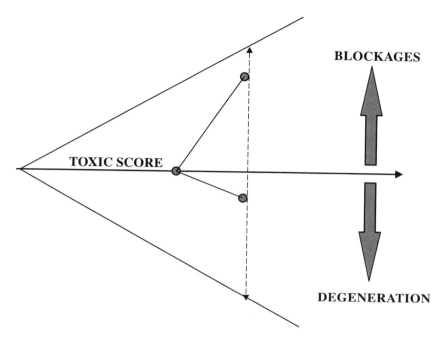

**FIGURE 16.5** The Integrated Bioenergetic Score Index of Roy Martina.

maximum effect. The energy vampires will try to drain you, but in order to protect yourself, you have to develop that condition of connected reservation — you are attached but not part of or affected by the patient. This enables you to see the patient for what he or she truly is, his or her state of grace.

During times of energetic fatigue, a doctor tends to start treating the patient piecemeal (an old pattern) or will use quick suppressive therapy. When this starts to occur it is time for a break, a decrease in the patient load, or a change in the office routine. Once you have made the energetic emotional commitment to a patient, the contract does not change. This contract is not of this reality, and you will be held to it. If a patient is draining, using you, or abusive at any level, you need to dismiss the patient and place him or her in the care of another practitioner.

There are times when you may become very uncentered and doubt your sanity, but the patients always bring you back, because what you see clinically and the results that occur are real, to you and the patient, and that's all that counts.

Up until now there has been very little corroboration of the use of Integrated Medicine and its results. We, at all times, have to have covered the regular allopathic path of examination and assessment, because it is integrated, not alternative medicine we are practicing. The selection of modalities at times will be clear-cut, but at other times will be problematic, and we must always err on the conservative side to afford the patient the best care possible. Integrated Medicine is an ongoing experiment in one sense, but the patient should not become the guinea pig. The offhanded use of one or another miracle cure (and there is a new one every week) is to be deplored.

## PATIENT ISSUES

Almost all of my patients are self-referred by word of mouth. HMO patients are authorized through their primary care doctors, or if their primary is obstructive, they can appeal and self-refer. We send out a cover letter and comprehensive medical questionnaire (Figure 16.6) to each new patient

TRIAD MEDICAL CENTER INC

Kietzke Plaza
4600 Kietzke Lane, Suite M-242
Rerro, Nevada 89502
(702) 829-2277

**PATIENT INFORMATION**　　　Date _____

Please complete all sections of this form.

PLEASE PRINT

## PERSONAL INFORMATION _____

LAST NAME _____　　HOME TEL. # _____
FIRST NAME/S _____　　BUSINESS TEL. # _____
ADDRESS _____ _　　REFERRED TO TRIAD BY _____
CITY _____　　SOCIAL SECURITY # _____
STATE _____ZIP _____　　RELIGIOUS PREFERENCE _____
BIRTHDATE _____　　RESPONSIBLE PARTY _____
SEX　　Male　　Female　　　　　　NAME OF SPOUSE _____
MARITAL STATUS　　Single　Married　Divorced　　NAME OF PARENTS _____
　　　　　　　　　Widowed　Separated　　(if a minor)

## MEDICAL DATA _____

Are you allergic to medications (Penicillin, Vit. B-12, etc.)? _____
Are you allergic to Procaine, Lidocaine, Xylocaine or Novocaine _____
Do you have pets? _____ What kind? _____ Do they live in your home? _____
**Habits**
Do you drink coffee or regular tea? _____ How much? _____
Have you ever used alcohol? _____ How much and how often? _____
Do you smoke or did you ever use tobacco? _____ How much and for how long? _____
Have you ever used heroin, cocaine, LSD, POP, marijuana, etc.? Which ones and how
frequently? _____
Have you ever used sleeping pills and/or pain pills? _____ How often? _____
Do you handle chemicals? _____ Which ones and to what extent? _____
Do you exercise regularly? _____ What type and how often _____
Insurance Company _____

### Patient Information and Informed Consent _____

1. **Acknowledgement Notice to all Medicare Subscribers**
   Please be advised that Triad Medical Center and its physicians do not accept assignment for Medicare. Therefore, please be advised that Medicare may not cover the expenses for services they feel are medically unnecessary. Medicare does not recognize medical acupuncture, homeopathy or nutritional counseling, electro-acupuncture, chelation therapy or Sclerotherapy for tendons and ligaments.

   Although I may not be reimbursed for the above medical /surgical services, I desire said services to be performed by the physicians of Triad Medical Center, and I agree to pay for the above services if payment is denied by Medicare, now and in the future.

2. **General Disclaimer Regarding Non-Toxic Therapy**
   Homeopathy, acupuncture, electro-acupuncture, Chinese herbal therapy, nutritional counseling, bioenergetic medicine, food allergy testing, Sclerotherapy and some instrumentation may not be recognized by some insurance companies, the FDA or traditional medicine as reimbursable or acceptable. Nevertheless, in expressing my constitutional right of freedom of choice of medical care, I choose to be diagnosed and treated by the physicians of Triad Medical Center.

   **RELEASE OF INFORMATION** I hereby authorize release of my medical information to the physician(s) I have been referred to by the physician(s) of Triad Medical Center, or any person designated by me, and to my Insurance carriers.

   I have read, understood and agree to the above statements.
   Patients signature: _____ **Date:** _____
   Parent / Guardian, if minor:

**FIGURE 16.6** Comprehensive Medical Questionnaire sent to patients prior to their first visits.

## MEDICAL DATA

TRIAD MEDICAL CENTER

**CHIEF COMPLAINT AND MAJOR PROBLEMS**

**PREVIOUS DIAGNOSIS**

1.
2.
3.
4.
5.
6.
7.
8.
9.
10.

Have you consulted another Doctor about these problems?
If yes, Doctor s name and diagnosis:

List of previous illnesses/hospitalizations or surgeries

Year

1.
2.
3.
4.
5.
6.
7.
8.
9.
10.

List any medicine, homeopathics, vitamins, minerals or herbs you are taking below:

Medicine/Supplement          Dosage          Year

## ADDITIONAL DATA

Occupation _____     Education _____

Test Year

1. _____ Complete physical exam
2. _____ Chest X-ray
3. _____ Kidney X-ray
4. _____ G.I. X-ray
5. _____ Colon X-ray
6. _____ Gallbladder X-ray
7. _____ Electrocardiogram
8. _____ TB test
9. _____ Sigmoidoscopy
10. _____ CAT/NMR scan
11. _____ Heart catheterization

Year     Immunizations (Adult)

1. _____ Tetanus
2. _____ Influenza
3. _____ DPT
4. _____ Other

Family History
HEALTH

| | GOOD | POOR | DECEASED | AGE AT DEATH AND CAUSE | MEDICAL PROBLEMS |
|---|---|---|---|---|---|
| 1. Yourself | | | | | |
| 2. Father | | | | | |
| 3. Mother | | | | | |
| 4. Brothers & Sisters | | | | | |
| 5. Spouse | | | | | |
| 6. Children | | | | | |

**FIGURE 16.6 (Continued)** Comprehensive Medical Questionnaire sent to patients prior to their first visits.

that has to be filled in prior to the first visit. I do not screen the new patients, as I believe strongly in offering service to all people of the community. Many clinics will have patients fly in from afar and spend a week being treated. I strongly discourage anyone outside of the northern Nevada and eastern California foothills as patients, as I think it is bad medicine. I have a 100-mile exclusionary perimeter, except for supporting old patients who have moved out of the area and cannot find a comparable practitioner.

TRIAD
MEDICAL
CENTER
INC

ENERGETIC HISTORY PLEASE CHECK

A.  Mark your favorite:        1.  FLAVOR          2.  SEASON              3.  COLOR
                                   Sour                Spring                  Blue
                                   Bitter              Summer                  Red
                                   Sweet               Indian Summer           Yellow
                                   Spicy               Fall /Autumn            White
                                   Salty               Winter                  Black

B.  At what time of the day or night are your symptoms worse?  _____

C.  Do you prefer to be inside?      _          D.  Do weather changes effect you?
        or to be outside?            _              _  Yes How?  _____
                                                    _  No       _____

E.  Do you sleep well? _ Yes _ No  If no, elaborate.  _____
    _____

F.  What is your energy level?  worst  1   2   3   4   5   best
G.  What makes your symptoms better?  _____
                        worse?  _____
H.  What was the most significant medical or emotional occurances in your life?  _____
    _____

I.  On a scale of 1 - 10, what do you rate your present stress level?  _____
    What are the stressors in your life?  _____
J.  What is your greatest fear?  _____
K.  What really makes you happy?  _____

**NUTRITIONAL HISTORY**
A. What do you eat and drink for.   1.  Breakfast     _____
                                                      _____
                                    2.  Lunch         _____
                                                      _____
                                    3.  Dinner        _____
                                                      _____
                                    4.  Snacks        _____
                                                      _____

B.  What do you crave to eat?  _____
C.  Do you have any food allergies?   Yes _   What are they?  _____
                                      No _                    _____
D.  Do you have any digestive problems?  _____
E.  Do you have regular bowel actions?  _____
F.  Do you feel sleepy or tired after eating?  _____
G.  Are you able to fast without symptoms?  _____

**ALLERGIC HISTORY**

Do you suffer from any of the following sypmtoms:
    _  asthma        _  fatigue              _  trouble with:   perfumes
    _  rashes        _  headache                               gasoline fumes
    _  hives         _  itchy eyes                             paints, chemicals
    _  hay fever     _  nasal congestion                       smoke
    _  arthritis     _  sinusitis            _  trouble with weight

**FIGURE 16.6 (Continued)** Comprehensive Medical Questionnaire sent to patients prior to their first visits.

Most patients are pretty well informed before they arrive, but I think they are probably preselected for the practice by their referring friends. We treat the young and the old, but have a cutoff below the age of two, and have as a prerequisite, an active pediatric relationship for hospitalizations and other services we do not provide. We try to treat whole families because it makes sense in terms of the holistic pathology and dynamics that occur within most families.

Education is a primary part of the practice. Most of the *patient education* needed is in regard to the emotional component of disease, and the relationship and interconnectedness of all symptoms.

## Medical Data
Mark an X next to any of the following which you have had or now have:

| | | | |
|---|---|---|---|
| _ Anemia | _ Dental Problems | _ Heart Disease | _ Poison - Ivy/Oak |
| _ Allergies | _ Diarrhea - Chronic | _ Head Injury | _ Polyps - Site |
| _ Asthma | _ Digestion Problems | _ Herpes - Location | _ Pancreatitis |
| _ Arteriosclerosis | _ Dysentery | _ Hair Loss | _ Psoriasis |
| _ Arthritis | _ Deafness | _ Hay Fever | _ Phlebitis |
| _ Attention Def. Disorder | _ Drug Addiction | _ Hearing Impairment | _ Polio/Paralysis |
| _ Acne | _ Diverticulitis/osis | _ Hypoglycemia | _ Pneumonia |
| _ Alcohol Problem | _ Diabetes Mellitus | _ Hyperlipidemia | _ Rheumatic Fever |
| _ Appendicitis | _ Eating Problem | _ BloodCt~olesterol/Fats~ | _ Ringworm |
| _ Bronchitis | _ Emphysema | _ Impetigo | _ Strep Throat |
| _ Back Pain | _ Epstein Barr Virus | _ Ingrown Toenails | _ Stomach Ulcers |
| _ Baldness | _ Ear Infections | _ Injuries, serious | _ Scarlet Fever |
| _ Bladder Infection | _ Eye Problems | _ Jaundice, Yellowing | _ Stroke |
| _ Bleeding Tendency | _ Eczema | _ Kidney/Bladder Disease | _ Sexual Dysfunction |
| _ Bloating | _ Eructions | _ Liver Trouble | _ Shingles |
| _ Boils | _ (Burping/Belching) | _ Meningitis | _ Sinusitis |
| _ Bowel Condition | _ Endocrine/Glandular | _ Mental Illness | _ Skin Infections |
| _ Blood Disease | _ Trouble | _ Menstrual Cramps | _ Sore Throat |
| _ Blood Transfusion | _ Epilepsy | _ Migraines | _ Styes |
| _ Cirrhosis (Liver) | _ Fistula/Fissures | _ Mouth Sores | _ Suicide Attempt |
| _ Colds - Recurrent | _ Gall Bladder Disease | _ Measles (Rubella) | _ Syphilis |
| _ Colitis -   Irritable Bowel, | _ Fractures | _ Multiple Sclerosis | _ Scarlet Fever |
|                 Spastic | _ German Measles (Rubella) | _ Mumps | _ Salivary Gland Problem |
| _ Constipation | _ Excess Gas | _ Mononucleosis | _ Thyroid Problem |
| _ Chronic Fatigue | _ Gonorrhea (Clap) | _ Neck Strain | _ Tuberculosis |
| _ Concussion | _ Gout | _ Nose Bleeds | _ Toxic Chemical Poisoning/ |
| _ Cancer | _ Goiter | _ Nervous Breakdown |      Exposure |
| _ Convulsions/Seizures | _ Hyperactivity | _ Neuralgia/Neuritis | _ Tumors |
| _ Congenital Defect | _ High Blood Pressure (HT) | _ Obesity | _ Visual Problems |
| _ Candida/Yeast Infection | _ Heart Attack | _ Palpitations | _ Voice Problems |
| _ Cataracts | _ Heart Murmur | _ Prostate Problems | _ Venereal Disease |
| _ Chicken Pox | _ Heart Condition | _ Parasites (Worms) | _ Warts |
| _ Dandruff | _ Hernia - Location | _ Pain - Chest, Sciatic, | _ Weight Loss/Gain |
| _ Dyslexia | _ Hemorrhoids |      Muscular, Abdomen, | _ Whooping Cough |
| _ Depression | _ Hepatitis |      Headache | |
| | _ Headaches | | |

**FIGURE 16.6 (Continued)** Comprehensive Medical Questionnaire sent to patients prior to their first visits.

Patients usually learn for the first time that we are partners in the healing process, and that they have to take responsibility for their diseases and handle them in a prospective way. We also spend time explaining the homeopaths and herbs, which many patients have not had before, and we have a special instruction room for that activity. The possibility of homeopathic and herbal aggravations is explained and what to do if such a reaction occurs. We have a bibliography of useful books and web sites for the more compulsive and inquisitive patients.

Communication with the patient is perhaps the single most important medical and relation-building activity in a practice. All messages are answered within in an 8-hour time frame, the more urgent ones are screened to be answered immediately or within the hour. This is especially important in an integrated practice, where patients are experiencing energetic movements and new sensations that may be very foreign to them. We are experimenting with contact via e-mail and the Triad Website, which is under construction. Each doctor at the clinic carries a beeper and is available 24 hours a day, 7 days a week. Patients, especially if new, are encouraged to call in with any strange or new experiences, a sign of the body changing. This provides good information for us as to how their biology is responding and reacting. It enables us to build a reactive profile of sensitivity and organ weakness and preferences for each individual patient. Our old patients are very good about calling in only on important issues. We require that all patients have a primary caregiver of some kind for hospital admissions, as we only have hospital privileges on request for medical acupuncture.

## THE INTEGRATED OFFICE AND STAFF

The Integrated Medical office is no different from any other doctor's office, with only a couple of added nuances. The physical plant has to be warm and receptive. What we are servicing is the body, mind, and soul; the office has to reflect that ambiance. Our office is decorated in light rose and teal with a Southwest theme and lots of plants. The reception counter always has fresh flowers. Our wall decor is composed of paintings, wall hangings, photographs, and pottery. My office has a wolf motif, my acupuncture rooms have African wildlife paintings. We have small fountains in the treatment rooms and dimmed lighting. The reception area is open to the waiting room, no little cubbyholes with glass partitions.

The staff has to be mature and stable. We are dealing with serious problems and whole lives. The staff has to be educated about, and believe in, the philosophy of the office and the modalities practiced there. Most of them have experienced acupuncture at least once, and all have had the miracle of homeopathy and a well-crafted Chinese herb work on them. They can speak to the patients from experience. All our staff are very empathetic and have been taught that the patient's attitude and state of mind at any time are part of the pathology to be treated and are never to be judged. The staff is very good at explaining all aspects of this new medical experience to patients on their initial phone calls, and emphasizes the inclusivity of this practice of medicine with the patients' doctors. Patients are encouraged to discuss their experiences and treatment with their doctors and to have their doctors contact us at any time — we and our patients have nothing to hide.

## THE INTEGRATED PHARMACY

The Integrated Medical office is almost forced to keep its own supply of homeopathics, herbs, and nutritionals because of the state of nonstandardization that exists in the market place. All suppliers are inspected by one of us. We tour the plant, talk to the technicians, and only use suppliers that have been passed the GMP (Good Manufacturing Practices) standards. We need to have very strong control of the quality of what we are giving our patients. All the lines we use are professional lines. We will often compound our own mixtures for individual patient needs.

The pharmacy needs to be in compliance with all local and federal laws. To accomplish this end of compliance, we have a software program that tracks every patient and all the medications that patient has been given for the last 10 years. It prints out a label for the medication each time it is dispensed, identical to the label on the drugs from a pharmacy; prints out a superbill for the medication; tracks refills; and updates the inventory. It also tracks both physician and seasonal usage, so that we can order medications in advance of the flu season or the allergy season. We are continually updating our inventory and trying new mixtures and supplements as they arrive on the market. We also keep samples of regular drugs for muscle testing before we use any new drug that is being promoted on the market. Based on energetic testing, we warned our patients about the Lung disharmony produced by the diet drug combination Phen Fen, long before it all came crashing down. We have also warned our male patients about the use of Viagra with cardiac problems.

In ten years of practice we have had almost no herb–drug interactions of note, due to energetic testing of the combinations before prescribing.

## PROFESSIONAL ISSUES AND RELATIONS

Our relations with doctors in the community are, for the most part, cordial. We respect them and we get good enough results for them to respect us. If we share patients, we are very careful to inform them of what is being done, even if they don't understand why we are doing it. It is just like any other group of professionals, the good doctors are happy to see their patients improving at our hands, and we have respect for their opinions and attitudes as befits professionals. We have a group of specialists to whom we refer, and when they get into trouble, they refer back. I have honorary privileges at one large hospital and I am allowed, on application by any patient, to practice medical acupuncture if requested. I am allowed to visit any of my own patients in any of the hospitals and have access to their medical notes. We are called upon to speak all the time and have a very good rapport with the press and television.

The State of Nevada, Board of Medical Examiners, has condoned and included medical acupuncture, herbology, homeopathy, and therapeutic nutrition in its list of medical specialities, and these activities are counted as CME. The State of Nevada also has a Board of Homeopathic Medical Examiners that controls unlicensed M.D.s, that is, M.D.s who practice homeopathy but are not licensed to practice medicine in the state. We also have a state Oriental Medicine Board that regulates non-M.D. acupuncturists. Our relation with that board has always been somewhat adversarial. Other states have adopted their own versions of regulation. Arizona lumps all alternate practitioners, M.D.s and non-M.D.s, into one category overseen by one board. Some states do not allow M.D.s to practice acupuncture if they have not passed the non-M.D. acupuncture exam.

The major problems facing Integrated Medicine throughout the country are the lack of certified education, problems with credentialing, and no real Board of Integrated Medicine. Joseph Helms, M.D. has, through the American Academy of Medical Acupuncture, instituted a proficiency exam and is in the process of trying to establish a specialty board.

Up until this year (2000), malpractice insurance was not a problem. It was cheap and easy to obtain. But, with the new popularity of alternative medicine, and the woeful lack of training, the insurer's experience with alternative medicine has turned sour and the premiums have skyrocketed.

## INTEGRATED MEDICINE, HMOs, AND MANAGED CARE

We were lucky to be approached by two large HMOs in the mid-1990s to join their plans. This was not due to any altruism on their part, but to subscriber requests, and resulted in one large employer's picking the one HMO over another due to our availability. Our relationship with these two HMOs (together with 80,000 members) was difficult at first. They did not understand what we did, kept on treating us as general practitioners, and could not understand why it took me 20 minutes to see a patient with chronic sinusitis. Their computer programs did not allow for our mode of care. However, with perseverance and lots of communication, we have both settled into a harmonious relationship, and half of our patients now belong to an HMO. The one HMO, at one stage, tried to put us on capitation, but we were so popular as general practitioners that the other doctors started to complain. Also, we could beat capitation every time with our home kits and reactive medical profile of each patient, telling us whether or not we needed to see them. The HMOs will, in general, pay for the office visit, even if it is a bit longer than customary, and, in our case, will pay a discounted rate for homeopathics, herbs, and nutritionals. They do not pay for over-the-counter (OTC) nutritional, just as they won't for regular OTC drugs. We have to get authorization for visits, but in the long run we save them so much money through fewer hospitalizations, expensive multidrug use, and surgeries, that we have very little trouble. Whenever they try to decrease the Integrated Medicine component of a program, the members put up such a fuss (and believe me, they are vocal), that any change soon dies in favor of hassling someone else. Many HMOs and insurance carriers will cover some form of Integrated Medicine, be it chiropractic, acupuncture, or massage. Some states, such as Washington, mandate coverage.

We do see Medicare patients but, as Medicare regards acupuncture, homeopathy, herbs, or nutrition as fraudulent, we bill our services as a noncovered service. The visit is then denied and the secondary insurer will pick up the cost according to the provisions of the plan.

# 17 Example of the Integrated Management of a Disease: Acute and Chronic Sinusitis

## OVERVIEW

**Definition and symptoms** — Acute and chronic sinusitis is an inflammation or infection of the paranasal sinuses that causes a feeling of congestion, mucoid or mucopurulent nasal discharge, postnasal drip, cough, local pain, and headache with fatigue and malaise.

**Embryology and esoteric anatomy and physiology** — The sinuses are part of the endoderm, together with the bowel, liver, pancreas, and lungs. Anything affecting one part of the endoderm, affects it all. In TCM the sinuses are considered part of the Lung, which is in the same energetic line as the Spleen, Stomach, and Large Intestine. The Stomach, Large Intestine, and Small Intestine acupuncture meridians all either end or begin in the area overlying the maxillary sinuses. The Kidney and Bladder meridians overlie the frontal and ethmoidal sinuses.

**Etiology and risk factors** — The majority of cases are chronic with acute exacerbations. The predisposing and etiological factors include, in order of importance:

1. **Allergic diathesis** — usually food or environmental allergies. Food allergies include dairy, wheat, corn, sugar, yeast, and soybeans. Environmental allergies include pollens of trees, grasses, weeds, and some bushes. Dust, animal fur and epithelium, smoke, perfumes, and mold fill out the remainder.
2. **Infections** — viral, bacterial, and fungal infections. Look for rhinovirus, enterovirus, Coxsackie A and B, Coronavirus, Echovirus, Respiratory Syneytial Virus (RSV), influenza, and parainfluenza viruses. Bacteria include Streptococcus pneumoniae, H. Influenzae, and Branhamella catarrhalis. Anaerobes are rarely found. Fungal cultures will be positive in 30 to 40% of recalcitrant cases — mainly Candida species, Mucor and Aspergillus.
3. **Bowel dysbiosis** — large bowel symptoms including chronic constipation, diarrhea, irritable bowel, or even chronic colitis in almost all cases of chronic sinusitis. Most have a yeast overgrowth dependent on multiple antibiotic usage, birth control pills, or excessive sugar and carbohydrate ingestion.
4. **Physical issues** — deviated septum, foreign body, small osteomeatal complex, and large nasal polyps. These must be ruled out with appropriate investigations.

## PHYSICAL AND ENERGETIC EXAM

**Physical** — Allergic and Kidney Yin deficient patients will have dark rings under their eyes (allergic shiners). Red or scaly rashes or seborrhea in the area of the corners of the mouth or around the nasal alae (LI-20) or inner aspect of the eyebrows (BL-2) reveal the associated organ dysfunction. The maxillary and frontal sinuses should be palpated to elicit discomfort or pain. The Large Intestine, Spleen, and Lung meridians should be palpated for tender acupoints (LI-10, LI-11, SP-6, SP-9, ST-36, ST-40).

The *tongue* will be swollen and pale with Spleen Dampness, red and dry with Kidney Yin deficiency, and coated yellow (Heat, acute) or white (Cold, chronic) showing Phlegm forming.

The *ears* will demonstrate fluid (chronic picture) or be acutely irritated (acute picture). Pharynx will show irritation with postnasal drip (either colored, Hot; or clear/pale, Cold).

Palpation of the *abdomen* will reveal it to be bloated and tender over the colon. Evidence of yeast elsewhere in the body includes dermatophytoses, onychomycosis, and fungal infections of the ears with itching.

**TCM** — due to invasion by either Wind, Cold, Heat, Fire, or toxins of the Lung and by extension, into the nose. If the mucus is clear, the invasion is by Wind-Cold; if purulent, by Wind-Heat. Nasal stuffiness and obstruction is a result of Lung Qi stagnation. A dry obstructed nose is caused by a deficiency of Lung Yin. Redness, swelling, and erosion of the nose are due to lung heat. Sneezing with nasal drip is due to Lung Qi deficiency.

**MSA** — high readings: Lymph, Sinus, Large Intestine, Allergy, Liver, and Kidney. Test for bacteria, viruses, fungi, and allergens. Test bowel for dysbiosis and food allergy.

## TREATMENT AND FOLLOWUP

### Root Treatment

1. **Homeopathy**
   - Tuberculinum bovinum 200C (Cel) — x 3 doses on three successive days, especially patients with cat and milk allergy, who are prone to lung involvement.
   - Medorrhinum 200C (Cel) — x 3 doses the following month.
   - These miasmatic therapies should be given in an intercurrent manner, between acute attacks and before the spring or fall allergy season.
2. **Probiotics**
   - Enterogenic capsules (Tyl) — 2 caps 3x/day in between meals if yeast overgrowth is moderate.
   - Candid complex (Tyl) — 2 caps 3x/day in between meals if yeast overgrowth is severe.
3. **Chinese Herbs and Acupuncture** — The underlying root causes of sinusitis (usually a heat presentation) arise in Lung, Spleen, and Stomach Qi deficiency and Dampness. Herbs are needed to tonify the Qi organ deficiencies.
   Chinese herbs:
   - Lung Qi Deficiency — Astra 8 (HC), Resilience (CMS), Tri Myco Gen (K'an), Herbal Sentinel Yang or Yin (EW).
   - Spleen or Stomach Qi Deficiency — Astra 8 (HC), Six Gentlemen (HC), Soothe the Center (EW), Prosperous Farmer (K'an), Strengthen Spleen+Disperse Qi (CMS), Ginseng and Astragalus (Zand), AL-113 (PRO).
   Acupuncture:
   - Tonify Lung Qi — LU-9, BL-13, ST-36.
   - Tonify Spleen and Stomach Qi — LI-4, LI-20, ST-36, ST-40, SP-3, SP-6.
   - Spleen–Stomach Distinct Meridian — ST-30+SP-12 (Access Points) to ST-1 (Return Point). Use EA: Neg to Pos, 2 and 8 Hz for energy tonification; 100 Hz for energy movement of acute problems that need dispersing.
4. **Diet**
   - Reduce simple sugars and carbohydrates in the diet.
   - No wine, beer, or fortified alcohols.
   - Increase protein in diet, especially in the morning to stabilize blood sugar.
   - Reduce dairy and all allergenic foods in diet.

5. **Allergy Desensitization** — Use the ALR-G-ANSR (IM) the season before the allergy season for that patient. You can use the technique during the acute allergy manifestation, but it is more difficult and may take more treatments. Abstain from foods that are refractory to desensitization procedures.

6. **Therapeutic Nutrition**
   - Pantothenic Acid (B5) (Doug) — 500 mg daily to support adrenals.
   - Ester C (Doug) — 2 to 5 gm daily, or
   - Pycnogenol (Doug) — 25 to 50 mg daily.

7. **Emotional Connectors** — Sinusitis is associated with sadness due to its Lung connection. Rhinitis is a metaphor for crying. Make patient aware of the issue and let him or her determine its significance.

## ACUTE TREATMENT

1. **Acupuncture** is important for relieving the Qi blockage (pain) locally in the face; to unblock the meridians affecting the Large Intestine, Small Intestine, and stomach for maxillary sinusitis; and, the Bladder and Gall Bladder meridians for ethmoidal, sphenoidal, and frontal sinusitis. Acupuncture around the ear will help congested ears and restore eustachian tube function. Basic TCM treatment consists of face points of the Bowel and Bladder, with heat-reducing points for the Lung and Large Intestine (Figure 17.1).

| Local Points | Distal Points |
|---|---|
| LI-20 | LI-4 |
| ST-2/3 | ST-45 |
| BL-2 | BL-67 |
| YinTang (EX-1) | — |

Additional Points according to symptoms may be selected as follows:

| | | | |
|---|---|---|---|
| LU-7 | Wind Invasion | LU-9 | Deficient Lung Qi |
| LI-4 | Nasal Problems | TH-5 | Wind Heat |
| ST-36 | Def. Defensive | ST-40 | Retained phlegm |
| ST-44/5 | Stomach Fire | LR-2 | Liver Fire |
| SP-10 | Allergy | EX-2 | TaiYang Headaches |

   a. Points for *congested ears*: GB-2, GB-8, TH-17, TH-19. You can use EA, crossing wires in an "x" pattern.
   b. *French energetics* — Use Tai Yin-Yang Ming circuit or deep drainage of Spleen–Stomach for maxillary sinusitis. Add Tai Yang–Shao Yin circuit for frontal, ethmoidal, or sphenoidal sinusitis.
   c. *Auricular Acupuncture* — Sympathetic, nose, liver, Large Intestine, and allergy points.
   d. *YNSA* — Yin and Yang sensory points for nose on the forehead (Yin = 1 cm lateral from the midline and 2 cm inferior from the "A1" point, or 3 cm inferior to hair line).
   e. *KHA* — Nose point on midline, mid-anterior aspect of terminal phalanx of middle finger (K-A28).

2. **Chinese Herbs**
   - *Cold pattern* — Clear or white mucus in cold patient — Minor Blue (Green) Dragon Formula (HC) (Z)(GF), Blue Green Lung Clearing Formula (K'an), Jade Screen (EW), Xiao Qing Long Tang (K'an), Blue Earth Dragon (7F).

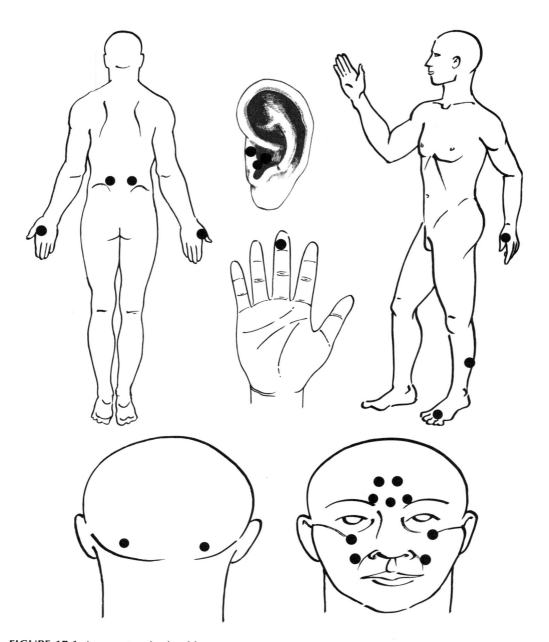

**FIGURE 17.1** Acupuncture in sinusitis.

- *Heat pattern* — Yellow or green-brown purulent mucus with Heat and Toxic symptoms
  — Puraria N (Z), Nasal Tabs (HC), Xanthium Relieve Surface (HC), NA — 551
  (PRO), Welcome Fragrance (EW), Bi Yin Pian (MAY).

3. **Neural Therapy** — Novocaine or Procaine SC injection of the face in the acupuncture
   points BL-2 (supraorbital nerve), Yin Tang (EX-1), Tai Yang (EX-2, Sphenopalatine
   Ganglion and Maxillary Nerve), ST-2 (Infraorbital Nerve), LI-20, area between bony
   and cartilaginous part of the nose laterally (Anterior Ethmoid Nerve), ST-5 (Mental
   Nerve), GB-20 (Greater Occipital Nerve). Additional injections into trigger points in the

sternocleidomastoids, trapezius, and temporalis muscles are sometimes indicated for relief. Nasal insufflation of local anesthetic may also be of some use.

## HOMEOPATHY

There are many constitutional single remedies that have allergy, hay fever, nasal congestion and discharge, and sinusitis as part of the total patient picture. Main polycrests include: Pulsatilla, Arsenicum album, Nux vomica, Natrum muriaticum, and Silica. These may be given in high potency, 200C for 3 daily doses as a constitutional remedy (Boiron, Dolisos or B+T), or in a 6C or 12C as a 2 x/day, or daily dose, respectively.

Of more use is *composite homeopathy*, in which all acute sinusitis remedies are given in one shotgun dose. Acute symptomatic remedies include: Arnica, Aurum metallicum, Bryonia, Eucalyptus globulus, Euphorbium resinifera, Hydrastis canadensis, Kali bichromium, Kali iodatum, Kali muriaticum, Sticta pulmonaria, and Viola odorata (Nasal 1 — IM). Remedies for nasal polyps include Cadmum sulphate, Calcarea carbonica, Formica rufa, Lemnor minor, Phosphorus, Sanguinaria nitricum, Sulphur, and Teucrium (Nasal 2 — IM). Homeopathic remedies for allergy, liver detox, associated bacteria, viruses, fungi, and bowel dysbiosis could also be used concurrently.

## WESTERN APPROACH

**Antibiotics** — Evidence-based medicine does not support the general use of antibiotics in either acute or chronic sinusitis. In fact, the overuse of antibiotics is the very thing that will cause chronicity of the process, as the antibiotics will cause dysbiosis in the bowel, which in turn will disturb the Large Intestine meridian and weaken the maxillary energy and immunity. The one class of drugs that is not used enough are the antifungals, with between 40 to 60% of sinuses showing positive fungal cultures.

**Antihistamines and decongestants** — Issues of tachyphylaxis and side effects on urinary retention in older patients and increasing blood pressure make use of these drugs somewhat difficult and shortsighted at best. Occasionally a patient will not open up his or her sinuses with acupuncture or neural therapy, and a short overnight use of decongestants would seem prudent. The concomitant drying up of the nasal mucosa should be obviated with a saline nasal or homeopathic nasal spray.

**Nasal steroid sprays** — These are indicated only if allergic rhinitis is a causative factor. This problem should have been dealt with in allergy desensitization under ALR-G-ANSR.

## INTEGRATED TREATMENT

In general, in *chronic sinusitis* you end up treating allergies (foods, inhalants, and petrochemicals) and bowel dysbiosis, and using a homeopathic composite remedy (Sinus 1 or 2 from IM). You may use some constitutional acupuncture and some root tonifying Chinese herbs as well. Diet will play an important part in intercurrent therapy.

In *acute sinusitis* you need to use local acupuncture to the face or neural therapy and an acute Chinese herbal prescription and possibly composite homeopathy (Sinus 1 and Sinus Nasal Spray from IM). Use of antibiotics is generally unwarranted.

## CONCLUSION

In conclusion, the world at large is becoming more connected and economically interdependent. One country cannot start a war, or burn a field or toxic dump without affecting everyone around and downstream. We are but a microcosm of our surroundings as are bodies. All disease is an interconnected and integrated manifestation of the whole. Please treat it as such.

# References

1. Young, A.M., *The Reflexive Universe*, Robert Briggs Associates, Mill Valley, CA 1976, xxiii.
2. Bohm, D. and Peat, D. F. *Science, Order and Creativity*, Bantam Books, New York, 1987, Chapter Four.
3. Rossi, E. L.,*The Psychobiology of Mind-Body Healing*, W. W. Norton and Company, New York, 1986.
4. Kuhm, T.F., *The Structure of Scientific Revolutions*, Second Edition, 11, 2, University of Chicago Press, Chicago, 1970.
5. Engel, G. L., The need for a new medical model: a challenge for biomedicine, *Science*, 196, 4286, 129, 1977.
6. Tiller, W. A., *Science and Human Transformation*, Pavior Publishing, Walnut Creek, CA, 1997, chap. 6.
7. Capra, F., *The Web of Life*, An Anchor Book, Doubleday Publishers, New York, 1996.
8. Capra, F., *The Tao of Physics*, Shambhala Publications, Boulder, CO, 1976.
9. Williams, R. J., *Biochemical Individuality*, University of Texas Press, Austin, 1979.
10. Bland, J. S., The Institute for Functional Medicine, Publications from HealthComm International, Gig Harbour, 1999.
11. Woolf, S. H., Clinical practice guidelines in complementary and alternative medicine: an analysis of opportunities and obstacles, *Arch. Fam. Med.*, 6, 149, 1997.
12. Eisenberg, D. M. et al, Unconventional medicine in the United States: prevalence, costs and patterns of use, *N. Eng. J. Med.*, 328 (4), 246, 1993.
13. Eisenberg, D. M. et al., Trends in alternative medicine use in the United States, 1990-1997: results of a follow-up national survey, *JAMA*, 280 (18), 1569, 1998.
14. Miller, L. G., Selected clinical considerations focusing on known or potential drug-herb interactions, *Arch. Int. Med.*, 158, 2200, 1998.
15. Nevada State Board of Medical Examiners, letters to author, December 1998.
16. Coulter, H. L., *Divided Legacy: The Conflict Between Homeopathy and the American Medical Association*, North Atlantic Books, Berkeley, CA, 1973.
17. Hawking, S. W., *A Brief History of Time*, Bantam Books, New York, 1988.
18. Schrodinger E., *What Is Life?*, Cambridge University Press, New York, 1967.
19. Morowitz, H. J., *Energy Flow in Biology*, Academic Press, New York, 1968.
20. Robbins, John, *Diet for a New America*, Stillpoint Publishing, Walpole, NH, 1987.
21. Gleick, J., *Chaos*, Viking Press, New York, 1987.
22. Briggs, J. and Peat, D. F., *Turbulent Mirror*, Harper and Row, New York, 1989.
23. Lipsitz, L. A., Loss of "complexity" and aging, *JAMA*, 267, 13, 1806, 1992.
24. Yeargers, E. K., *Basic Biophysics for Biology*, CRC Press, Boca Raton, FL, 1992.
25. Goldberger, A. L. et al., Chaos and fractals in human physiology, *Scientific American*, 43, 1990.
26. Coffey, D. S., Self-organization, complexity and chaos: the new biology of medicine, *Nature Medicine*, 4, 8, 882, 1998.
27. Diamond, W. J., *An Alternative Medicine Definitive Guide to Cancer*, Future Medicine Publishing, Tiburon, 1997.
28. Becker, R. O., *Cross Currents*, Jeremy P. Tarcher, Los Angeles, 1990.
29. Becker, R. O. and Selden, G., *The Body Electric*, William Morrow and Company, New York, 1985.
30. Nordenstrom, B. E. W., *Biologically Closed Electrical Circuits*, Nordic Medical Publications, Stockholm, 1983.
31. Zaren, A., *Materia Medica: Core Elements of the Materia Medica of the Mind — Volumes I and II*, Ulrich Burgdorf Publishing, Gottingen, 1993.
32. Sarno, J. E., *Healing Back Pain*, Warner Books, New York, 1991.
33. Sarno, J. E., *The Mind Body Prescription*, Warner Books, New York, 1999.

34. Jensen, M. C. et al., Magnetic resonance imaging of the lumbar spine in people without back pain, *N. Eng. J. Med.*, 331, 2, 69, 1994.
35. Groddeck, G., *The Meaning of Illness*, International Universities Press, New York, 1977.
36. Simon, G. E. et al., An international study of the relation between somatic symptoms and depression, *N. Eng. J. Med.*, 341, 18, 1329, 1999.
37. Wessely, S. et al, Functional somatic syndromes: one or many? *Lancet*, 354, 936, 1999.
38. Reston, J., Now about my operation in Peking, *New York Times*, 26, 1,6, July 26, 1971.
39. Beinfield, H. and Korngold, E., *Between Heaven and Earth*, Ballentine Books, New York, 1991.
40. Maciocia, G., *The Foundations of Chinese Medicine*, Churchill Livingstone, Edinburgh, UK, 1989.
41. Klinghardt, D., American Academy of Neural Therapy, Seattle, WA, telephone: 1-800-844-8251.
42. Blumenthal, M., The Complete German Commission E Monographs, American Botanical Council, Austin, TX, and Integrative Medicine Communications, Boston, MA, 1998.
43. Stux, G. and Pomeranz, B., *Acupuncture — Textbook and Atlas*, Springer-Verlag, Berlin, 1987.
44. Helms, J., *Acupuncture Energetics*, Medical Acupuncture Publishers, Berkeley, CA, 1995.
45. Seem, M., *Acupuncture Imaging*, Healing Arts Press, Rochester, VT, 1990.
46. Pischinger, A., *Matrix and Matrix Regulation*, Haug International, Brussels, Belgium, 1991.
47. Bland, J.S., *Genetic Nutritioneering*, Keats Publishing, Los Angeles, 1999.
48. D'Adamo, P. J., *Eat Right 4 Your Type*, Putnam Publishing Group, New York, 1997.
49. Fuchs, N. K., *My Mother Made Me Do It*, Lowel House, Los Angeles, 1989.
50. Wolever, T. M., The glycemic index, flogging a dead horse, *Diabetes Care*, 20, 452–56, 1997.
51. Maciocia, G., *The Practice of Chinese Medicine*, Churchill Livingstone, London, 1994, p. 777.
52. Mussat, M., *The Physics of Acupuncture*, Librairie Le François, Paris, 1983.
53. Hiroshi Nakazawa, 700 Geipe Rd. #204, Baltimore, MD 21228. Phone (410) 744-8505.
54. Goodman, L.S. and Gillmans, A.G., *The Pharmacological Basis of Therapeutics*, 9th ed., McGraw-Hill, New York, 1996.
55. Stebbins, J., Electrotherapy, Paper presented at CAAOM Meeting, San Francisco, CA, 1996.
56. Hahnemann, S., *Organon of Medicine*, Sixth Edition, J.P. Tarcher, Inc., Los Angeles, 1982.
57. Linde, K. et al, Are the clinical effects of homeopathy placebo effects? A meta-analysis of placebo controlled trials, *Lancet*, 350, 834–843, 1997.
58. Linde, K. et al., Critical review and meta-analysis of serially agitated dilutions in experimental toxicology, *Hum. Exp. Toxicol.*, 13, 481–492, 1994.
59. de la Fuye, R., *Traité d'Acupuncture*, Librairie Le François, Paris, 1956.
60. Selye, H., *The Stress of Life*, McGraw-Hill, New York, 1956.

## RESOURCES

All resources may be found on the website: www.integratedmedicines.com.

# Index

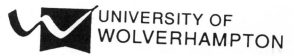
UNIVERSITY OF
WOLVERHAMPTON

LR/LEND/001

**Harrison Learning Centre**
City Campus
University of Wolverhampton
St Peter's Square
Wolverhampton WV1 1RH
Telephone: 0845 408 1631

Telephone Renewals: 01902 321333
This item may be recalled at any time. Keeping it after it has
been recalled or beyond the date stamped may result in a fine.
See tariff of fines displayed at the counter.

– 5 NOV 2004

– 4 NOV 2005

0 8 NOV 2006

2 8 SEP 2007

1 2 NOV 2007

1 1 JAN 2008

– 9 MAY 2008

– 3 NOV 2008

3 0 JAN 2009

– 8 FEB 2010

2 7 DEC 2017

2 3 JAN 2018

See tariff of fines displayed at the Counter.        (L2)